PORTFOLIO

OF

THE PRODUCT BULLETINS

CLINICIANS MANUAL

BY

ROYAL LEE D.D.S. AND VITAMIN PRODUCTS COMPANY

THE PRODUCT BULLETINS

Published by Therapeutic Food Company
Copyright 1949 all rights reserved under international and Pan American copyright convention. No portion of this book may be reproduced without written permission from the publisher.

Second edition 1951

Third edition 1959
Published by Lee Foundation for Nutritional Research

Fourth edition 1999
Published by International Foundation for Nutrition and Health.

Fifth edition 2001
Published by International Foundation for Nutrition and Health.

Six edition 2010
Published by International Foundation for Nutrition and Health.

 Copyright 1999-2010 International Foundation for Nutrition and Health. All Rights Reserved

All rights for reprinting and republishing by the Lee foundation of Nutritional Research were granted to the International Foundation for Nutrition and Health. No part of this manual shall be reproduced, stored in a retrieval system, or transmitted by any means, electronic, mechanical, photocopying, recording, or otherwise, without written permission from the publisher. No patent liability is assumed with respect to the use of the information contained herein. Although every precaution has been taken in the preparation of this book, the publisher assumes no responsibility for errors or omissions. Neither is any liability assumed for damages resulting from the use of the information contained herein.

Published and Distributed
By
International Foundation for Nutrition and Health:
3963 Mission Blvd.
San Diego, CA 92109
(858) 488-8932 Phone
(858) 488-2566 Fax
www.ifnh.org
ISBN -0-9713314-8-0

INTRODUCTION

When you started out in practice, most of us were only interested in a protocol: what's the protocol for congestive heart failure; what do you do for high blood pressure; or what do you do for diabetes? After all, that's the model that pharmaceutical companies have conditioned us to reference: just use the protocol, don't the reason why.

As I went through this manual, I found myself excited all over again and impressed with the in-depth knowledge that is put forth. Today, everyone tries so hard to make one size fit all, but Dr. Lee and other nutritional pioneers tried to make us look at the big picture by understanding function and giving us numerous methods of cross-referencing any issue.

The original text of this manual came from clinical notes for practitioners produced by the Therapeutic Food Company. Later, these one-to-two-page annotations were published into a single volume by the Therapeutic Food Company and the Vitamin Product Company, firms owned by Dr. Lee.

A court ruling against Dr. Lee, stating that food could not be described as therapeutic, forced the closure of those companies as well as the Endocardiograph Company. In an attempt to save the educational materials within the companies, prior to his 1961 Supreme Court hearing, Dr. Lee assigned the copyrights of all of his materials to the Lee Foundation for Nutritional Research. For more information regarding the Lee foundation go to ifnh.org.

Dr. Lee originally established the Lee Foundation for Nutritional Research under a state charter as a nonprofit organization back in 1941. The purpose of the Lee Foundation was to engage in research and to coordinate and communicate nutritional breakthroughs from laboratories around the world. The Foundation was the world's largest clearinghouse for nutritional information for doctors, agriculturists and homemakers. During its existence, the Lee Foundation disseminated hundreds of thousands of pieces of research materials and books on health and nutrition.

Of interest are the original dates of these articles by the Therapeutic Food Company. The articles represented a comprehensive knowledge of vitamins from a whole food perspective during a period when the major manufacturers had not yet inundated the public with synthetic substitutes. Only after World War II did the entire scenario of synthetic vitamins come to the forefront. In other words, we think the information included in this book represents the finest and most unprejudiced facts about vitamins at the time of writing. Today, much of this information is still relevant regarding the uses of vitamin complexes found in real whole-food.

In re-publishing this book, the International Foundation for Nutrition and Health (IFNH) has taken great lengths attempting to put forward not only the knowledge, but also the design of the original publication. We have come as close as possible to re-creating this classic work in the same typography and format as the original. Some of you might notice a difference in the labeling of some of the products. Unfortunately, because of government regulations, Standard Process was forced to alter the original labeling and formulation to comply with government regulations. A classic example is the use of "ascorbic acid" when identifying vitamin C complex. Obviously, ascorbic acid is not the whole food complex of vitamin C.

In keeping with the spirit and philosophy of Dr. Lee, IFNH is proud to be entrusted with the stewardship of this manual and the many others published by the Lee Foundation for Nutritional Research. It is our commitment at the International Foundation for Nutrition and Health to make available these priceless works to today's practitioner in an effort to enlighten the public of the therapeutic value of whole natural foods.

Note: It is highly recommended that you read the original preface on the following page to better understand the atmosphere that the nutritional pioneers found themselves operating under. IFNH has updated the names of the products to clarify some of the material. Sometimes there is confusion because a product has a different name depending on the company that produced it. We have provided a list of name changes and discontinued products for further reference.

It has been over 15 years since I reviewed this manual in such detail. With each page you can't help feeling like you have Dr. Lee as your personal mentor, nurturing your growth and knowledge in the use of clinical nutrition. This manual is just one of the many reasons why we hold in our archives numerous heartfelt letters of gratitude from those whom Dr. Lee had taken the time to mentor and how, through his efforts, their lives were changed. As Dr. Lee once said "This information isn't to be possessed, it's to share".

Enjoy the journey.

John R. Brady III

Director IFNH

PREFACE

In reading this original Preface printed by Dr. Lee and the THERAPEUTIC FOOD COMPANY you can't help snickering at Dr. Lee's dry sense of humor, knowing some of his legal headaches and frustration that he must have been enduring.

Some of the information offered herein on the effects of malnutrition and its prevention and relief has not yet been accepted by the consensus of medical opinion. UNDER THIS CIRCUMSTANCE, TO COMPLY WITH FEDERAL LAW, WE CANNOT DISTRIBUTE THIS LITERATURE TO ANY PERSON OTHER THAN TO A LICENSED MEMBER OF THE HEALING ARTS.

NOTE: Literature given to the physician must be true and not misrepresent. Literature for the general public, however, must conform to the consensus of medical opinion, whether that be true or false (Food and Drug Law of 1938).

THEREFORE: All suggestions made in this book (which legally are subject to labeling laws) are purely for *EXPERIMENTAL PURPOSES*. We are not permitted by federal law to make any other kind, unless they are accepted as being in accord with the consensus of "medical opinion." They do represent, however, schedules established as a result of our acting as a clearinghouse of nutritional information since 1930.

It is obvious that where nutritional deficiencies exist their correction is essential to the recovery of the patient. It is also obvious that regardless of the form of other therapy that may be used, the correction of nutritional deficiencies is a basic and indispensable feature of treatment where it is required. Only the practical experience of a physician can be the final guide in selecting nutritional factors. This list of recommendations, to be used in conjunction with other therapeutic measures or alone as the physician may decide, is offered as the collection of data from doctors in acting as a clearinghouse for nutritional information.

A Word of Caution

Note that these statements apply only to natural complexes and we doubt that they can apply to any synthetic products. The first principle of nutrition is to get *all* the factors needed in the maintenance of the human body. This is unlikely to happen when the nutritional integrity of the vitamin is confused with its chemical integrity. This is a specialized field of research and requires a laboratory staff who has made a special study of the problems involved, who has devised and built the exclusive machinery necessary to concentrate and prepare the food source extracts that carry these vital elements which are unavailable otherwise; whose research activities have developed methods for extracting, dehydrating, fractionally separating and sterilizing these extracts, all at temperatures below body heat; whose research activities have brought forth in the last 15 years *four* new vitamins (vitamins F_1, F_2, E_2 and E_3, not as yet accepted by the medical consensus of opinion); a laboratory which was capable in 1930 of making a multiple essential food product known as **CATALYN**. (Seventeen organic trace minerals were in **CATALYN** years before the spectrograph was perfected to the point of finding them.)

We are indebted to the large number of doctors who have generously contributed their experience in the use of these factors by reporting case histories to us. This has made possible this compilation. In every sense it represents "*our* consensus of opinion" to the best of our ability to report it.

Your continued cooperation in reporting case histories regarding the use of nutritional entities will enable us to improve our recommendations and be of widespread benefit. Case History Forms are available on request for this purpose when desired.

For complete information regarding specific aspects of nutritional factors in respect to diagnosed conditions see listings in the *Therapeutic Food Manual*. For specific aspects of the nutritional factors of signs and symptoms use *Mastering Nutrition with the Symptom Survey*. Both of these books can be extremely helpful when you consider the average patient comes to you with complaints about pathology and disease or signs and symptoms.

PORTFOLIO OF PRODUCT BULLETINS

INTRODUCTION — This manual is designed primarily as a practical clinical reference source for the doctor who is considering use of physiological remedies as offered by the THERAPEUTIC FOODS COMPANY. In addition, however, it serves as a study manual for consideration of various biochemical problems which are encountered by all doctors regardless of therapeutic entities applied.

INSTRUCTIONS FOR USE — In view of the unique construction of this book, i.e., the strict categorizing of information-it is well for the reviewer to familiarize himself with its contents so that he may employ it to its fullest capacity.

OUTLINE OF CONTENTS

HEADING OF PAGE — This gives the name of the product (and directly beneath, the catalog or order number if any). An alphabetical index is provided at the front (Page VI) of the book for ready reference.

LABEL — This lists exact labeling information at the original time of printing. Naturally this information is subject to change as improvements in formulas are made, but the overall status here is relatively stable. The purpose of providing this information is to assist the doctor in patient management where the labeling information would be a problem with which the patient may be concerned. *Obviously some of the labeling of Standard Process products has been changed to conform with government regulations.*

TISSUE OR FUNCTION SUPPORTED — The most general application of the product is given; this, in most cases, provides an easily understandable explanation of the use of the product in terminology acceptable to the lay person.

CLINICAL CONSIDERATIONS — This is a practical check-list of clinical signs and symptoms which experience has shown to be applicable to the use of the product concerned. The possible etiological background is also given under this heading, as well as a subheading "Symptom Characteristics" which is an overall means of evaluating the symptoms previously listed so that ramifications of their implications may be employed.

LABORATORY TESTS — These are tests which are ordinarily performed by an outside laboratory, the significance of which may be useful in evaluating the biochemical problem under consideration.

CLINICAL TESTS — The tests in this manual are usually performed in the doctor's office, often as a part of routine physical examinations. The purpose of listing these tests is to show how they may be applied to nutritional diagnosis. More information on these tests and others are all part of the CCWFN certification program. To learn more about the Nutritional Exam and foundational approach, go to ifnh.org.

GENERAL CONSIDERATIONS — Provides information intended to give a broader scope of understanding of the therapeutic possibilities of the product. It is primarily useful in clinical research and where additional information is desired.

CLINICALLY ASSOCIATED CONDITIONS — This section lists, according to disease categories and rationale previously given, conditions that indicate a product may prove beneficial in the support of treatment. It is useful in examining the results of therapy and for exploring, .to a greater extent, the therapeutic possibilities of the whole food concentrates.

Note: The above outline follows the usual sequence of consideration encountered in practice during a clinical exam. IFNH has updated the names of the products in an effort to clarify some of the material. Sometimes there is confusion when a product will have a different name depending on which one of Dr. Lee's company's it originated from. Please check the list of name changes and discontinued products on the following page.

See Subject Index at End of Book

TABLE OF CONTENTS

FRONT OF BOOK:

Introduction…………………………………	History and Overview	I
Preface……………………………………..	An Introduction and Premise	III
Portfolio of Product Bulletins……………..	explanation of The Page Layout	IV
Outline of Contents………………………..	Explanation of Information Supplied	V
Index of name changes……………………..	Quick Reference	VI
Index of Product Bulletins…………………	Alphabetical Listings of Products	VII

PRODUCTS (Pages 1-192)
The products appear in the same order as listed on Standard Process order forms.

DISCONTINUED PRODUCTS (Pages 193-199)
These products have been carried over in the new alphabetical version for reference purposes.

BACK OF BOOK:

Special Formulas (Pages 201-205)

Associated Products: (Pages 207-210)
This section lists the Basic Products and their relation to other products, so that, for example, if Cardio-Plus is being considered, the fact that it contains C, E_2, G and Cardiotrophin will be evident. Or when G, for example, is being considered, that it will be evident that G is also contained in Drenamin and Cardio-Plus.

Drugs And Whole Food Support (Pages 211-218)

Optimal Times To Take Nutritional Supplements (Page 219)
This section is just what it says a quick reference to help the practitioner understand when they can get the best results.

Rich Food Sources Of Nutrients (Pages 221-223)
This section is an excellent patient handout. Today, diet and lifestyle are a must for success.

Clinical and Laboratory Test (Pages 225-238)
This section supports the practitioner in the understanding the value of the nutritional exam and a functional approach to health, the normal lab tests are also included but we would recommend the practitioner getting <u>Mastering Nutrition with Blood Chemistry Quick Reference Guide</u> for quick and easy reference.

Subject Index: (Pages 239-243)
This is an index of symptoms and clinical tests which are listed under the following headings in the Product Bulletins: 1) Clinical Considerations, and, 2) Clinical and Laboratory Tests.

IFNH Information
This section contains a clinical reading list as well as more information on the whole foods certification program (CCWFN). IFNH has been supporting practitioners in the therapeutic use of whole food nutrition since 1994.

STANDARD PROCESS – NAME CHANGES

Old Name	New Name
Acidophilus Yeast	Lactic Acid Yeast
Adrenamin	Drenamin
Allorganic Trace Minerals	Trace Minerals B12
Anterior Pituitary	E-Manganese
Anti-Coryza	Congaplex
Anti-Gastrin (Capsules/Powder)	Gastrex
Anti-Pyrexin	Antronex
Betalco	Betacol
Betaris	Betafood
Calcifood A	Calcifood
Calciphade Powder	Discontinued
Calciplex	Calsol
Carbamide	A-C Carbamide
Cerodyn	Cyrofood
Cerol	Wheat Germ Oil Perles
Chlorophyll Aqueous Capules	Discontinued
Comfrey Pepsin E3	Okra, Pepsin & E3
Complex	Cataplex *

Example: ACP Complex — Cataplex ACP

Old Name	New Name
Cyroplex	Catalyn
Cyruta A	Cyruta-Plus
Cytotrophin	PMG
Cyofood D	Discontinued

Example: Kidney Cytotrophin — Renatrophin PMG
Spleen Cytotrophin — Spleen PMG

Old Name	New Name
Drenaplex	Drenamin
EFF Plus	Super-EFF
Eflex Perles	Cataplex F Perles
Vitamin F Ointment	USF Ointment
Fenucom	Fen-Gre
Ferroplus	Ferrofood
GEC (Cardioplex)	Cardio-Plus
Glucroplex	Cataplex GTF
Lecithin Perles	Soy Bean Lecithin
Manganese Phytate B12	Manganese B12
Minaplex	Organic Minerals
Nucleo Protein	Discontinued
Ostogen Wafers	Biost
Oculotrophin	Iplex
Organic Iodine	Prolamime Iodine
Parathyroid	Cal-Ma Plus
Phosphade	Phosfood Liquid
Potassium Bicarbonate	Discontinued
Prostex	Prost-X
Protedyn	Protefood
Protemere	Nutrimere
Protomorphogen	PMG

Example: Bone Protomorphogen — Ostrophin PMG

Old Name	New Name
Rutaplex	Cyruta
Ruta-Plus	Cyruta-Plus
Sodium Citrate	Discontinued
Symphytum	Okra, Pepsin & E3
Vermidase	Zymex II
Vitamin-	Cataplex*

Example: Vitamin E — Cataplex E
Vitamin A-C Complex — Cataplex AC

*CATAPLEX is the Standard Process term for the vitamin-mineral-enzyme complex as it occurs in nature in whole foods.

INDEX OF PRODUCT BULLETINS

Alphabetical

1. Intro and table of contents
2. A-C Carbamide, 1
3. A-F Betafood, 5
4. Antronex, 7
5. Arginex, 9
6. Betacol, 11
7. Betafood, 15
8. Betaine Hydrochloride, 17
9. Bio-Dent, 19
10. Biost, 21
11. Cal-Amo, 25
12. Calcifood, 27
13. Calcium Lactate, 29
14. Calsol Wafers, 33
15. Cardio-Plus, 35
16. Cardiotrophin, 37
17. Catalyn, 39
18. Cataplex A, 41
19. Cataplex A-C, 43
20. Cataplex A-C-P, 45
21. Cataplex B12, 49
22. Cataplex B, 51
23. Cataplex C, 53
24. Cataplex D, 55
25. Cataplex E2, 57
26. Cataplex E, 59
27. Cataplex F, 61
28. Cataplex F Perles, 63
29. Cataplex G, 65
30. Chlorophyll Complex, 69
31. Chlorophyll Ointment, 71
32. Cholacol II, 73
33. Cholacol, 75
34. Choline, 77
35. Collinsonia Root, 79
36. Congaplex, 81
37. Cyrofood, 83
38. Cyruta, 85
39. Cyruta Plus, 87
40. Dermatrophin PMG, 89
41. Di-Sodium Phosphate, 91
42. Drenamin, 93
43. Drenatrophin, 95
44. Ferrofood, 97
45. For-Til B_{12}, 99
46. Gastrex, 101
47. Hepatrophin, 103
48. Inositol, 105
49. Iplex, 107
50. Lactic Acid Yeast, 109
51. Mammary PMG, 111
52. Manganese Phytate-B12, 113
53. Min-Tran, 115
54. Myotrophin PMG, 117
55. Neurotrophin PMG, 119
56. Niacinamide-B6, 121
57. Okra, Pepsin & E3, 123
58. Orchex, 125
59. Orchic PMG, 127
60. Organic Bound Minerals, 129
61. Ostrophin, PMG, 133
62. Ovatrophin PMG, 135
63. Ovex, 137
64. Pancreatrophin PMG, 139
65. Parotid PMG, 141
66. Phosfood Liquid, 143
67. Pituitrophin PMG, 145
68. Pneumotrophin PMG, 147
69. Prolamine Iodine, 149
70. Prostate PMG, 151
71. Prost-X, 153
72. Protefood, 155
73. Renatrophin PMG, 157
74. Ribo-Nucleic Acid, 159
75. Soybean Lecithin, 161
76. Spleen PMG, 163
77. Super-EFF, 165
78. Thymex, 167
79. Thymus PMG, 171
80. Thytrophin PMG, 173
81. Trace Minerals B12, 177
82. USF Ointment, 179
83. Utrophin PMG, 181
84. Vasculin, 183
85. Wheat Germ Oil Perles, 185
86. Zymex, 187
87. Zymex II, 189
88. Zypan, 191

INDEX OF PRODUCT BULLETINS

Alphabetical

89. DISCONTINUED ITEMS
90. Chlorophyll Aqueous Capsules, 193
91. Cyrofood D, 195
92. Nucleo Protein, 196
93. Potassium Bicarbonate, 197
94. Sodium Citrate, 199
95. Special Formula Products, 201-205
96. Associated Products, 207-210
97. Drugs and Whole Food Support, 211-218
98. Optimal Times to Take Nutritional Supplements, 219
99. Nutrient Sources of Whole Natural Foods, 221-223
100. Clinical and Laboratory Tests, 225-238
101. Subject Index, 239-243

PORTFOLIO

OF

THE PRODUCT BULLETINS

CLINICIANS MANUAL

BY

ROYAL LEE D.D.S. AND VITAMIN PRODUCTS COMPANY

A C CARBAMIDE

Label: (Carbamide is found in blood and all tissue fluids.) For nutritional use internally where deficiency may exist, and for external use in 2% solution to promote healing. Dosage ¼ to ½ teaspoonful in water.

Tissue or Function Supported Carbamide (urea) metabolism.

CLINICAL CONSIDERATIONS
Prominent Clinical Signs And Symptoms

Symptoms:

1. Kidney-Bladder Symptoms (Diminished urination, pain, burning, itching on urination, etc.)
2. Water Balance (Fluid retention, dehydration, "pressure" headaches, edema)
3. Sweat Gland Activity (Excess or diminished perspiration: use with salt)
4. Gastritis (Local inflammation in gastrointestinal tract, ulcers, colitis, etc.)
5. Low Protein Diets
6. Acidosis Symptoms (Tachycardia, irregular respiration, hyperirritability, anoxia)
7. Allergic Reactions
8. Local Application (Skin lesions, ulcers, festers, etc., as wet poultice)
9. Glaucoma

Possible Etiological Background:

Carbamide reduces the electrical conductivity of water. Its physiological effects can perhaps best be understood by its influence in protein metabolism. According to various investigators, it acts in this respect to denature protein compounds. This means that it alters the affinity of the protein molecule for any mineral salts which may be conjugated with it. This effect materializes by denaturing the calcium-protein complex, releasing into the blood free ions of calcium phosphate, which react with sodium bicarbonate always present, to afford calcium bicarbonate and sodium phosphate, both important blood buffers. Chemically, Carbamide is carbon dioxide combined with ammonia. As such, it must be considered as a blood buffer salt, for while neutral in itself, it can release ammonia for neutralizing acids if urease is present, an enzyme that catalyzes this reaction.

Symptom Characteristics: The most common clinical indication is disturbance in the ventilation, and even when this is mild, the patient often expresses gratification of "being able to breathe better" after Carbamide is administered. Otherwise, characteristics follow the patterns set by protein metabolism, fluid balance and acid-base disorders.

Laboratory And Clinical Tests None known. (Urea Clearance Test shows nothing of urea metabolism, simply the ability of the kidney to expedite its excretion, and indication of kidney impairment—**Arginex** would be indicated.)

Administration	**Dosage:** One teaspoonful per day. This may be divided into two half teaspoonfuls. Another method is to add a pinch of drinking water.
	Effect: Diuresis may be produced. Results, according to above described symptoms, are usually satisfactory and noticeable clinically within a few days.
	Note: Formula for heat prostration, low blood volume and excessive sweating is according to Klein (See Lee Foundation Reprint No. 96), "A New Theory of Diet and Coronary Thrombosis," to which Carbamide is added, as follows: equal parts of orange juice and water with one level teaspoonful of salt (Organic Sea Salt [Commissary] preferred), to which is added one teaspoonful of Carbamide. One or two glasses per day. If symptoms of edema occur, discontinue and use **Arginex**.
	One or two glasses per day are usually sufficient to produce observable clinical results. The solution simulates Ringer's Solution, but employs natural ingredients which favor absorption and control of osmotic pressures in most cases. Proportions are important, and for this reason, patient should be instructed to use a standard measuring spoon for the accuracy of measurement required.
Administration	**Side Effect:** When the above solution is used, most cases are benefited, but a few will be aggravated, which, of course, should be reason for discontinuation of this avenue of approach. However, since so many seemingly "contraindicated" cases of edema respond favorably, the alternative remains to make a therapeutic test at the clinical level. We have seen cases where edema of the ankles of many years standing have been brought under control by this method where every other approach attempted had failed.

A C CARBAMIDE

Synergists:	Activity Contributed:
Vitamin F Complex	Calcium Diffusing Influence
Arginex	Enzyme activator important in urea metabolism
Renafood	kidney detoxification and support

GENERAL CONSIDERATIONS

The nutritional effects of **Carbamide** may be listed as follows:

1. Promotes osmotic transfer of tissue fluids.
2. Acts as a physiological diuretic.
3. Acts as a blood buffer salt.
4. Acts to denature proteins.

We may rationalize clinical application as follows:

1. Disturbances in osmotic transfer of tissue fluids (water balance) may result in either hydration (edema) or dehydration (emaciation). This needs to be considered not only from the viewpoint of total amounts of fluids present, but also in relation to the location of these fluids within the bodily compartments—i.e., the balance between the tissue fluids (intracellular) and the blood volume (extracellular). Largely changes within these compartments—with the kidney acting in accordance to them—a more or less constant hydrostatic pressure is maintained throughout the body. **Carbamide** is an important factor in this balance, acting in this respect as a common denominator in these changes. Many diseases are associated with such changes, as premenstrual depression (edema), glaucoma, migraine headaches, shock and heat prostration, ascites, edema, uremia, and vasomotor disturbances (hypo- and hypertension).

2. Acts to combat acidosis by reason of its chemical constituents which are ammonia and carbon dioxide, reflected clinically in benefits in the respiratory mechanism.

3. **Carbamide** is synthesized by the liver and reduced by the kidney or excreted as urea. As such, it may be considered an important "vehicle" in the metabolic intermediate processes designed to rid the body of wastes.

4. It is the only substance to our knowledge which reduces the electrical conductivity of water (all other mineral salts increase its conductivity). This is an important factor in "desensitizing" reactions which occur in the allergic state-denaturing of proteins.

5. Topical application should be considered in requirements involving inflammatory conditions of the skin, healing effects (cell proliferating factor) having been reported in this respect, simulating here the action of chlorophyll.

6. It is useful in gastritis (inflammation of gastrointestinal tract), particularly where acids or strong chemicals have produced a necrotizing effect. NOTE: Children are particularly vulnerable to accidents involving the swallowing of strong chemicals. We know of one case where a child had swallowed a strong industrial solvent which, after removal by hospital procedure, left the child with an extremely irritated intestinal tract which was almost immediately relieved after **Carbamide** was added to the drinking water.

7. **Carbamide** has also been reported to be of value in the relief of pain in Muscular Dystrophy.

CLINICALLY ASSOCIATED CONDITIONS

GASTROINTESTINAL-URINARY
    <u>Stomach and Intestine</u>
        Colitis, Mucous
    <u>Kidney and Bladder</u>
        Cystitis
        Nephritis

NERVOUS AND PSYCHOGENIC
    <u>Functional</u>
        Colitis, Ulcerative
        Headaches
        Ulcers, Gastric
    <u>Metabolic</u>
        Tranquilizing Effects

A C CARBAMIDE

CLINICALLY ASSOCIATED CONDITIONS

NERVOUS AND PSYCHOGENIC
- <u>Mentality</u>
  - Brain, Dysfunction of
- <u>Vasomotor</u>
  - Heat Prostration

METABOLIC DISORDERS
- <u>Water-Balance</u>
  - Ascites
  - Dropsy
  - Edema
- <u>Respiratory</u>
  - Bronchitis

EXOGENIC DISORDERS
- <u>Toxic</u>
  - Nightmares
- <u>Inflammation</u>
  - Sciatica

MALE DISORDERS
- Prostate Disease

A C CARBAMIDE

A C CARBAMIDE

CLINICALLY ASSOCIATED CONDITIONS

NERVOUS AND PSYCHOGENIC
- <u>Mentality</u>
  - Brain, Dysfunction of
- <u>Vasomotor</u>
  - Heat Prostration

METABOLIC DISORDERS
- <u>Water-Balance</u>
  - Ascites
  - Dropsy
  - Edema
- <u>Respiratory</u>
  - Bronchitis

EXOGENIC DISORDERS
- <u>Toxic</u>
  - Nightmares
- <u>Inflammation</u>
  - Sciatica

MALE DISORDERS
- Prostate Disease

AF BETAFOOD

Label: Each tablet contains 1,500 IU of Vitamin A with concentrates of factors from alfalfa, carrot, beef kidney and fish liver lipoids, Vitamin F derived from essential unsaturated fatty acids (arachidonic, linolenic, linoleic) from flax and beef lipoids. **Betafood** from dehydrated beet leaf juice. Suggested dosage: 2 tablets per meal or as directed.

Tissue or Function Supported: Vitamins A and F deficiency states, liver and gallbladder stasis.

CLINICAL CONSIDERATIONS
Prominent Clinical Signs and Symptoms

Symptoms:

1. Signs of Liver Disease (Such as prominence of veins on chest and abdomen venous congestion indigestion, constipation, etc.)
2. Gallbladder Symptoms (Nausea, flatulence, jaundice, intolerance to fats or gas-producing foods)
3. Hypoglycemic Symptoms (Symptoms occurring before or after meals such as tremors, headaches, faintness, irritability, tachycardia and craving for sweets)
4. History of Hepatitis (Weakness or lowered resistance following attack)
5. Liver Cirrhosis (Alcoholism)

Possible Etiological Background:

Vitamins A and F act to promote liver function, Betafood is probably associated with intermediate processes involving conversion of blood fat to sugar. The latter effect logically concerns itself with the viscosity of the bile, fats (cholesterol) being eliminated via the bile route. The congestion of the liver as a sequela of the fat-sugar imbalance is also rationally applied to these effects. Note that of an elevated blood fat and an elevated blood sugar, the former is most likely to result in the arteriosclerotic changes which are characteristic of the diabetic syndrome and are of great concern where cholesterol problems are being considered.

Symptom Characteristics: The pattern generally-though not always-follows the clinical picture of indigestion, the vague symptoms of liver disease and hypoglycemic reactions being two important conditions which may or may not be evidenced as gastrointestinal complaints

Laboratory Test

Tests:
a. Cholesterol
b. Glucose Tolerance Test
c. Gallbladder X-Ray
d. Liver Function Tests

Need Shown By:
a. Elevated values, cholesterol being eliminated via the bile route.
b. Curve deviations show deficits in carbohydrate metabolism.
c. Evidence of stones
d. (See Product Bulletin No. 9)

Clinical Tests

Tests
a. Palpation
b. Observation

Need Shown By
Tenderness, palpable liver, abdominal hyperirritability.
Evidence of venous congestion.

Note: **AF Betafood** is often used where intolerance is noted to fat-soluble vitamins or other reactions occur. In many of these cases the incapacity is due to an inability of the liver to manage the products produced by increased detoxification processes. For these reasons, **AF Betafood** is often given where desensitization of the patient is desired before attempting more active channels of detoxification. Therefore this product may be immediately recommended in all cases where a tentative diagnosis is in the working stage and until a specific diagnosis is obtained.

AF BETAFOOD

Administration	**Dosage:** 3 to 9 per day depending upon the symptomatic picture, higher in more acute conditions
	Effect: Relief from gallbladder symptoms is usually evident within a few days, dependent upon adequate dosage. Cholesterol-type problems may be expected to show response in two or three weeks, dependent upon chronicity and degree of degeneration which has occurred. Hypoglycemic symptoms are often relieved immediately if taken during an attack.
	Side Effect: None known.

<u>**Synergists:**</u>
Zypan
Choline
Lecithin Perles

<u>**Activity Contributed:**</u>
Gastric catalyst
*Anti-cholic factor and physiological detergent
*Emulsifying action

*Both augment the effect of bile

GENERAL CONSIDERATIONS

The nutritional effects may be listed as follows:
1. Aids in decongestion of liver and gallbladder drainage by reducing bile viscosity and thus promotes elimination of toxic materials and cholesterol via the bile route.
2. Provides precursors for conversion of blood fat to sugar and thus promotes reduction of excess blood fat and control of hypoglycemic symptoms.
3. Acts as a tonic to promote liver and kidney function by reason of it's A and F vitamin components and is a source of betaine, a factor in liver detoxification and other intermediate processes.

Possibly through the above mechanisms, this product has proved useful in decreasing sensitization reactions particularly where food allergy or intolerance to certain foods is encountered

CLINICALLY ASSOCIATED CONDITIONS

GASTROINTESTINAL-URINARY	NERVOUS AND PSYCHOGENIC	METABOLIC DISORDERS
<u>Stomach and Intestine</u>	<u>Functional</u>	<u>Acid-Base Balance</u>
Achlorhydria	Dysphagia	Ketosis
Alimentary Canal Flora	<u>Metabolic</u>	<u>Allergies</u>
<u>Liver and Gallbladder</u>	Alcoholism	Asthma
Biliary Stasis	<u>Vaso-Motor</u>	Sneezing Attacks
Digestion Faulty	Dizziness	<u>Body Weight</u>
Gallbladder Disease	METABOLIC DISORDERS	Appetite Excessive
Hepatitis	<u>Intermediate Processes</u>	Obesity
Jaundice	Carbohydrate Metabolism	Psoriasis
Indigestion, Acute	Diabetes Mellitus	Telangiectasis
Liver Disease	Cholesterol Metabolism	OTHERS
	Reactions to Foods	Sedimentation Rate
	<u>Collagen</u>	Psoriasis
	Arcus Senilis	Telangiectasis
	Arteriosclerosis	

ASSOCIATED PRODUCTS:

Cataplex A	(See **Cataplex A-C-P** see page, 45)
Cataplex F	(See **Cataplex F** see page, 61)
Betafood	**Betafood** does not contain the A and F Complexes, but contains proportionately higher amounts of the bile-thinning factor and has a more potent effect in this respect. Useful where this effect is to be augmented or when for some reason, the A and F Complexes are not desired

ANTRONEX

Label: Each tablet contains 10 mg of Yakriton from beef liver. A liver extract that is opposed in its biological significance to thyroxine. For experimental use in hypertension, allergic states and as a natural anti-histaminic. Dosage 1 to 3 per day or as directed.

Tissue or Function Supported	Synergistic to liver detoxification mechanisms.

CLINICAL CONSIDERATIONS
Prominent Clinical Signs And Symptoms

<u>Symptoms:</u>

1. Hypertension
2. (Headaches, insomnia and related symptoms).
3. Hyperthyroidism
4. (Tachycardia, mental symptoms related to).
5. Allergies
6. (Skin rashes, etc.)
7. Hyperirritability
8. (Nervous tension, headaches, insomnia)
9. Toxemia
10. (Toxic manifestations of epilepsy, eclampsia, drug addiction, drug poisoning, etc.).
11. Liver Disease
12. (Gynecomastia, edema, ascites, venous congestion, redness of palms of hands, etc.).
13. Cerebral Pressure Symptoms
14. (Described as "surge of blood in the head", often associated with hypertension)

<u>Possible Etiological Background:</u>

Antronex may be generally described as "the liver detoxification hormone". Insofar as we are able to clinically determine, its physiological effect seems to consist of causing more blood to flow through the liver, a hyperemia of physiological importance. This effect may be used to rationalize its benefits in the symptoms listed since the distribution of blood is changed in the vascular network. Hence, increased flow of blood through the portal system, less in the peripheral channels. The increase of blood through the liver may also account for its increased activity in detoxifying such substances as excess histamine, both sex and thyroid hormones and other factors such as drug toxicity mentioned. In this respect, Antronex acts to promote detoxification in liver overload, just as Arginex aids in kidney overload. He same mechanism is also useful in the more profound liver diseases such as in fatty degeneration where the detriment is in incomplete oxygenation and in fibrosis where blood supply becomes increasingly important upon a functional basis alone.

Symptom Characteristics: Aside from detoxification need which is usually obvious from evidence of the history, the most common indication is in that of blood volume deviations usually evidenced by cranial symptoms (such as headache, pressure, etc.)

	Test:	Need Shown By:
Laboratory Tests	Blood Volume	Ratio of red cells to plasma is method used, although this may not be practical for our purposes in this case.
Clinical Tests	a. Postural Blood Pressure Test	May indicate disturbance in portal circulation shown by drop in standing position.
	b. Blood Pressure Level	Indicated in elevated diastolic pressure as well as elevated systolic pressure.
	c. History	History of hypertension, headaches of toxic origin.

Administration	**Dosage:** Should not exceed one or two tablets per day in initial stages until tolerance is determined; see "Side-Effects" below.
	Effect: Usually beneficial effects are immediate in headaches and insomnia when due to this cause; hypermetabolic states such as hyperthyroidism and hypertension require long-term therapy
	Side Effects: Response of the low blood pressure or hypothyroid case may be negative due to its effect in lowering the blood pressure. Most of its side-effects, of which vertigo is the most characteristic, may be explained on the basis of the blood volume factors outlined above.

ANTRONEX

Synergists:
a. Orchex
b. Calcium Lactate and (Cataplex F)
c. Betacol

Activity Contributed:
Physiological Tranquilizer
Hypermetabolic states
Liver Conditions

GENERAL CONSIDERATIONS

The nutritional effects of Antronex may be listed as follows:

a. Physiological anti-histamine factor.
b. Blood pressure lowering factor.
c. Liver detoxifying factor.
d. Synergist of thyroxine.

Its clinical application may be rationalized as follows:

Mechanism of action is apparently by producing a hyperemia of the liver thus increasing blood supply to this organ. This action enables the liver to perform increased activity, particularly in its detoxification function.

This effect tends to bring about a temporary change in the blood volume, increasing the blood in the portal circulation, thus shunts blood from other channels, particularly the cerebral circulation. Evidence of such changes of circulation are seen in relief of "pressure headaches" and in insomnia where the cerebral pressure may be high, preventing normal circulation in the head and a source of much discomfort to the patient as well as a potential danger from the increased pressure.

CLINICALLY ASSOCIATED CONDITIONS

GASTRO-INTESTINAL-URINARY
   <u>Liver and Gallbladder</u>
      Liver Disease
NERVOUS AND PSYCHOGENIC
   <u>Functional</u>
      Chorea
      Epilepsy
      Headaches
   <u>Metabolic</u>
      Tranquilizing Effects
   <u>Vaso-Motor</u>
      Hypersensitivity

NERVOUS AND PSYCHOGENIC
   <u>Lesions</u>
      Cerebral Palsy
   <u>Allergies</u>
      Anti-Histamine Effects
      Sneezing Attacks
EXOGENIC DISORDERS
   <u>Toxic</u>
      Delirium
      Nightmares
GLANDULAR
      Gynecomastia

ARGINEX

Label: Enzyme complex from rice polish and beet leaf biologically processed with special yeast strains. Suggested dosage: 2 to 6 tablets per day, or more as may be directed by physician.

Tissue or Function Supported: Intermediate processes involving urea metabolism which support liver and kidney function where toxic overload places stress on these organs.

CLINICAL CONSIDERATIONS
Prominent Clinical Signs And Symptoms

Symptoms:

Symptoms of kidney-bladder disorders
(Pain in area of kidneys or bladder may radiate through dorsal region to liver area) burning on urination; uremia, uriniferous odor of breath, itching of skin from "salty" (residue) perspiration; edema, ascites, dropsy, etc.; toxemia, body odor, pasty skin, biliousness; liver disease, enlargement, diminished urination, veinous congestion, etc.

Possible Etiological Background:

Apparently a factor in metabolizing urea for excretion by reason of its enzyme arginase, acting as a physiologic diuretic thus promoting the elimination of toxins and influencing the osmotic transfer of tissue fluids.

Symptom Characteristics: We would consider Arginex a valuable adjunct in all problems involving the liver and kidneys, particularly where this is evidenced by systemic manifestations involving the detoxification mechanisms and fluid balance.

Laboratory Tests	Test: Urinalysis	Need Shown By: Cells, casts, albuminuria, etc.

Clinical Test — CONCENTRATION AND DILUTION TEST

A. Concentration Phase: First night: At supper patient is restricted to one glass of fluid; thereafter no food or drink is given until the end of the test. Patient remains inactive as possible. Before going to bed patient empties bladder and specimen is discarded. On arising, patient passes a urine specimen which is saved. Second and third specimens are collected one and two hours later, recording exact time of voiding. After third specimen patient may have food and drink.

B. Dilution Phase: Second Night: A regular supper is eaten; no food or drink is allowed thereafter; patient is as inactive as possible. On awakening in the morning, patient empties bladder and specimen is discarded. After this urination, patient is given 5 glasses of fluid to drink within 45 minutes (water or lemonade). Urine is collected at 1, 2, 3 and 4 hours after patient has started drinking. These specimens saved. After 4 hour specimen, patient may have food and drink.

PROCEDURE: Specific gravity for each specimen is measured with urinometer. Range should be 1.026 or over for concentration phase; about 1.003, gradual increase for dilution phase. Failure to show this range indicates some sort of disorder of the kidney tubules. Arginex and other kidney support is indicated.

Administration	**Dosage:** Initial dosage should be at least 6 per day, later reduced to 1 to 3 per day.
	Effect: May be spectacular in some cases. In most cases a satisfactory clinical response may be expected where indicated.
	Side Effect: Usually none are observed.

Synergists:
a. AC Carbamide
b. Chlorophyll Complex (perles)
c. Phosfood
d. Zymex

Activity Contributed:
Physiological diuretic
Detoxification effect
Aids diuresis in some cases
Intestinal detoxification factor

ARGINEX

GENERAL CONSIDERATIONS

Toxic overload from many conditions may cause inability to eliminate the increased metabolic wastes. This places stress on both kidney and liver function for which Arginex is indicated.

Arginex promotes physiological diuresis in indicated cases. It apparently aids in metabolizing urea for excretion by its enzyme arginase. As such it should be considered in all cases where Carbamide is indicated or where Carbamide has been shown to benefit the patient, arginase being the basic physiological factor required in these cases. This is a common occurrence on low protein diets.

CLINICALLY ASSOCIATED CONDITIONS

GASTRO-INTESTINAL-URINARY
   <u>Liver and Gallbladder</u>
      Liver Disease
   <u>Kidney and Bladder</u>
      Albuminuria
      Nephritis
      Uremia
NERVOUS AND PSYCHOGENIC
   <u>Functional</u>
      Epilepsy
      Migraine Headaches
   <u>Vaso-Motor</u>
      Blood Pressure Changes
      Heat Prostration
METABOLIC DISORDERS
   <u>Intermediate Processes</u>
      Diabetes Mellitus
   <u>Collagen Diseases</u>
      Arthritis, Rheumatoid
      Gout

METABOLIC DISORDERS
   <u>Acid-Base Balance</u>
      Acidosis
      Ketosis
      Urine, pH of
   <u>Water Balance</u>
      Ascites
      Dropsy
      Edema
   <u>Respiratory</u>
      Emphysema
EXOGENIC DISORDERS
   <u>Toxic</u>
      Burns, Systemic
      Delirium
      Eclampsia
   <u>Inflammation</u>
      Tonsillitis

BETACOL

Label: Alcohol soluble factors from Beet Molasses, mineral fractions from Sugar Cane juice, Tillandsia, and the specific lipoproteins of the chromatin of Beef Liver. 1 to 2 capsules per day or as directed.

Tissue or Function Supported	A complex of nutritional factors which experience has shown to be beneficial in support of liver function, activating and aiding restoration of liver tissue.

CLINICAL CONSIDERATIONS
Prominent Clinical Signs And Symptoms

Symptoms:	Possible Etiological Background
1. Venous Congestion (Prominence of veins on chest and abdomen, hemorrhoids, varicosities, etc.).	Stasis in portal circulation routes.
2. Arthritis (Joint pains, rheumatic swellings, inflammation).	Failure of detoxification mechanisms.
3. Paresthesia (Burning or itching sensations, particularly on soles of feet).	Neurological involvement probably secondary to toxic manifestations.
4. Erythema (Red, flushed skin areas, particularly palms of hands)	(Same as 3, above)
5. Gastro-Intestinal Complaints (Indigestion, constipation, flatulence, nausea, etc.)	Biliary incompetency.
6. Stool Variations (Variations in color, presence of undigested foods, etc.).	
7. Water Balance (Edema, ascites, swollen ankles, bloating, etc.)	(Same as 5 above)
8. Biliousness (Malaise, headaches, constipation, etc.)	Portal circulation involvement.
9. Appearance (Pasty color of skin, telangiectasis, capillary breakdown, etc.)	Biliary stasis.
10. Kidney Disease	Circulatory disturbances.
	Protein metabolism.

Laboratory Tests	Most Frequently Used Tests: a. Urine for Presence of Bile b. Icterus Index c. Van Den Berg Reaction d. Cephalin-Cholesterol Flocculation Test 1. Galactose Tolerance Test	Indications for Tests of Liver Function: Dilated veins over chest or abdomen; indigestion symptoms; enlarged liver or spleen; jaundice or ascites; oliguria; leukocytosis; decreased serum albumin.
Clinical Tests	1. Observation 2. Palpation 3. Blood Pressure 4. Phonocardiograph 5. History	Clinical findings of the above mentioned abnormalities. Enlargement of liver or spleen Elevated diastolic pressure is considered by some as significant. Usually liver disease is concomitant with congestive heart failure. History of jaundice, hepatitis or chronic kidney disease.
Administration	**Dosage:** This is important and various dosages are required depending upon patient's tolerance and clinical response, generally 1 to 3 per day. Note that some patients may not be able to tolerate even one capsule per day (taken at one time), and in this case, the capsule should be divided into 2 o 3 doses gradually increasing, as normalcy of liver function is brought about. **Effect:** Some types of arthritis, particularly low-back pain type, may show immediate results. In specific liver diseases and metabolic disorders, response is in proportion to acuteness and chronicity and amount of degeneration present. Use of synergists listed below is very important where liver degeneration is the problem	

BETACOL

Administration **Side Effects:** These are most likely to occur in those cases with the most advanced degeneration and thus acts as a means of estimating the extent of derangement. Reactions, such as nausea, may occur in some types of biliary stasis. This is not difficult to predetermine as it is usually associated with the classical symptoms of gallbladder disease. These reactions may usually be mitigated or avoided by the use of AF Betafood, which, through its bile thinning effect, aids in the control of the increased liver activity brought about by the use of Betacol. In all cases of doubt as to tolerance of Betacol, use AF Betafood for at least 10 days before administering Betacol. Di-Sodium Phosphate augments this effect.

<u>Synergists:</u>	<u>Activity Contributed:</u>
1. Choline	Physiological detergent; anticolic
2. Zypan	Gastric secretion catalyst
3. AF Betafood	Bile-thinning effect
4. Di-Sodium Phosphate	Liver stimulant

GENERAL CONSIDERATIONS

Discussion: The etiological background of liver dysfunction should be brought into focus in two major categories, as follows:
1. Where response to selected therapy is slow or failing.
2. In most chronic, degenerative diseases.

While liver involvement is present in most chronic disease, the screening of patients requiring specific liver support presents a problem which must be answered. The following suggests a screening process useful in determining the most needful of these cases:
1. Evidence of venous congestion by signs of dilated veins showing over chest and abdomen, also hemorrhoids and varicose veins would come in this category.
2. Kidney pathology. Since kidney pathology may rest largely on deviations I protein metabolism, over which the liver has primary control, all kidney cases require liver support on this basis. Clinical results bear out this statement.
3. Most chronic diseases involving the degenerative processes, and, specifically wasting diseases and disturbances in water balance, edema and ascites, require specific liver support. This would include most cases of congestive heart failure.

CLINICALLY ASSOCIATED CONDITIONS

GASTRO-INTESTINAL-
URINARY
  <u>Liver and Gallbladder</u>
    Constipation
    Hepatitis
    Jaundice
    Liver Disease
  <u>Kidney and Bladder</u>
    Albuminuria
    Nephritis
NERVOUS AND
PSYCHOGENIC
  <u>Functional</u>
    Epilepsy
  <u>Metabolic</u>
    Alcoholism
  <u>Vaso-Motor</u>
    Dizziness
    Shock
METABOLIC DISORDERS
  <u>Growth and Repair</u>

Aging Processes
<u>Collagen Diseases</u>
  Arcus Senilis
  Arteriosclerosis
  Arthritis
  Bones, Pain in
  Cataracts
<u>Acid-Base Balance</u>
  Ketosis
<u>Water Balance</u>
  Ascites
  Dropsy
  Edema
<u>Blood</u>
  Anemia, Pernicious
  Epistaxis
<u>Allergies</u>
<u>Body Weight</u>
  Appetite Decreased
  Obesity
EXOGENIC DISORDERS

  <u>Toxic)</u>
    Delirium
    Eclampsia
    Halitosis
  <u>Traumatic</u>
    Sedimentation Rate
VASCULAR DISORDERS
  <u>Circulatory Diseases</u>
    Hemorrhoids
    Phlebitis
    Varicose Veins
SKIN CONDITIONS
  Acne
  Psoriasis
  Telangiectasis
GENETIC DISORDERS
  <u>Female</u>
    Pregnancy Schedule
SPECIFIC DEFICIENCY
  <u>Glandular</u>
    Gynecomastia

BETACOL

DISCUSSION: As has been stated, the outstanding clinical picture presented in liver failure is circulatory collapse, marked by venous congestion, ascites and edema and various other changes in the vascular network. However, a specific enumeration of hepatic functions may prove helpful as a reference. According to Best and Taylor (Physiological Basis of Medial Practice) these are as follows:

a. Blood formation in the embryo; storage of Vitamin B12
b. Fibrinogen production
c. Prothrombin production
d. Heparin production
e. Iron and copper storage
f. Blood volume regulation. Liberation of a depressor antidiuretic principle.
g. Reticulo-endothelial activity (Kupffer cells)
h. Protein metabolism, deamination, amino acid synthesis, urea, uric acid and hippuric acid synthesis.
i. Detoxification.
j. Fat metabolism
k. Heat production
l. Carbohydrate metabolism
m. Formation of Vitamin A from carotene

The importance of pancreatic activity in respect to liver function should be emphasized; proteolytic enzymes of pancreas making methionine available from dietary protein.

ASSOCIATED PRODUCTS:

Heratrophin: Useful where effects of **Betacol** produce side-reactions. (See "Side-Effects" under administraiton this bulletin).

BETAFOOD

Label: The soluble components of green beet leaf juice, dehydrated in high vacuum to conserve betaine content. One or two tablets three times a day, swallowed with water. For nutritional use to supply the trace mineral content from beet greens.

Tissue or Function Supported: Intermediate processes, primarily carbohydrate and fat metabolism.

CLINICAL CONSIDERATIONS
Prominent Clinical Signs And Symptoms

Symptoms:

1. Gallbladder Symptoms (Intolerance to fats or gas-producing foods; nausea, flatulence, jaundice, etc.).
2. Portal hypertension (Signs of liver disease such as veins showing on chest and abdomen-venous congestion).
3. Hypoglycemic symptoms, (Craving for sweets, eating of which relieves symptoms).
4. Hypercholestrolemia (Also high blood fat remaining elevated for prolonged period)
5. Liver insufficiency (Acholic stool, constipation).
6. Biliary stasis (Interference with bile flow).

Possible Etiological Background

The empirical use of beet leaf juice in gallbladder disorders has long been known. We now believe this can be rationalized on the basis of the naturally occurring betaine-highest when grown on ammonia rich soils. Apparently the intermediate process concerning conversion of blood fat to sugar and its utilization is concerned. This logically concerns itself with bile viscosity and liver function, the high blood fat following meals being cause of not only discomforting symptoms but probably contributing to the reported deleterious effects in arteriosclerosis. Recall that the diabetic characteristically has an elevated cholesterol reading.

Symptom Characteristics: Usually associated with the gallbladder syndrome-though not always-since deviations in fat and carbohydrate metabolism may be concerned with their deviated clinical manifestations.

Laboratory	**Tests Test:** a. Cholesterol b. Glucose Tolerance Test c. X-Ray d. Liver Function Tests	**Need Shown By:** Hypercholesterolemia Curve deviations Gallstones See **Betacol** Bulletin
Clinical Tests	a. Palpation b. Observation	Liver margin, tenderness Venous congestion
Administration	**Dosage:** Two with each meal in gallbladder-liver dysfunction, two tablets at time of occurrence usually aborts a hypoglycemic attack..	
	Effect: The effect is potentiated by the simultaneous administration of **Choline** and, where indicated, **Zypan** or **Betaine Hydrochloride**. Symptomatically satisfactory in a high percentage of gallbladder cases	
	Side Effect: Minimal side-effects are noted for the reason that **Betafood** is not a biliary stimulant, but rather lowers bile viscosity and contributes thus to its control.	

Synergists:
a. Choline
b. Zypan or Betaine Hydrochloride

Activity Contributed:
Anti-colic factor and physiological detergent.
Gastric catalyst

GENERAL CONSIDERATIONS

High blood fat following meals is certainly one of the most important considerations in the management of the gallbladder patient. This tends to become prolonged and excessive, not only in the gallbladder patient, but also in the geriatric subject. Physiological support of the fat-sugar conversion mechanism is certainly, therefore, a valued contribution to their economy. Betafood as such is a completely physiological remedy and, where effective, may be safely used for as long as desired. Small, frequent meals should be advised for this type of patient.

BETAFOOD

GENERAL CONSIDERATIONS

The use of synergistic products, Choline and Zypan or Betaine Hydrochloride, will contribute considerably in the management of these patients when administered as indicated.

The prevalence of hypercholesterolemia with its attendant arteriosclerotic syndrome plus the high incidence of liver and gallbladder dysfunction provides a wide-spectrum range for the use of Betafood and its synergists. Note that even though these may exist only on a subclinical level, the possibility of their existence lies within the category of most chronic and degenerative diseases.

CLINICALLY ASSOCIATED CONDITIONS

GASTROINTESTINAL-URINARY
    Stomach and Intestine
        Alimentary Tract Flora
    Liver and Gallbladder
        Biliary Stasis
        Gallbladder Disease
        Hepatitis
        Jaundice
        Liver Disease
METABOLIC DISORDERS
    Intermediate Processes

Carbohydrate Metabolism
    Diabetes Mellitus
    Cholesterol Metabolism
Acid-Base Disorders
    Ketosis
Body Weight
    Obesity
OTHERS:
    Sedimentation Rate
    Psoriasis
    Telangiectasia

BETAINE HYDROCHLORIDE

Label: Each tablet contains: 2 grains Betaine HCL, 2 grains Pepsin 1:3000, one-half grain Ammonium Chloride U.S.P. USE: To supply Hydrochloride Acid in Achlorhydria. Dose: Two Tablets after each meal or as directed.

Tissue or Function Supported	Diminished gastric secretion, achlorhydria or hypochlorhydria.

CLINICAL CONSIDERATIONS
Prominent Clinical Signs And Symptoms

Symptoms:

1. Appetite changes (Loss of taste for meat, eating when not hungry, etc.)
2. Malassimilation (Protein, calcium and iron deficiency states).
3. Flatulence (Lower bowel gas).
4. Indigestion (2 to 3 hours after eating, fullness but no pain characteristic).
5. Increased metabolic demands (Pregnancy, stress situations, prolonged fever).
6. Vomiting and diarrhea (HCL loss by these routes).
7. Pernicious anemia (Achlorhydria is pathonomonic).
8. Demineralization (Either from excess use of alkalizers or from long-standing salt-free diets.

Possible Etiological Background:

Physiological explanations of the mechanisms of gastric secretions lag far behind clinical evidence of their efficacious application, thus experience in use of hydrochloric acid in practice constitutes an essentiality for fullest spectrum of application. By and large this consists of making a Therapeutic Test in most subjects suspected of diminished gastric secretion. When the factors are known and properly observed, the findings are quite positive clinically in most cases. Unfortunately, laboratory methods, even though practical, may not reveal the limited range of mild insufficiency, but rather tend to show the extremes of achlorhydria and hyperacidity. The "intangible" middle range, which consists the majority of those in need, practically remains to be diagnosed by the clinical test method. The importance of this test is shown by statements from many authorities that gastric secretions diminish almost in ratio to the aging process. See "Achlorhydria" in Clinical Trophology (Therapeutic Food Manual)

Symptom Characteristics: Anemia, loss of taste for meat, and gastrointestinal symptoms are most common findings. See "Zypan" in product bulletin for further details.

Laboratory Tests	Remarks: While gastric analysis may be used, the inconvenience and expense to the patient is considerable, compared with the Therapeutic Test described above. For further information see "Achlorhydria", Clinical Trophology.
Clinical Tests	See above: Diagnex (Squibbs) is a relatively simple test which may be useful.
Administration	**Dosage:** Symptomatic response is criterion of levels required. This should be regulated to time of indigestion symptoms, thus if symptoms occur before administration 3 or 4 hours after meals and after administration 5 or 6 hours after meals, it simply shows that the fermentation process has been delayed and that dosage needs to be increased. It is the number of tablets per meal, not per day, which is important. Thus, 3 tablets with evening meal, for example, may produce appreciable results, whereas, 3 tablets t.i.d. may not be discernible.
	Effect: Relief from gatsrointestinal symptoms when from this cause is usually immediate, or within a few days; in absence of gastrointestinal symptoms-amenias and emaciation, for example-long term use is required.
	Side Effect: The various reactions which occur have a specific diagnostic value. For complete information on this subject see "Achlorhydria", Clinical, Trophology

Synergists:	Activity Contributed:
Pancreatrophin	Protomorphogen
Cal-Amo	Anti-alkalosis factors
Cholacol	Bile salts
Cholacol II	Adsorbent
Okra, Pepsin E3	Mucilaginous colloids

BETAINE HYDROCHLORIDE

GENERAL CONSIDERATIONS

The primary indication for **Betaine Hydrochloride Tablets** is achlorhydria-diminished-gastric secretions. When favorable response is obtained from this product, it should lead the clinician to investigate the possibilities of diminished secretions of the pancreas and liver. **Zypan**, containing Betaine Hydrochloride and pancreas factors, then becomes the product of choice. This may be assisted in its effects by, Pancreatrophin. We may list further associated products and concomitant conditions as follows:

    Cholacol (Bile salts and Collinsonia)---------Cholecystectomy or constipation

    Cholacol II (Montmorillonite)-----------------Adsorbent in intestinal toxemia

    Okra, Pepsin E3 (Mucilaginous colloids)---Gastritis

Pituitrophin has been shown to contribute favorably to many types of digestive disorders. Recall also that diminished gastric secretions inhibit the absorption of calcium, protein and iron and that these factors may need to be supplied as **Bio-Dent Tablets** (calcium), **Protefood** (protein) and **Ferrofood** (iron). Overalimentation should also be considered, small, high-quality foods at frequent intervals being given preference over large meals, the digestive capacity being limited by the quality and quantity of food it may handle at any one time. See "LOW STRESS DIET" for further information in this regard.

CLINICALLY ASSOCIATED CONDITIONS

GASTROINTESTINAL-URINARY
    <u>Stomach and Intestine</u>
        Achlorhydria
        Alimentary Canal Flora
        Flatulence
    <u>Liver and Gallbladder</u>
        Biliary Stasis
        Gallbladder Disease
        Constipation
METABOLIC DISORDERS
    <u>Blood</u>
        Anemia, Pernicious
        Anemia, Secondary

METABOLIC DISORDERS
    <u>Body Weight</u>
        Obesity
EXOGENIC DISORDERS
    <u>Toxic</u>
        Halitosis
    <u>Inflammatory</u>
        Diarrhea
FEMALE CONSIDERATIONS
    Pregnancy Schedule

BIO-DENT TABLETS

Label: Each tablet contains the equivalent of 3 gr. of fresh veal bone (processed without heat, in accordance with Pat. No. 2,374,219), and 1 mgm. of organically combined manganese. Carrier Material: Defatted wheat germ. Binder: Licorice Root Extract. This product is sold for use as a part of the nutritional pattern of a human diet to promote normal health of teeth and bones. It has no drug use known to us in the dosage recommended. Suggested Dosage: 6 to 12 tablets per day or as directed by physician or dentist. Tablets may be chewed to assure complete assimilation.

Tissue or Function Supported	Source of nutrients intended to support growth and repair of bone, teeth, and related structures, such as ligaments and tendons. Contains enzyme factors, minerals and proteins(particularly tryptophane and methionine) and bone tissue determinants.

CLINICAL CONSIDERATIONS
Prominent Clinical Signs And Symptoms

Symptoms:

1. Bone deformities (Exostosis "spurs", osteoarthritis of spine, hip joints, knees, particularly).
2. Lack of motility (stooped posture and gait, ligament and tendon disorders).
3. Dental problems (Caries, loose teeth, reabsorption of gums, tender, sore gums).
4. Arteriosclerotic changes (Mental changes of aged, increased changes in connective tissues, osteoporosis of aged, etc.).
5. Protein, mineral, enzyme, deficiency states (Insomnia, restlessness, cramps, emaciation, chronic fatigue, increased irritability and others).
6. Blood dyscrasias (Anemias and related blood problems).
7. Spinal lesions (Disc lesions, integrity of supporting tendons, membranes, capsules, etc.).

Possible Etiological Background:

It is perhaps well to recall that bone is a dynamic tissue in spite of its apparent static nature, it being a storehouse for not only calcium and phosphorus, but also of proteins and enzymes. As such it is a potent food source and like all such foods is highly perishable, being particularly susceptible to heat or cooking which materially detracts from its food value. The maintenance of this high nutritional value depends, therefore, upon low heat methods of processing, **Bio-Dent Tablets** meeting this qualification. Thus, rare amino acids, specific bone nutrients, raw material for fibrocartilagenous structures are supplied by this product as well is included in the processing, a nutrient source of the central factors of the hemopoietic system. **Bio-Dent Tablets** are made from veal spine and ribs--meat, marrow and all—therefore contains the specific factors for these tissues. (**Biost**, in powder form, is available also where these factors are desired and has the advantage of being able to be added to other foods in the diet. **Bio-Dent**, in tablet form, has the advantage of convenience of use where cooperation may be lacking in use of the powdered form, expediency of use being the criterion for selection of each product.)

Symptom Characteristics:	Usually involve changes in teeth, bone and connective tissue, but specificity is unimportant since this product adds important nutrients to all normal diets.	
LaboratoryTest	Most Frequently Used Tests: a. X-Ray Examination b. Hypoproteinemia	Indications for Tests: a. Osteoporosis b. Decreased total serum protein
Clinical Tests	Tests a. Postural Examination b. Starch test	Need Shown By a. Stooped or bent legs when walking. B. decreased range of motion in tendons,(Achilles, fasia lata, Spine
Administration	**Dosage:** See label above for dosage and uses with the Page Food Plan (Refer to the back of the book).	
	Effect: Immediate clinical observation of results are not ordinarily to be expected since structural changes are usually involved, as would apply to arthritis, for example. Rapid results may be obtained in more functional types of disorders such as insomnia, restlessness, hyperirritability, etc.	
	Side Effect: These seldom occur and when they do may be considered as an indication for **Calcium Lactate**, the ionizable form of calcium more directly concerned with the relief of calcium deficiency symptoms.	

BIO-DENT TABLETS

<u>Synergists:</u>   <u>**Activity Contributed:**</u>
a. Ostogen   A source of biologically active uncooked veal bone calcium-protein-enzyme complex which supplies phosphatase and other bone factors.
b. Catalyn   To supply additional synergistic vitamin and trace mineral complexes which may not be adequately provided in the dietary.

Note: While practically the whole array of nutritional factors are concerned with calcium metabolism in one way or another, the ionized forms, of which **Calcium Lactate** is one of the most important, may be the only ones to relieve calcium deficiency symptoms such as muscle cramps, blood clotting mechanisms and nervous irritability. For this reason, **Calcium Lactate** should be reviewed and if symptoms of this nature are present, it should be administered simultaneously with **Bio-Dent Tablets**.

GENERAL CONSIDERATIONS

Bio-Dent may be considered an important protective food in practically all problems related to bone, teeth, and connective tissues; the rare amino acids present, ordinarily lost in cooking, make it useful in protein metabolism; and the determinant factors of bone and bone marrow make it specific for these tissues. It thus aids in the formation and repair of bone, teeth and fibrocartilaginous tissues such as fascia, ligaments, and tendons, as well as having a beneficial influence on the blood forming organs.

The known amino acids of which **Bio-Dent** is a good source are tryptophane and methionine. The former, in a recent test in children, stopped tooth decay; the latter, methionine, is known to be important in eclampsia, liver cirrhosis, liver enlargement and liver necrosis. It is also a good source of lysine, the amino acid needed in the diet in greatest amounts, the deficiency of which, in human subjects, results in fatigability and irritability. The combined deficiency of lysine and tryptophane, is one cause of corneal vascularization, simulating the riboflavin deficiency reaction, not affected by riboflavin treatment. References for above statements: **Biost** (formerly known as **Calcifood A**) product sheet, Form no TG 239 ®, Therapeutic Foods Company.

The exception to **Bio-Dent**, as a source of calcium, is where alkaline calcium to form calcium bicarbonate, the ionized blood calcium is desired. T his is in cases of acute infection (and symptoms as described above) where the calcium is to aid Vitamin C in controlling the infective agent, in the stimulation of phagocytosis. Lime water or the proprietary Kalak water are other forms of alkaline calcium.

CLINICALLY ASSOCIATED CONDITIONS

NERVOUS AND PSYCHOGENIC
  <u>Functional</u>
    Insomnia
  <u>Metabolic</u>
    Torticollis
  <u>Mentality</u>
    Backwardness in children
METABOLIC DISORDERS
  <u>Growth and Repair</u>
    Bones, Healing of
    Caries
    Gums, Receding of
    Teething
  <u>Intermediate Processes</u>
    Calcium Metabolism

METABOLIC DISORDERS
  <u>Collagen Diseases</u>
    Arcus Senilis
    Arteriosclerosis
    Arthritis, Hypertrophic
    Bones, Pain in
    Bursitis
    Disc Lesions
    Ligaments, Deformity of
  <u>Acid-Base Disorders</u>
    Alkalosis
  <u>Blood</u>
    Anemia
    Leukopenia

EXOGENIC DISORDERS
  <u>Inflammation</u>
    Periodontoclasia
    Denture Irritation
SPECIFIC DEFICIENCY DISEASES
    Conjunctivitis
    Pellagra

ASSOCIATED PRODUCTS:
Ostogen: This is an extract from **Biost** containing primarily the enzyme phosphatase and rare amino acids and is useful where higher concentrations of these factors are desired. (See Page, 21)
Biost: We feel that the best nutritional purposes are served by **Biost**, but that where patient management presents a barrier to the powder form that **Bio-Dent** provides the second best means of administration of these essential food factors. (See Pages, 19, 21)
Ostrophin PMG: Contains factors of **Ostogen** and **Cytotrophic Extracts of Bone**

BIOST

Label: A biologically active, fresh dehydrated veal bone, powdered with the addition of defated cereal germ to absorb the excess fat from the bone marrow. Contains approximately 50% of fresh veal bone, in a carrier of cereal germ. Hydrous natural crystalline calcium sulphate is added to afford non-phosphate soluble calcium. Each heaping teaspoonful contains 166 I.U. Vitamin D from fish liver lipoids (1/3 adult minimum daily requirement). Non-phosphate assimilable calcium 900 mg. per ounce. Intended to supply the elements necessary to build teeth and bone in palatable and most assimilable form.

Use in milk shakes, malted milks, fruit juice, breakfast cereal, as a spread for sandwiches blended with peanut butter, in salad dressings, and in ice cream in place of gelatin or other bodifiers.

Recommended daily maximum schedule: 2 to 3 teaspoonfuls for adults; 1 to 2 for children 4 to 12 years of age; infants, ½ to 1 level teaspoonful in milk.

Tissue or Function Supported	Source of nutrients specific in support of growth and repair of teeth and related structures such as ligaments and tendons. Contains enzyme factors, minerals and proteins (particularly, tryptophane and methionine) and bone tissue determinants.

CLINICAL CONSIDERATIONS
Prominent Clinical Signs And Symptoms

Symptoms:

1. Bone deformities (Exostoses "spurs", osteoarthritis of spine, hip joints, knees, particularly).

2. Lack of motility (Stooped posture and gait, ligament and tendon disorders).

3. Dental problems (Caries, loose teeth, reabsorption of gums, tender, sore gums).

4. Arteriosclerotic changes (mental changes of aged, increased changes in connective tissues, osteoporosis of aged, etc.).

5. Protein, mineral, enzyme deficiency states (Insomnia, restlessness, cramps, emaciation, chronic fatigue, increased irritability and others).

6. Blood dyscrasias (Anemias and other picture problems).

7. Spinal lesions (Disc lesions, integrity of supporting tendons, membranes, capsules, etc.).

Possible Etiological Background

Lack of specific bone nutrients and determinants.

Fibrocartilagenous structures requiring specific nutrients which may be lacking in diet.

Rare amino acids as well as other factors important here, particularly tryptophane, commonly lost when cooked in presence of sugar.

Accelerated metabolic disturbances from malnutrition resulting in premature senility in which minerals, enzymes and proteins found in Biost provide important bulwark.

Deficiency of nutrients of which calcium and phosphorus with their metabolizer, Vitamin D, play important role.

Intimate relationship of the nutrient source with the hemopoietic system.

Biost is made from veal spine and ribs-meat, marrow and all-therefore contains factors specific for these tissues.

Symptom Characteristics: Usually involve structural changes of bone and connective tissue. General deficiency states are also to be considered, specificity being unimportant since this product is an important food in all normal diets.

Laboratory Tests	Test: a. X-Ray Examination b. Hypoproteinemia	Need Shown By: Osteoporosis or exostoses Decreased total serum protein
Clinical Tests	a. Postural Examination b. Stretch Tests	Stooped or bent legs when walking Decreased range of motion in tendons, (Achilles, fascia lata, spine, etc.)

BIOST

Administration	
	Dosage: See label above for dosage and uses in diet.
	Effect: Immediate clinical observation of results are not ordinarily to be expected since structural changes are usually involved, as would apply to arthritis, for example. Rapid results may be obtained in more functional types of disorders such as insomnia, restlessness, hyperirritability, etc.
	Side Effect: These seldom occur and when they do may be considered as an indication for **Calcium Lactate**, the ionizable form of calcium more directly concerned with the relief of calcium deficiency symptoms.

<u>Synergists:</u>   <u>Activity Contributed:</u>
a. Bio-Dent   These supply bone factors also in other forms:
b. Cyrofood   Bio-Dent in Tablet form; Cyrofood in combination with other nutritional factors which generally supply essential food complexes.

Note: While practically the whole array of nutritional factors are concerned with calcium metabolism in one way or another, the ionized forms, of which Calcium Lactate is one of the most important, may be the only ones to relieve calcium deficiency symptoms such as muscle cramps, blood clotting mechanisms, and nervous irritability. For this reason, the product bulletin on Calcium Lactate should be reviewed and if symptoms of this nature are present, it should be administered simultaneously with Biost.

GENERAL CONSIDERATIONS

Biost may be considered an important protective food in practically all problems related to bone, teeth, and connective tissues; the rare amino acids present, ordinarily lost in cooking, make it useful in protein metabolism; and the determinant factors of bone and bone marrow make it specific for these tissues. It thus aids in the formation and repair of bone, teeth, and fibrocartilagenous tissues such as fascia, ligaments, and tendons, as well as having a beneficial influence on the blood forming organs.

The known amino acids of which **Biost** is a good source are tryptophane and methionine. The former in a recent test in children stopped tooth decay, the latter, methionine, is known to be important in eclampsia, liver cirrhosis, liver enlargement, and liver necrosis. It is also a good source of lysine, the amino acid needed in the diet in greatest amounts the deficiency of which in human subjects results in fatigability and irritability. The combined deficiency of lysine and tryptophane is one cause of corneal vascularization, simulating the riboflavin deficiency reaction, not affected by riboflavin treatment. References for above statements: Biost (formerly Calcifood A) product Bulletin, form no. TG 239 ®, Therapeutic Foods Company.

The exception to **Biost**, as a source of calcium, is where alkaline calcium to form calcium bicarbonate, the ionized blood calcium, is desired. This is in the cases of acute infection (and symptoms as described above) where the calcium is to aid Vitamin C in controlling the infective agent, in the stimulation of phagocytosis. Lime water or the proprietary Kalak water are other forms of alkaline Calcium.

CLINICALLY ASSOCIATED CONDITIONS

NERVOUS AND PSYCHOGENIC
   <u>Functional</u>
      Insomnia
   <u>Metabolic</u>
      Torticollis
   <u>Mentality</u>
      Backwardness in Children
   <u>Lesions</u>
      Cerebral Palsy
METABOLIC DISORDERS
   <u>Growth and Repair</u>
      Bones, Healing of
      Dental Caries
      Gums, Receding of
      Teething
   <u>Intermediate Processes</u>
      Calcium Metabolism

<u>Collagen Diseases</u>
   Arcus Senilis
   Arteriosclerosis
   Arthritis, Hypertrophic
   Arthritis, Rheumatoid
   Bones, Pain in
   Bursitis
   Cataracts
   Disc Lesions
<u>Dypuytren's Contracture</u>
   Hernia
   Ligaments, Deformity of
   Peyronie's Disease
<u>Acid-Base Disorders</u>
   Alkalosis
<u>Blood</u>
   Anemia
   Leukopenia

BIOST

CLINICALLY ASSOCIATED CONDITIONS

EXOGENIC DISORDERS
   Inflammation
      Periodontoclasia
      Denture Irritation
EXOGENIC DISORDERS
   Inflammation
      Traumatic
      Strictures
VASCULAR DISORDERS
   Circulatory Diseases
      Intermittent Claudication

   Circulatory Diseases
      Leg Ulcers
      Phlebitis
      Varicose Veins
   Heart Disorders
      Myocarditis
GENETIC
   Female Disorders
      Amenorrhea
      Uterine Congestion
SPECIFIC DEFICIENCY DISEASES
      Conjunctivitis
      Pellagra

ASSOCIATED PRODUCTS:

Ostogen Wafers: This is an extract from Biost containing primarily the enzyme phosphatase and rare amino acids and is useful where higher concentrations of these factors are desired. (See Biost, Page, 21) for details.

Bio-Dent Tablets: Contains Biost factors, but in tablet form. We feel that the best nutritional purposes are served by Calcifood A, but that where patient management presents a barrier to the powder form that Bio-Dent provides the second best means of administration of these essential food factors. (See Page, 19)

Ostrophin PMG: Contains factors of Ostogen Wafers and Cytotrophic Extracts of Bone Cytotrophin. (See Page, 133)

Note: *Sometimes there is confusion when a product will have a different name depending on which one of Dr. Lee's company's it originated from. Please check the list of name changes in the front of the book.*

BIOST

CAL-AMO

Label: Each tablet contains 1.5 grains of Ammonium Chloride, 1.5 grains of Glutamic acid hydrochloride, 1.4 grains of Calcium Phytate, and .8 grains of Magnesium Glycerophosphate. For the treatment of nutritional alkalosis. Usual dosage: 1 or 2 tablets with each meal. Keep tightly closed, this product attracts moisture.

Tissue or Function Supported	Factors tending to combat nutritional alkalosis.

CLINICAL CONSIDERATIONS
Prominent Clinical Signs And Symptoms

Symptoms:

1. Hyperventilation (Excessively deep and rapid respirations).
2. Vomiting (Continued loss of HCl from stomach).
3. Hyperadrenia (Excessive sodium retention, excess cortisone administration).
4. Excessive alkaline salts (Sodium bicarbonate [soda], and other preparations used in hyperacidity).
5. Joint pains (Bursitis, also creaking joints)
6. Low-Salt Diets (Long-term without chloride replacement).
7. Allergic states (also menopause and menstruation symptoms associated with other alkalosis symptoms).
8. Edema (Particularly "swollen" hands, feeling of stiffness as a result).
9. Radiation therapy.

Possible Etiological Background:

Alkalosis
Biochemical changers as follows:

a. Excessive carbonic acid loss from pulmonary alveoli..
b. Relative increase in extracellular fluid alkalinity.
c. Urinary output of acid phosphate decreased, alkaline phosphate in increased.
d. Urinary ammonium falls.
e. HCl loss from vomiting.
f. Increased ingestion of alkaline salts such as sodium bicarbonate.
g. Increase in serum carbonic dioxide, serum sodium increased while serum potassium and chlorides fall.
h. Above (g.) encountered in excess administration of cortisone, adrenal hormones.
i. Increased alkali reserve results in patients receiving X-Ray and radium therapy. Serum phosphate and chloride are decreased and pH is diminished

Symptom Characteristics:		The signs are those of tetany in varying degrees. Mild symptoms which should arouse suspicion are restlessness, excitability, numbness and prickling sensations.
Laboratory Tests	Test: CO2 Combining Power	Need Shown By: Increase is usually manifestation of alkalosis.
Clinical Tests	a. Chvostak's Sign b. Diastolic Tolerance Test c. Urine pH	Spasm produce by tapping facial muscles. Blood pressure held at diastolic level from 1 to 3 minutes produces tetany of hand muscles (prickling, numbness, claw-like grip, etc.). Strongly alkaline, persistent.
Administration	**Dosage:** In indicated cases should be higher for first six weeks, up to 6 per day, later reduced to symptomatic levels, or 1 or 2 per day.	
	Effect: depends upon degree of alkalinity and dosage administered, generally three weeks should be allowed before expecting full effects of therapy.	
	Side Effects: These would include the reactions of acidosis which **Cal-Amo** may, of course, aggravate. Acidosis symptoms include: indigestion immediately following meals (hyperacidity), tachycardia, fever blisters or cold sores, shortness of breath during exercise or emotional stress and others. Should these symptoms result from **Cal-Amo** administration, discontinue use until acidosis symptoms have been corrected. **Calcium Lactate** and **Sodium Citrate** is indicated (1 teaspoonful of **Sodium Citrate** and 12 **Calcium Lactate** tablets daily for a few days).	

CAL-AMO

Synergists:	Activity Contributed:
a. Renatrophin	Most important organ in acid-base balance.
b. Drenamin	Regulation of sodium-potassium balance.
c. Thytrophin	Regulation of calcium-phosphorus balance.

GENERAL CONSIDERATIONS

Alkalosis may be a predisposing factor in the following conditions:

a. Allergic states
b. Achlorhydria and hypochlorhydria
c. Respiratory embarrassment (hyperventilation)

The rationalization for clinical application is as follows:

1. Allergies, migrating pains (bursitis), joints that creak when moved (particularly cervical vertebrae), burning and tingling sensations, and many other vague symptoms may be associated with alkalosis.

2. Hyperventilation is a recognized sign (breathing exercises aggravate symptoms).

3. Clinical findings of alkalosis often accompany sex hormone imbalance, being especially prevalent in the menopause and during the latter stages of pregnancy (achlorhydria frequently accompanying the latter).

4. A deficiency of the chloride ion brought on by self-imposed salt restriction or protracted low-salt diets is a common occurrence.

5. The well-known effects of ammonium chloride as a diuretic apply from a nutritional viewpoint, the chloride ion being deficient, so that we include edema from this cause in our considerations of the deficient patient. Note: Enzyme-blocking diuretics do not correct this deficiency, but may, on the other hand, aggravate it, so that nutritional support becomes increasingly important where these substances are being employed.

CLINICALLY ASSOCIATED CONDITIONS

NERVOUS AND PSYCHOGENIC
   Vaso-Motor
      Hypotension
METABOLIC DISORDERS
   Intermediate Processes
      Salt Metabolism
   Collagen
      Bursitis
   Acid-Base Balance
      Alkalosis
   Water Balance
      Edema
   Respiratory
      Bronchitis

EXOGENIC DISORDERS
   Traumatic
      Cancer, relief of pain in
      Pain, Nutritional Aspects
GENETIC
      Leucorrhea
      Vaginitis
GLANDULAR
      Adrenal Insufficiency
SPECIFIC NUTRITIONAL DISEASES
      Cheilosis

Note: *Sometimes there is confusion when a product will have a different name depending on which one of Dr. Lee's company's it originated from. Please check the list of name changes in the front of the book*

CALCIFOOD WAFER

(OSTOGEN WAFERS C-Y 1733)

Label: Each wafer contains 150 mgm extract from fresh veal bone, and 6 mgm of organically combined manganese. Carrier Materials: Sea salt, milk solids, cereal germ. Mfg. Under U.S. Pat. No 2, 374, 219. Dose: 2 to 4 wafers daily or as directed. Use: To provide biologically active uncooked veal bone protein-enzyme factors.

Tissue or Function Suopprted	Source of rare amino acids and contains enzyme phosphatase which is found only in uncooked foods.

CLINICAL CONSIDERATIONS
Prominent Clinical Signs And Symptoms

Symptoms:

1. Bone and Joint Symptoms (Arthritis, joint pains, ligamentous problems, pain in bones, etc.).
2. Connective Tissues (Supportive tissue as irritated gums, loose teeth, receding gums).
3. Calcium Utilization (Osteoporosis, rheumatoid arthritis, osteomyelitis, etc.).
4. Circulation Symptoms (Headaches,
5. Varicose veins, hemorrhoids, veinous congestion).

Possible Etiological Background:

Apparently **Ostogen Wafers** promote the calcium and protein metabolizing systems of the body through its rare amino acids and enzyme content a faulty metabolism brought on, we believe, by deficiency of raw foods in the diet bringing on kindred clinical pictures as demonstrated by Dr. Pottenger

Symptom Characteristics: In a wide range of connective tissue diseases this product may be considered as a useful adjunct. Generally, calcium utilization problems and loss of integrity of the ligamentous structures are concerned.

Administration	**Dosage:** 1 to 4 per day..
	Effect: May be rapid in case of loss of integrity of the tooth socket, gum tissue lesions and some types of pain in the bones; arthritic lesions, bone repair and other similar problems may require long term use.
	Side Effect: None known..

Synergists:	Activity Contributed:
a. Calcium Lactate	Source of ionizable calcium
b. Bio-Dent	Bio-Dent Biologically active uncooked veal bone factors

Note: **Ostogen Wafers** contain the amino acids, enzymes and bone determinants in highly concentrated form, but depends upon the diet to supply calcium and phosphorus; therefore, above synergists should be used as indicated.

	Test:	Need Shown By:
Laboratory Tests	X-Ray	Bone porosity, "spurs," etc.
Clinical Tests	Observation	Bleeding, spongy gums, joint motility, venous congestion, etc.

GENERAL CONSIDERATIONS

1. Utilization of calcium, phosphorus and protein is promoted by **Ostogen Wafers** and their use is indicated where such supplementation is being used but response is lacking. This is particularly applicable where patient is lacking raw foods in the diet.
2. Phosphatase is found in highest amounts in growing bone and its use is valuable as an adjunct wherever evidence of need for repair of bone is encountered.

CALCIFOOD WAFER

3. This product has been found useful in sore, receding, or spongy gums, as well as joint pains, loose teeth, and other conditions where one would expect its rare amino acid content is the active factor

CLINICALLY ASSOCIATED CONDITIONS

NERVOUS AND PSYCHOGENIC
- <u>Functional</u>
  - Headache
  - Migraine Headaches
- <u>Metabolic</u>
  - Torticollis
- <u>Collagen Diseases</u>
  - Bursitis
  - Disc Lesions
  - Ligaments, Deformity of
- <u>Blood</u>
  - Anemia
  - Leukopenia
- Varicose Veins

METABOLIC DISORDERS
- <u>Growth and Repair</u>
  - Bones, Healing of
  - Gums, Receding of
- <u>Intermediate Processes</u>
  - Calcium Metabolism

EXOGENIC DISORDERS
- <u>Circulatory Diseases</u>
  - Buerger's Disease
  - Hemorrhoids
  - Intermittent Claudication

ASSOCIATED PRODUCTS:

Biost: See Associated Products, **Biost** Product Bulletin, (See Page, 21).

Bone Cytotrophin: May be used interchangeably with **Calcifood Wafer,** (See Page, 28).

Note: *Sometimes there is confusion when a product will have a different name depending on which one of Dr. Lee's company's it originated from. Please check the list of name changes in the front of the book*

CALCIUM LACTATE

Label: Each tablet contains 5 grains Calcium Lactate, 1 grain Calcium-Magnesium Phytate. Carrier Material: Milk Powder. To supply Calcium and Magnesium in approximate balance required in human nutrition. Dose: 1 to 4 tablets per day, best assimilated on an empty stomach. Take 15 minutes before breakfast, or as directed.

Tissue or Function Supported	Source of diffusible calcium for maintenance of ionized calcium levels in calcium deficiency states involving such vital processes as: Muscle contraction — Blood coagulation; Nerve transmission — Membrane permeability

CLINICAL CONSIDERATIONS
Prominent Clinical Signs And Symptoms

Symptoms:	Possible Etiological Background:
1. Tachycardia	Glandular hyperactivity, toxemia, acidosis, or fever.
2. Cramps (intestinal, muscular, or menstrual)	Lowered threshold of irritability involving neuromuscular system.
3. Coughing (Worse at night, also insomnia)	Apparently diffusible calcium level is lowered along with decrease in metabolism occurring at night.
4. Hemorrhage (Nosebleed, excessive mense, bleeding gums, etc.)	Blood coagulation.
5. Increased secretions (Saliva, urine, tears, sweating, sinus drainage)	Nervous control of autonomic nervous system; membrane permeability.
6. Fever (Infections)	Toxemia

Symptom Characteristics: Usually associated with increased metabolism.

Laboratory Tests Discussion: As much as 50% of the blood calcium may be in the ionized state. Ionized calcium is not measurable by usual laboratory methods used to determine calcium-phosphorus ratios. Therefore, the broad calcium may appear to be "normal" by these methods, yet the patient may be deficient in the ionized calcium form. (The ionized calcium is though to more closely approximate the blood protein level.)

Clinical Tests

Test:	Need Shown By:
a) Phonocardiograph	Diminished height of second sound
b) Pulse rate
c) Temperature	Increase
d) Respiration rate
e) Postural Blood Pressure	Failure to show rise when standing
f) Sulkowitch Reagent Test	Increased or decreased excretion
g) Reflex Tests	Hyperirritability

Administration

Dosage: The amount required is regulated by the acuteness of the situation. As high as 18 per day may be required in the initial stages, later reduced to symptomatic levels.

Effect: Usually rapid, often within 20 minutes where specific symptoms are being observed. Muscular or menstrual cramps usually respond immediately on sufficient dosage when from this cause.

Side Effect: Few known and these are usually absent. Phosphorus deficiency may be suspected when they do occur. Joint stiffness, constipation, vertigo, and headaches have been reported in this category, common also to hypothyroidism.

Synergists:	**Activity Contributed:**
1. Cataplex F	Calcium diffusing influence
2. Cataplex D	Absorption promoting influence, raises blood calcium levels.
3. Nutrimere	Low blood proteins being considered in relation to ionized blood Calcium levels

CALCIUM LACTATE

GENERAL CONSIDERATIONS

These follow the same general pattern as the vital processes listed above, some of the more important of which are:

a. Tetany and other spasmodic states.
b. Acid-base disorders (indicated in both)
c. Hemorrhage
d. Hyperirritability
e. Infection, fever and toxemia
f. Increased metabolic demands associated with elevated blood phosphorus levels (See Note Below).

Note: Elevated blood phosphorus levels are associated with increased metabolism, which may be brought about by such conditions as the following:

1. Glandular hyperactivity (particularly thyroid)
2. Toxic conditions, such as fevers and infections
3. Hypertension
4. Pregnancy (particularly the last trimester)
5. Neurasthenia

When the thyroid is overactive experimental animals are known to loose up to 250% more than normal amounts of calcium. The classical symptoms of hyperthyroidism are related to calcium deficiency states, as follows:

a. Tachycardia
b. Tremors
c. Instability

CLINICALLY ASSOCIATED CONDITIONS

GASTROINTESTINAL- URINARY
   <u>Liver and Gallbladder</u>
      Biliary Stasis
      Gallbladder Disease
   <u>Kidney and Bladder</u>
      Albuminuria
      Cystitis
      Urinary Incompetence
NERVOUS AND PSYCHOGENIC
   <u>Functional Disorders</u>
      Asthenia
      Autonomic Unbalance
      Chorea
      Dysphagia
      Hyperirritability
      Nervous strain
      Sweat Gland Activity
   <u>Metabolic</u>
      Legs, weakness of
      Tremors, Muscular
   <u>Vasomotor</u>
      Blood Pressure Changes
      Heat Prostration
      Hypotension
      Shock
METABOLIC DISORDERS
   <u>Growth and Repair</u>
      Bones, Healing of
      Caries
      Gums, Receding of
      Healing, Promotion of
      Nails, Integrity of
      Osteoporosis
      Teething
   <u>Intermediate Processes</u>
      Calcium Metabolism
      Cramps
      Protein Metabolism
      Drowsiness
   <u>Acid-Base Disorders</u>
      Acids, Craving for
      Acidosis
      Alkalosis
   <u>Blood</u>
      Epistaxis
      Leukopenia
   <u>Respiratory</u>
      Bronchitis
      Emphysema
      Coughs, Chronic
   <u>Allergies</u>
      Antihistamine Effects
      Hives
   <u>Body Weight</u>
      Obesity
EXOGENIC DISORDERS
   <u>Infections</u>
      Brucellosis
      Febrile Diseases
      Lymph Node Infections
      Pneumonia
      Rheumatic Fever
      Vincent's Infection
   <u>Virus Infections</u>
      Colds, Flu, Grippe
      Earache
      Herpes Simplex
      Herpes Zoster
      Lumbago
   <u>Toxic Disorders</u>
      Burns, Systemic Effects
      Eclampsia
      Poison Ivy and Oak

CALCIUM LACTATE

CLINICALLY ASSOCIATED CONDITIONS

EXOGENIC DISORDERS
- Inflammation
    - Mastitis
    - Denture Irritation
    - Sinusitis
    - Tonsillitis
    - Gingivitis
    - Periodontoclasia

VASCULAR DISORDERS
- Circulatory Diseases
    - Bed Sores
    - Leg Ulcers

SKIN DISORDERS
- Dermatitis
- Purpura
- Skin Irritations

GENETIC DISORDERS
- Female Disorders
    - Abortion
    - Dysmenorrhea
    - Endocervicitis
    - Menopausal Symptoms
    - Menstruation Symptoms
    - Pregnancy Schedule

SPECIFIC DEFICIENCY
- Glandular
    - Adrenal Insufficiency
    - Goiter

ASSOCIATED PRODUCTS

Notes: That insofar as Calcium Lactate is concerned, we are referring only to the ionizable or diffusible form of calcium, which is the type ordinarily used to correct calcium deficiency symptoms. However, other nutritional factors are concerned and the products which follow are considered to be improvements over the Calcium Lactate formula where these specific factors are indicated.

Min-Tran: This is a balanced mineral formula containing calcium lactate and Pacific sea kelp. The naturally occurring potassium and iodine act in coordination with calcium, to replace minerals which are likely to occur in nervous states, particularly those associated with the hyperthyroid case. (See Page, 115)

Cataplex D: The Vitamin D is supplied in a base of calcium lactate and is particularly beneficial where parathyroid problems are concerned. We have also found this product of benefit in osteoporosis and in some types of arthritis. (See Page, 55)

Note: *Sometimes there is confusion when a product will have a different name depending on which one of Dr. Lee's company's it originated from. Please check the list of name changes in the front of the book*

CALCIUM LACTATE

CALSOL

Label: Soluble Food Calcium – Contains the calcium-magnesium salt of inositol, phosphoric acid (cereal source) and calcium glycerophosphate with carbamide as physiological buffer. Because of ready solubility these tablets may be swallowed whole with water. 2 to 12 per day or as directed by physician.

Tissue or Function Supported	Vegetable source calcium beneficial for soft tissues.

CLINICAL CONSIDERATIONS
Prominent Clinical Signs And Symptoms

Symptoms:
1. Hyperirritability (Insomnia, muscle cramps, restlessness)
2. Hyperperistalsis (Colitis, frequent bowel movements, gas ains)
3. Sphincter Spasms (Biliary stasis, pyloric spasms, delayed emptying time of stomach)
4. Muscular Symptoms (Soreness, weakness)

Possible Etiological Background

Where a balanced calcium-phosphorus supplement for long-term usage is desired, being particularly beneficial for soft tissues and comparable with the requirements of vegetarianism, Calsol is the product of choice. It produces a marked quieting effect on the nerves in susceptible cases. The sustained beneficial effects usually experienced are, no doubt, due to its balanced formula and ready solubility.

Symptom Characteristics: Manifestations are primarily neurological involving both the voluntary and autonomic nervous system insofar as the muscular action of the receptor organs is concerned. Clinically, its indications include practically all of the situations ordinarily considered in the calcium deficiency syndrome.

Laboratory Tests	Test: Sulkowitch Reagent	Need Shown By: Normally a high alkaline diet as frequently encountered in vegetarians will show a clear solution indicating low blood pressure.
Clinical Tests	None known	
Administration	**Dosage:** Enough", being a balanced food calcium, dosage occupies a wide range of application, 6 to 12 per day being adequate in most cases.	
	Effect: In sufficient dosage this product is often effective in such conditions as insomnia and colitis where all else fails and as such is an important adjunct in most programs designed to induce a tranquilizing effect by physiological means..	
	Side Effect: None known	

Synergists:	Activity Contributed:
Cataplex D	Calcium Absorption Factor
Cataplex F	Calcium Diffusing Factor
Zypan	pH Factor (Calcium is absorbed best in acid environment)

GENERAL CONSIDERATIONS

The clinical problems faced by the clinician where specific calcium or phosphorus therapy is instituted, are very great indeed and are undertaken, as a matter of fact, only to produce the immediate benefits where a severe unbalance exists. The specific therapy is, of course, engendered with potentially greater benefits in correction of unbalances or where specific deficiencies exit of a particular fraction, but it also may be the means of accentuating an already unbalanced condition. While this is seldom the case, all types of calcium deficiency being the rule, we do encounter cases where Calsol is the best tolerated calcium supplement for these reasons.

W e have found calcium therapy where Calsol is particularly effective in the range of certain neurological involvements, particularly in the following conditions: extra-systoles, colitis, biliary stasis (sphincter control) and intestinal hyperperistalsis.

CALSOL

GENERAL CONSIDERATIONS

We would therefore list **Calcium Lactate, Bio-Dent, Calcifood** and **Phosfood** as supplying higher amounts of specific calcium metabolizing factors (See respective Product Bulletins for details), and Calsol in contrast as a balanced calcium metabolizing formula. This rationale suggests the following applications:

A. Where general calcium supplementation is desired in connection with multiple essential foods such as **Cyro-Yeast, Catalyn** or **Cyrofood**, and, of course, useful when sued by itself.
B. As an adjunct where specific calcium therapy, as described above, is being used, to be continued after specific unbalances or deficiencies have been corrected.
C. As a tranquilizing alternative in neurological conditions as previously described and in all cases where intolerance or incomplete results have been experienced upon specific calcium supplementation.

Note: The Sulkowitch Reagent Test usually shows a low blood calcium on high alkaline ash diets (common in vegetarianism) indicating need for Calsol, which is also comparable with vegetarian principles. In this case, however, hydrochloric acid administration (**Zypan** or **Betaine Hydrochloride** Tablets) may be necessary since calcium is best absorbed in an acid medium. **Phosfood** and **Lactic Acid Yeast** also contribute to the production of acidity required.

Where restless at night or insomnia is concerned, 3 to 6 tablets before bedtime is beneficial since the effect is then reflected in the lower metabolic rate usually present during sleep.

CLINICALLY ASSOCIATED CONDITIONS

GASTRO-INTESTINAL-URINARY
    Stomach and Intestine
        Colitis
    Liver and Gallbladder
        Biliary Stasis
NERVOUS AND PSYCHOGENIC
    Functional
        Insomnia
        Salivary Disorders
    Metabolic
        Tranquilizing Effects
    Mentality
        Brain, Dysfunction of
METABOLIC DISORDERS
    Collagen
        Rheumatoid Arthritis

EXOGENIC
    Toxic
        X-Ray burns
    Inflammatory
        Periodontoclasia
VASCULAR DISORDERS
    Circulatory
        Tinnitus Aurium
    Heart Disorders
        Myocarditis
SPECIFIC DEFICIENCY DISEASES
    Goiter
    Cheilosis

CARDIO-PLUS

Label: This formula contains extracts form Yeast, Sprouted Grains, Calf Brain (G), and specific determinant factors of Beef Heart muscle (**Cardiotrophin**), in addition to a concentrate which is a phospholipid synergist of alpha-tocopherol from beef chromatin (E2). Two tablets contain 1 mg of Riboflavin and 12 mg of Niacin (1/3 daily adult requirement of each) in addition to the above mentioned associated factors. Dosage: 3 to 9 tablets per day, or as directed.

Tissue or Function Supported	Nerve and muscle cells.

CLINICAL CONSIDERATIONS
Prominent Clinical Signs And Symptoms

Symptoms:

1. Neuromuscular Disorders (Paralysis, muscular atrophy, weakness, loss of muscular control, coordination, etc.)
2. Heart Disorders (Congestive heart failure, history of coronary disease, cardiac symptoms)

Possible Etiological Background:

Note: For complete discussion of related nutritional factors see "Heart" and "Neuromuscular Disorders" in the Manual of Clinical Trophology. Also see **Cataplex G** and **Cataplex E2** Bulletins discussed in this book.

Symptom Characteristics: The musculature, nervous system, coronary circulation or extrinsic factors such as hypertension, liver disease, etc. may be involved. While cardiac indications are looked upon as being most common indication, the extent of use should not be restricted to cardiac involvements as the entire neuromuscular structure is concerned.
(Note: A product named "Myotrophin" which is the same as "Cardiotrophin" is supplied where the doctor may desire to avoid cardiac inference).

	Test:	Need Shown By:
Laboratory Tests	a. Creatine Urine (Pathologically)	Found in wasting muscular diseases.
	b. Sedimentation Rate	Increased in tissue breakdown.
Clinical Tests	Endocardiograph	Coronary insufficiency (decreased diastolic interval)

Administration	**Dosage:** Determined by acuteness and chronicity of the case. In cardiac cases, one tablet per day should be used until tolerance is determined then increased proportionately to serve the purpose of the three formulas included, i.e., three times as many Cardio-Plus tablets must be given as would be given if E2, G and Cardiotrophin were used separately.
	Effect: Most cases complaining of muscular weakness obtain a definite tonic effect, from the use of this formula. Its specific effects, such as in heart conditions, must be determined by the use of the Endocardiograph or other diagnostic means.
	Side Effect: These rarely occur, but, when they do occur, reactions such as tachycardia may be attributed to disturbance in potassium or sugar metabolism (both closely related and acted upon by muscular changes). See "Synergists" below.

Synergists:	Activity Contributed:
Organic Minerals	Potassium source (*)
Calcium Lactate	Source ionizable calcium (**)
Betafood	Sugar metabolism factor

(*) The transfer of sugar to the muscle cell is accompanied by a utilization of serum potassium, the action of insulin being one of the few therapeutic agents known to temporarily reduce serum potassium.

(**) Calcium is the counterbalancing factor for potassium.

CARDIO-PLUS

GENERAL CONSIDERATIONS

The **Cardio-Plus** formula, consisting of **Vitamin E2**, **Vitamin G Complex** and **Cardiotrophin**, is the result of very favorable clinical reports received from each of these as related nutritional factors.

We may list its nutritional effects as follows:
1. Enzymatic tranquilizing effect (cholinesterase precursors of **Vitamin G Complex**).
2. Contributes to muscular tonicity (particularly cardiac muscle).
3. Provides influential factors generally beneficial to muscle metabolism and as such contributes to utilization of potassium and sugar which are needed as "raw materials" for muscular activity.
4. The protomorphogen effect of **Cardiotrophin** contained, acts to combat excess Natural Tissue Antibodies, and is thus helpful in most types of degenerative heart disease.

Clinical rationalization for use is suggested as follows:
A. In general, we may use **Cardio-Plus** wherever we find muscular problems as it acts as a potentiator of nutrition to the muscle cell.
B. It imparts a tonic effect in most patients, particularly the geriatric groups.
C. It increases the activity of muscle metabolism (ordinarily brought about through exercise) and thus has a beneficial effect in elevated blood sugar levels.

Note: Most diabetics are similarly benefited by exercise.

CLINICALLY ASSOCIATED CONDITIONS

NERVOUS AND PSYCHOGENIC
   Functional
      Asthenia
   Metabolic
      Neuromuscular Disorders
   Vasomotor
      Blood Pressure
METABOLIC DISORDERS
   Intermediate Processes
      Diabetes Mellitus
VASCULAR DISORDERS

Heart Disorders
      Angina Pectoris
      Heart Abnormalities
      Myocarditis
EXOGENIC DISORDERS
   Infection
      Rheumatic Fever
   Traumatic
      Sedimentation Rate

ASSOCIATED PRODUCTS

Cataplex E2:   (See Page, 57)
Cataplex G: (See Page, 65)

Note: Heart Cytotrophin, Cardiotrophin and Myotrophin are the same Cytotrophic Extracts available under trade names shown here. These various trade names for the same muscle extract are made available for esthetic reasons, where for obvious reasons, the doctor would prefer the product available under these names which indicate their use in various conditions.

CARDIOTROPHIN PMG

(HEART CYTOTROPHIN)
(Also available under tradename Myotrophin)

Label: **Cardiotrophin**, Cytotrophic Extract of Beef Heart—A tissue extract intended to supply the specific determinant factors of the above mentioned organ and to aid in improving the local nutritional environment for that organ. For experimental use in cooperation with conventional Therapeutic methods. (One to three tablets per day, or as directed. (One per day should be maximum dosage for first week.

Tissue or Function Supported Muscle tissue, particularly cardiac, supplying nutrients for the local nutritional environment of muscle cells.

CLINICAL CONSIDERATIONS
Prominent, Clinical Signs, And Symptoms

Symptoms:
1. Loss of Muscle Integrity (Atrophy, weakness, tonus, prolapse, etc.)
2. Carbohydrate Metabolism (Failure of muscle cells to metabolize glucose-glycogen)
3. Cardiac Weakness (Decompensation or failure due to lack of muscle tonus, nutrition to cell)
4. Sedentary Occupations (Predisposing heart failure)
5. Circulatory Problems (Due to tonus of musculature of arterial coats)

Possible Etiological Background:

Cardiotrophin apparently assists the entire muscular system by influencing the nutritional aspect of selective absorption range of the muscle cell membrane. This selective range includes glucose uptake and is related to the important energy mechanism (ATP). Exercise is the usual activator of this system, being particularly significant in the case of the diabetic and potential heart rate failure patient. As such, **Cardiotrophin** provides a valuable remedy for these patients, particularly where such activity would be inadvised or otherwise unobtainable.

Symptom Characteristics: Important relation to carbohydrate metabolism via ATP mechanisms, as well as muscle integrity per se must be considered.

	Test:	Need Shown By:
Laboratory Tests	Creatine (urine)	Pathologically found in wasting muscular disease.

Clinical Tests   Endocardiograph Diminished, elongated first sounds, proportionately elevated second sounds.

Administration	**Dosage:** One tablet per day for first week or until level of tolerance is determined (see Side-Effects, below). Later level of administration depends upon the symptomatic level of response, observing exercise tolerance as indicator.
	Effect: A tonic effect is usual in indicated cases. Its specific effect upon heart integrity must be determined by Endocardiograph or ACG readings or other diagnostic means.
	Side Effect: These rarely occur. Reactions such as tachycardia may be attributed to disturbance in potassium-glucose metabolism. (The transfer of glucose to the muscle cell is accompanied by utilization of serum potassium, the administration of insulin being one of the few therapeutic means of reducing serum potassium temporarily. Calcium is one of the counterbalancing factors for potassium, NaCl another when serum potassium is in excess. In most cases, however, indications are potassium deficiency and **Organic Minerals** is the product of choice in this event. **Cardiotrophin** taken over a period of time may progressively lower the blood sugar level and hypoglycemia may be aggravated. This same effect, of course, is beneficial in hyperglycemia.

Synergists: | Activity Contributed:
a. Organic Minerals | Potassiium source (see remarks above)
b. Calcium Lactate | Ionizable calcium source (see above)
c. Betafood | Sugar metabolizing influence (see above)

CARDIOTROPHIN PMG

GENERAL CONSIDERATIONS

Clinical rationalization for use is suggested as follows:

1) As a potentiator of nutrition to the muscle cell, thus useful in muscular weakness, atrophy, etc. In this respect, myoneural junction disorder must also be considered. See "Myoneural Junction Disorders" in Clinical Trophology.

2) As a nutritional factor favoring the geriatric patient, its tonic effect being most evident in these patients.

3) As a nutritional factor in increasing the energy metabolism of the muscle cell via the ATP mechanisms, apparently in same relation as exercises, which to the limits of tolerance is beneficial both to the diabetic and congestive heart failure patient.

4) Because of its effects in carbohydrate metabolism, as a possible factor in conditioning the hyperkalemia patient, a finding in Addison's Disease, which may also result in heart block. See notes under Side-Reactions for details.

CLINICALLY ASSOCIATED CONDITIONS

METABOLIC DISORDERS
Intermediate Processes
Diabetes Mellitas

VASCULAR DISORDERS
Heart abnormalities

CATALYN

Label: Concentrates from alfalfa, carrot, beef and fish liver lipoids, yeast, wheat germ, rice bran, liver, mushroom, green peas (whole plant), biologically processed corn. Carrier Materials: Milk solids, wheat and oat flours. Each tablet contains: 400 U.S.P. units Vitamin A, 10 U.S.P. units Vitamin B1, 20 U.S.P. units Vitamin C, 100 U.S.P. units Vitamin D, 25 Sherman Borquin units (60 gamma) Vitamin G Riboflavin), 10 milligrams unsaturated fatty acids, with naturally occurring associated factors. For statement on percentage of daily Vitamin requirement per tablet see accompanying circular*. Chew 1 or 2 tablets after each meal or as directed.

Tissue or Function Supported   Multiple essential food concentrate containing nutritive factors of above mentioned foods, processed to maintain biological potency.

CLINICAL CONSIDERATIONS
Prominent Clinical Signs And Symptoms

Symptoms:
1. Chronic fatigue (Failure to meet ordinary requirements of daily activities)
2. Hypertension or Hypotension (deviations in blood pressure for no discernable reason)
3. Chronic Diseases (Particularly degenerative
4. diseases.)
5. Lowered Resistance (Susceptibility to infections, colds, flu, etc.)
6. Glandular Insufficiency (Endocrinopathies in general including liver disorders.)
7. Nutritional Response (Failure to respond to specific nutritional schedules.)
8. Prophylaxis (Wide spread conditions of
9. malnutrition.)

Possible Etiological Background
Philip Norman, M.D., prominent nutritional consultant, has stated that dietary excesses aggravate dietary deficiency states. By the same line of reasoning, **Catalyn** which is a combination of selected essential food concentrates, as described on the above label, acts as a nutritional "governor" to regulate diverse physiological mechanisms in situations where only one or two may be given specific nutritional support on a recommended program. Also, **Catalyn**, by covering the broadest possible spectrum of nutritional factors is one of the most useful multiple food products for prophylactic purposes, because it is an established basic nutritional concept to get ALL of the factors concerned in deficiency states. We must also consider that **Catalyn** is a valued source of trace minerals and in this product these minerals are organically combined with their naturally associated enzyme and protein complexes.

Laboratory and Clinical Tests Discussion: One of the greatest needs of practitioners in the healing arts today is the development of an adequate laboratory method of measuring of nutritional deficiency states. So far attempts in this direction have been feeble indeed, and, as a result, we must rely upon clinical results to show us the effectiveness of nutritional entities. **Catalyn** has been appraised by thousands of doctors on this basis and for over 30 years has remained one of their most valued nutritional products.

Administration	**Dosage:** Perhaps one of the most common mistakes in dosage is to believe that increasing the dosage will proportionately increase the result. Our experience over the years has shown that this is seldom the case and that the recommended dosage from 1 to 3 per day continued over a long period of time, produces the best results.
	Side Effect: These are almost too inconsequential to mention but we must consider that activation of the detoxification mechanisms may produce seemingly adverse reactions. In most cases this is simply a matter of interpreting the reaction and continued usage merits a confident appraisal.

Synergistic Products	Specific Function
a. Organic Minerals	Furnishes organic potassium and alkaline ash minerals
b. Calcium Lactate	Supplies diffusible calcium
c. Chlorophyll Complex (perles)	Chlorophyll Source

CATALYN

GENERAL CONSIDERATIONS

Catalyn, an especially processed natural food concentrate, differs from synthetic vitamin formulas in that it may safely be given in the most extremes of delicately balanced physiological mechanisms without fear of over dosage or of producing adverse reactions, as for example, in infants or enfeebled aged individuals.

While the controversy between synthetic and natural vitamins has been and probably will continue to be an issue with clinicians for some time to come, the evidence pointing to toxic effects of various ingredients (chemicals) included in synthetic formulas is very considerable and impressive to the cautious doctor. On the other hand, the natural broad spectrum of **Catalyn** can hardly be considered anything but harmless.

The potential benefits in either case must be decided by clinical observation upon known patients, using their objective symptoms and detectable responses as a method of judgement. In this respect, we believe, **Catalyn** will adequately provide conclusive evidence as to its inherent benefits to any fair-minded and astute clinical observer.

CLINICALLY ASSOCIATED CONDITIONS

As malnutrition is, we believe, in the etiological background of most common diseases, especially the degenerative varieties, we feel that **Catalyn**, as an essential multiple food concentrate is indicated in all such disorders, not necessarily a specific but to fortify the usual complex nutritional deficiency pattern which is usually present. Comments on Daily Vitamin Requirement

According to regulations of the Federal Security Administration, Food and Drug Department, issued November 22, 1941, to be effective May 7, 1942, all food products sold for their vitamin content must state in the labeling "the proportion of the minimum daily requirement for such vitamin supplied by such food when consumed in a specified quantity during a period of one day."

The following table gives this information:

1 **Catalyn** tablet supplies: 1/10 of the adult minimum daily Vitamin A requirement; 1/34 of this requirement for Vitamin B1; 1/30 of this requirement for Vitamin C; ¼ of this requirement for Vitamin D; and 1/32 of this requirement for Vitamin G. The daily requirement of Vitamins E and F and their necessity for human nutrition has not been determined or agreed upon by experts.

This table represents the opinion of the Government authorities as to the nutritional requirements of purified or synthetic vitamin factors (based on units obtained by animal test or by weight of the pure vitamin). These dosages, however, are quite at variance with those that have been found effective by physicians experienced in the use of this product' in our opinion, this is because it contains natural food concentrates rather than chemically pure vitamins. The range of dosage on the label is based on our opinion of the performance of natural concentrates, rather than chemically pure vitamins.

ASSOCIATED PRODUCTS

The multiple essential food factors of **Catalyn** are available in various forms and concentrations as follows:

Cyrofood Powder...................Most economical form, higher concentration of fiber.

Cyrofood Tablets...................Most economical form in tablets, more desirable for seniors. (See pages, 83)

CATAPLEX A

Label: Concentrates of Vitamin Factors from Alfalfa, Carrot, Beef Kidney, and Fish Liver Lipoids. Carrier Materials: Milk solids, wheat germ, rice bran, oat flour. Each tablet contains 1500 U.S.P. Units of Vitamin A with naturally occurring associated factors. Three tablets per day furnish the full adult minimum daily Vitamin A requirement (4000 U.S. P. Units). 1 to 4 tablets per day or as directed. For best results tablets should be chewed or dissolved in the mouth.

Tissue or Function Supported	General resistance and epithelial cells in deficiency states.

CLINICAL CONSIDERATIONS
Prominent Clinical Signs And Symptoms

<u>Symptom</u>
1. Cystitis (Pain in area of bladder)
2. Nephritis (Albuminuria)
3. Skin disorders
4. Eye conditions (night blindness)
5. Angitis (inflammation of blood or lymph vessel)
6. Periarteritis
7. Liver disease (Inability to metabolize carotene)
8. Thyroid disorders (Hyperthyroidism)
9. Hypertension (Reported benefits)
10. Kidney-Stones (Prophylaxis)
11. Gastritis

<u>Possible Etiological Background</u>
The integrity of the epithelial cells is largely under the influence of Vitamin A and the disorders mentioned here relate to epithelial structures. We may recall that not only the skin and vascular network are composed of epithelial cells, but also that epithelium consists of the functional as well as structural elements of many endocrine glands as well as the kidney and liver. Blocking of a lumen-such as a tear duct-could conceivably be due to loss of epithelial integrity in this channel. Also, we must consider that loss of epithelial integrity may lead to infection, due to the localized inflammation. The mechanical avenue for entrance of microorganism thus made possible may account for the reported benefits of Vitamin A in relation to general resistance.

Symptom Characteristics:	Usually associated with epithelial cells and structures.	
Laboratory Tests	<u>Test:</u> Urinalysis	<u>Need Shown By:</u> Albuminuria. Epithelial Cells (many)
Clinical Tests	a. Concentration b. Blood Pressure c. Palpation d. Pulse rate	(See Bray's "Clin. Lab. Methods") Hypertension Lymph nodes, dry, lumpy skin Tachycardia is most common indication of toxemia
Administration	**Dosage:** 3 to 6 per day, frequently used to fortify Cataplex A-C-P where additional Vitamin A is desired. (6 per day, initial dosage). **Effect:** Depends upon acuteness of situation. In acute nephritis or cystitis, relief may be within 24 to 48 hours; chronic conditions take much longer. Valued as prophylactic measure in nephritis cystitis, etc. **Side Effect:** Rare, but in few cases reported may be due to Vitamin A cholesterol-reducing effect, and, may become evident in hypocholesterolemia, such as is present in Addison's disease. Drenamin is indicated in these case..	
<u>Synergists:</u>	<u>Activity Contributed:</u>	
a. Cataplex E……………………	Vitamins A and E are cooperative	
b. Chlorophyll Complex (perles)……	Fat-soluble vitamin complex A,E,F & K	
c. Cataplex G…………………….	Cell proliferating influence	
d. Calcium Lactate………………	General beneficial effect where calcium is a factor	

CATAPLEX A

GENERAL CONSIDERATIONS

From a clinical viewpoint, the effects of Vitamin K may be considered primarily or related to the integrity of the epithelial cells. However, recall that epithelium not only composes the internal and external surfaces of the body, but also consists of the glandular epithelium as well, acting thus as secreting cell organisms. It is well to keep in mind that Vitamins A and E are both antagonistic and cooperative in their effects and that both must be present for normal physiological activity, i.e., a deficiency of one alone is seldom present.

Discussion

1) Vitamin A_2, as found in **Cataplex A** consists of a variety of sources of the Vitamin A complex, one of the more important factors being the kidney source Vitamin A. This mammalian source may account for clinical evidence of benefit in kidney problems not accounted for where fish liver oil sources alone are relied upon.

2) The ability of the liver to metabolize Vitamin A from ordinary dietary sources (carotene) may be the primary cause of deficiency where dietary intake of carotene is adequate. Not only should bile salts be considered here, but also that the general reserve power of the liver may be deficient calling for specific support of that organ.

3) Although dysfunction of the glandular system through Vitamin A deficiency states is not an easily traceable clinical entity, the consideration of this factor should enter into the analysis of most endocrinopathies.

CLINICALLY ASSOCIATED CONDITIONS

GASTROINTESTINAL-URINARY
   <u>Kidney and Bladder</u>
      Albuminuria
      Cystitis
      Kidney Stones
      Nephritis
   <u>Intestinal</u>
      Gastritis
NERVOUS AND PSYCHOGENIC
   <u>Functional</u>
      Photophobia
   <u>Vasomotor</u>
      Hypertension
METABOLIC DISORDERS
   <u>Growth and Repair</u>
      Eye Conditions
   <u>Intermediate Processes</u>
      Cholesterol Metabolism
   <u>Acid Base Disorders</u>
      Urine, pH of (kidney relation)
EXOGENIC DISORDERS
   <u>Infections</u>
      Lymph Node Infections

EXOGENIC DISORDERS
   <u>Inflammation</u>
      Mastitis
      Sinusitis
      Tonsillitis
      Gingivitis
   <u>Traumatic</u>
      Strictures
VASCULAR DISORDERS
   <u>Circulatory</u>
      Bed Sores
      Phlebitis
   <u>Heart Disorders</u>
      Myocarditis
SKIN CONDITIONS
      Dermatitis
      Eczema
      Purpura
GENETIC DISORDERS
      Endocervicitis
      Vaginitis
      Sterility

CATAPLEX A-C

Label: Vitamins A and C – Each tablet contains 750 U.S.P. units of Vitamin A and 100 U.S.P. Units of Vitamin C with naturally associated vitamin and enzyme factors from alfalfa, carrot, mushroom, green buckwheat leaf, bone marrow, beef kidney, and fish liver lipoids. Carrier materials: Rice bran, Oat flour, fresh bone flour, and anhydrous honey. – Six tablets per day furnish the full adult minimum daily requirements of Vitamin A (4000 U.S.P. units) and of Vitamin C (600 U.S.P. units). 3 to 6 tablets per day, or as directed. For best results tablets should be chewed or dissolved in the mouth.

Tissue or Function Supported   Source of factors beneficial to blood, epithelial and connective tissue, promoting resistance.

CLINICAL CONSIDERATIONS
Prominent Clinical Signs And Symptoms

Symptom	Possible Etiological Background
1. Pain in lower abdomen (area of the bladder)	Bladder irritation secondary to epithelial cell integrity.
2. Polyuria (also burning sensation)	Loss of epithelial integrity of kidney cells.
3. Infectious diseases (Fevers, cold, flu)	Phagocytosis (resistance factors).
4. Kidney disease (Nephritis)	Epithelial and connective tissue involvement.
5. Lymph node congestion (Swelling, "lumps," etc.)	Drainage impairment (lymphatics) due to loss of connective tissue integrity.
6. Skin disorders	Epithelial involvement.
7. Eye disorders	Vitamin A factors.
8. Glandular disorders	Epithelial cells compose most endocrine glands.

Symptom Characteristics: Usually associated with circulatory disorders involving congestion or stasis

Laboratory Tests Test: Urinalysis

Need Shown By:
a. Albuminuria
b. Epithelial cell; (many)
c. Specific gravity (below or stabilized at 1.010)

Clinical Tests
Pulse Rate — a. Tachycardia indicating toxemia
Temperature (elevated) — b. Indicating fever
Concentration and Dilution test for kidney function — c. Inability of tubules to concentrate urine
Palpation — d. Lymph node swelling

Administration

Dosage: At least 6 per day in initial stages, later reduced to 3 per day. In acute stages, one every hour may be required.

Effect: Depends upon acuteness of the situation. In acute nephritis or cystitis. Relief of symptoms may be within first 24 or 48 hours; in chronic conditions, results take much longer. Effect may depend upon synergistic support listed below.

Side Effect: These are rarely experienced. In the few cases reported, the vitamin A factor may be concerned. This may be due to the vitamin A cholesterol-reducing effect and may become evident as symptoms where a very low blood cholesterol is present, as possible in Addison's disease, for example. Drenamin is indicated in these cases.

Synergists:	**Activity Contributed:**
a. Cataplex G	Indicated cell-proliferating influence
b. Chlorophyll Complex (perles)	Detoxification, healing affect, prothrombin factor (vitamin K)
c. Calcium Lactate	Cell permeability
d. Arginex and Betacol	(See note below)

CATAPLEX A-C

Note: Kidney pathology has been described as being basically a protein metabolism problem. For this reason, **Betacol** or other liver supporting factors should be given in all kidney cases. Arginex is important in both liver and kidney overload in most cases.

GENERAL CONSIDERATIONS

*Apparent functions of Vitamin A: (1) the normal function and integrity of tissue of epiblastic origin; epithelial tissues (wound healing hastened, resistance to infection raised); and nervous system. (2) Necessary maintenance of normal cell metabolism, such as cell respiration and blood cell generation (platelets), (3) Necessary to the formation and integrity of periodontal tissue. (4) Promotes growth and feeling of well-being and longevity. (5) Essential to successful reproduction. (6) Prevents keratinization of tissues.

* Apparent functions of Vitamin C: (1) Essential to health and integrity of the endothelial tissues (raises resistance to infections). (2) Essential to proper development of teeth. (3) Essential to oxygen metabolism. (4) Regeneration of blood cells. (5) Maintains proper blood clotting time.

Taken from the "Vitamins and Their Clinical Application" pages 123 and 127.

One of the most spectacular reactions to the use of potent concentrates carrying the "natural synergists" will be observed in the effect of **Cataplex AC** tablets in acute infectious states. Often the phagocyte count is normal in 3 or 4 days, the patient symptom free in half that time.

CLINICALLY ASSOCIATED CONDITIONS

GASTROINTESTINAL-URINARY
- Kidney and Bladder
  - Albuminuria
  - Cystitis
  - Kidney stones
  - Nephritis

NERVOUS AND PSYCHOGENIC
- Functional
  - Photophobia
- Vasomotor
  - Blood pressure changes

METABOLIC DISORDERS
- Growth and Repair
  - Caries
  - Eye conditions
  - Gums, Receding of
  - Mouth-Tongue disorders
- Intermediate Processes
  - Cholesterol Metabolism
  - Oxygen Metabolism
- Collagen Diseases
  - Arcus Senilis
  - Arteriosclerosis
  - Cataracts

METABOLIC DISORDERS
- Acid-Base Disorders
  - Urine, pH of
- Water Balance
  - Edema
- Blood
  - Epistaxis
  - Leukopenia
- Respiratory
  - Bronchitis
  - Emphysema

EXOGENIC DISORDERS
- Infections
  - Febrile Diseases
  - Lymph Node Infections
  - Vincent's Infections
- Virus Infection
  - Colds, Flu, Grippe
  - Earache
  - Lumbago
- Toxic Disorders
  - X-Ray Burns
- Inflammation
  - Mastitis
  - Denture Irritation
  - Sinusitis
  - Tonsillitis
  - Gingivitis
- Traumatic
  - Strictures

VASCULAR DISORDERS
- Circulatory
  - Bed Sores
  - Cold Hands and Feet
  - Hemorrhoids
  - Intermittent Claudication
  - Leg Ulcers
  - Phlebitis

SKIN CONDITIONS
- Dermatitis
- Eczema
- Psoriasis
- Purpura
- Telangiectasia

GENETIC DISORDERS
- Female
  - Amenorrhea
  - Endocervicitis
  - Leucorrhea
  - Uterine Congestion
  - Vaginitis

CATAPLEX A-C-P

Label: Each serving contains 2, 250 IU of Vitamin A, 16.6 mg of Vitamin C, and Dehydrated Buckwheat juice (whole plant), exclusive of seed extract, with naturally associated vitamin and enzyme factors from Alfalfa, Carrot, Mushroom, Green Buckwheat Leaf, Bone Marrow, Beef Kidney and Fish Liver Lipoids. Carrier Material: Phytin, oat flour, fresh bone flour, and Anhydrous Honey. Serving Size: 3 tablets, 3-12 tablets per day.

Tissue or Function Supported — Source of factors beneficial to blood, epithelial and connective tissue, promoting resistance.

CLINICAL CONSIDERATIONS
Prominent Clinical Signs And Symptoms

Symptom	Possible Etiological Background
1. Pain in lower abdomen (area of the bladder)	Bladder irritation secondary to epithelial cell integrity.
2. Polyuria (also burning sensation)	Loss of epithelial integrity of kidney cells.
3. Infectious diseases (Fevers, colds, flu)	Phagocytosis (resistance factors).
4. Kidney disease (Nephritis)	Epithelial and connective tissue involvement.
5. Lymph node congestion (Swelling, "lumps", etc.)	Drainage impairment (lymphatics) due to loss of connective tissue integrity.
6. Skin disorders	Epithelial involvement.
7. Eye disorders	Specific Vitamin A factor.
8. Glandular disorders	Epithelial cells compose most endocrine glands.

Symptom Characteristics: Usually associated with circulatory disorders involving congestion or stasis.

Laboratory Tests

Test:	Need Shown By:
Urinalysis	a. Albuminuria
	b. Epithelial cells (many)
	c. Specific gravity (below or stabilized at 1.010)

Clinical Tests

Pulse Rate	Tachycardia indicating toxemia
Temperature (elevated)	Indicating fever
Concentration and Dilution	Inability of tubules to concentrate
Test for Kidney Function	urine (See Clinical Manual)
Palpation	Lymph node swelling

Administration

Dosage: At least 6 per day in initial stages, later reduced to 3 per day. In acute stages, one every hour may be required.

Effect: Depends upon acuteness of the situation. In acute nephritis or cystitis, relief of symptoms may be within first 24 or 48 hours; in chronic conditions results take much longer. Effect may depend upon synergistic support listed below.

Side Effect: These are rarely experienced. In the few cases reported, the vitamin A factor may be concerned. This may be due to the vitamin A cholesterol-reducing effect and may become evident as symptoms where a very low blood cholesterol is present, as possible in Addison's disease, for example. Drenamin is indicated in these cases.

Synergists:	Activity Contributed:
Cataplex G	Indicated cell-proliferating influence
Chlorophyll Complex (perles)	Detoxification, healing affect, prothrombin factor (vitamin K)
Calcium Lactate	Cell permeability
Arginex and Betacol	(See note below)

Note: Kidney pathology has been described as being basically a protein metabolism problem. For this reason, Betacol or other liver supporting factors should be given in all kidney cases. Arginex is important in both liver and kidney overload in most cases.

CATAPLEX A-C-P

GENERAL CONSIDERATIONS

The general nutritional effects may be listed as follows:
- a. Supplies specific Vitamin A factor of kidney tissue
- b. Promotes epithelial and connective tissue integrity
- c. Increases oxygen-carrying capacity of the blood
- d. Promotes phagocytosis (protective and resistance factors)

Note:
1. Cataplex A-C-P is indicated in all cases where there is an involvement of epithelial cells, the most common occurrence being in kidney pathology where the epithelium of the tubules is concerned, and, in endocrinopathies where the epithelial tissue of the glands are involved.

2. Helpful in supporting phagocytosis and is therefore indicated in toxic and infectious states. The protein-protective mechanism of the Vitamin C Complex insuring protection for the phagocytic activity, thus supporting the defense mechanisms of the reticulo-endothelial system.

3. The oxygen-conserving mechanisms are also supported by Cataplex A-C-P. This effect is beneficial in both frank heart disease and in sub-clinical cases where cardiac insufficiency is the problem.

CLINICALLY ASSOCIATED CONDITIONS

GASTRO-INTESTINAL-URINARY
  <u>Kidney and Bladder</u>
    Albuminuria
    Cystitis
    Kidney Stones
    Nephritis
    Uremia

NERVOUS AND PSYCHOGENIC
  <u>Functional</u>
    Photophobia
  <u>Vaso-Motor</u>
    Blood Pressure Changes

METABOLIC DISORDERS
  <u>Growth and Repair</u>
    Caries
    Eye Conditions
    Gums, Receding of
    Mouth-Tongue Disorders
    Osteoporosis
    Tumors, Fibroid

VASCULAR DISORDERS
  <u>Circulatory</u>
    Bed Sores
    Cold Hands and Feet
    Buerger's Disease
    Hemorrhoids
    Intermittent Claudication
    Leg Ulcers
    Phlebitis
    Tinnitus Aurium
    Leucorrhea
    Varicose Veins

VASCULAR DISORDERS
  <u>Heart Disorders</u>
    Angina Pectoris
    Myocarditis
  <u>Intermediate Processes</u>
    Cholesterol Metabolism
    Oxygen Metabolism
  <u>Collagen Diseases</u>
    Arcus Senilis
    Arteriosclerosis
    Cataracts
  <u>Acid-Base Disorders</u>
    Urine, pH of
  <u>Water Balance</u>
    Edema
  <u>Blood</u>
    Epistaxis
    Leukopenia
  <u>Respiratory</u>
    Bronchitis
    Emphysema

EXOGENIC DISORDERS
  <u>Infections</u>
    Brucellosis

SKIN CONDITIONS
    Dermatitis
    Eczema
    Psoriasis
    Purpura
    Telangiectasis

CATAPLEX A-C-P

CLINICALLY ASSOCIATED CONDITIONS

GENETIC DISORDERS
- Female
    - Amenorrhea
    - Endocervicitis
    - Uterine Congestion
    - Vaginitis
- Male
    - Prostate Disease
- Infections
    - Febrile Diseases
    - Lymph Node Infections
    - Pneumonia
    - Rheumatic Fever
    - Vincent's Infection
- Virus Infection
    - Colds, Flu, Grippe
    - Earache
    - Lumbago

Toxic Disorders
- X-Ray burns
- Inflammation
    - Mastitis
    - Denture Irritation
    - Sinusitis
    - Tonsillitis
    - Gingivitis
- Traumatic
    - Strictures

SPECIFIC DEFICIENCY
- Glandular
    - Goiter
    - Sterility
- Nutritional
    - Glossitis
    - Conjunctivitis

ASSOCIATED PRODUCTS

Cataplex A: Although **Cataplex A-C-P** is the usual product of choice, higher concentrations of A are available by the use of this product. Cataplex A has primarily to do with epithelial integrity and is of particular concern in nephritis, where the epithelium lining the kidney tubules is concerned.

Cataplex C: Cataplex C is used where the patient may not tolerate Vitamin A due to its cholesterol reducing effects. **Cataplex C** has been reported as producing a diuretic effect in some patients.

Cyruta Plus: This is the P fraction of the C Complex. It is useful in correction of capillary fragility, and, although **Cataplex A-C-P** is usually preferred, **Cyruta Plus** is available for those who prefer higher concentrations of this particular fraction. It is recommended in hypotension where the blood pressure lowering effects of **Cyruta** are not desired, yet capillary integrity is the problem. (See pages, 85-88)

Cataplex A-C: This formula was widely used before the improved **Cataplex A-C-P** was introduced which is now the usual product of choice. Cataplex A-C is still available where desired.

CATAPLEX A-C-P

CATAPLEX B12

(VITAMIN B$_{12}$)

Label: Each tablet contains 5 micrograms natural Vitamin B$_{12}$ with liver, stomach parenchyma, cereal germ and milk solids. A new product not yet officially recognized as important in human nutrition. Dose: 1 – 2 daily, or as directed.

Tissue or Function Supported: Hemopoietic system and general systemic effects.

CLINICAL CONSIDERATIONS
Prominent, Clinical Signs And Symptoms

Symptoms:
1. Chronic Fatigue
2. Anemia
3. Mental aberrations (Slowness of thought, depression, apathy, etc.)
4. Achlorhydria (or hypochlorhydria)
5. Emaciation
6. Symptoms of arthritis (Osteoarthritis and osteoporosis, other bone diseases)
7. General tonic effect (Alterative, particularly where anoxia is concerned)
8. Pernicious anemia (also other anemias)
9. Debilitation diseases
10. Gastritis
11. Urticaria (Rashes, angioneurotic edema, etc.)

Possible Etiological Background:
The function of Vitamin B$_{12}$ is still being debated. The following are some of the factors under investigation:

a. Nucleoprotein synthesis
b. Transformation of carbohydrates to fats.
c. Nitrogen balance
d. Synthesis of choline
e. Neurotrophic factors

While the etiological biochemistry of Vitamin B$_{12}$ remains somewhat obscure, clinical evidence is becoming increasingly ample as to its therapeutic effectiveness in a wide variety of disease conditions.

Symptom Characteristics: Aside from its well-known effect as an antianemia factor, B$_{12}$ seems to serve well where neurological aspects are concerned, particularly in relation to cerebral involvements, the effect here probably due to improvement in oxygenation mechanisms.

	Test:	Need Shown By:
Laboratory Tests	Red Blood Count	Macrocytic anemias
Clinical Tests	Tallqvist Scale	Percentage read from scale
	Tachycardia	When indicated by anemia

Administration	**Dosage:** Emphasis should be placed on low dosage, at least after initial stages; thus, 2 or 3 per day for a week or 10 days, then dosage may be as low as 2 or 3 per week.
	Effect: We have noted definite differences in the response of patients using S.P. **Vitamin B$_{12}$ Tablets** which we have failed to observe with other products. The stomach parenchyma is undoubtedly an important factor in our opinion.
	SideEffect: Vertigo, headaches and other symptoms related to neurological responses have been reported. This, we believe, is a matter of overdosage, where the above schedule has been exceeded. The remedy seems to be simply to discontinue use of the product in these cases. Such reactions are rare.

Synergists:	Activity Contributed:
a. Ferrofood	Antianemia Complex
b. Super-EFF	Cell protective phospholipids
c. Chlorophyll Complex	Antianemia Factor
d. Wheat Germ Oil Perles	Antioxidant

GENERAL CONSIDERATIONS

Specificity of clinical indications is rather difficult to establish in the case of **Vitamin B$_{12}$**, however, since it produces a remarkable tonic effect in a very large percentage of cases, every complaint of chronic fatigue should

CATAPLEX B12

GENERAL CONSIDERATIONS

merit a clinical test for response to B_{12}, and, by the same reason, clinical application of this vitamin should not be restricted to anemia, which it is best known to correct.

A wide variety of reports are available showing **Vitamin B_{12}** to have a very beneficial effect in mental conditions and in underdevelopment in children, weight gain and improvement in studies being characteristic. These findings lean heavily on the side of a much broader scope of application in pediatrics than has formerly been applied, perhaps assuming an importance in this respect equivalent to the time-honored use of cod liver oil.

The synergistic effects of **Wheat Germ Oil** in connection with **Vitamin B_{12}** are of particular note, the antioxidant effects of wheat germ oil, no doubt being the complimentary factor.

CLINICALLY ASSOCIATED CONDITIONS

NERVOUS AND PSYCHOGENIC
    Functional
        Asthenia
    Metabolic
        Tranquilizing Effect
    Mentality
        Backwardness in Children
        Brain, Dysfunction of
    Vasomotor
        Hypotension

EXOGENIC
    Inflammation
        Periodontoclasia

ASSOCIATED PRODUCTS:

Ferrofood:	(See Page, 97, Ferrofood)
Manganese B_{12}:	(See Page, 113, Manganese B_{12})
Trace Minerals B_6 :	(See Page, 177, Trace Minerals B_6)

CATAPLEX B

Label:	Contains 125 U.S.P. units of Vitamin B1 per wafer with naturally associated factors from yeast, cereal germ, beet juice and liver, with binder of milk solids. 3 wafers per day furnish the full daily adult minimum Vitamin B1 requirement (333 U.S.P. units). 1 to 4 wafers per day or as directed.
Tissue or Function Supported	Nerve integrity and cell energy reactions – oxidation mechanism accomplished enzymatically – concerned primarily with carbohydrate metabolism, particularly with oxidation of lactic acid and other intermediate processes.

CLINICAL CONSIDERATIONS
Prominent Clinical Signs And Symptoms

Symptom	Possible Etiological Background
1. Poor Muscular Tonicity (Lack of appetizer weakness of legs, muscular weakness, lack of stamina)	Inability to metabolize lactic acid accumulated during exercise
2. Lactic Acid Excess (Drowsiness after eating due to inability to oxidize products of fermentation)	Lactic acid excess due to unfavorable intestinal environment
3. Heart Symptoms (Enlargement, tachycardia, fibrillations)	Motor nerve conductivity
4. Edema ("Water-logged" tissues, diminished urination)	Vaso-dilation effect produced in lactic acid excess
5. Neurological Symptoms (Feeling of band around head, tenderness of calf muscles, hyperirritability, melancholia, etc.)	Nerve integrity.

Symptom Characteristics:	These follow the muscular and nervous patterns, weakness, drowsiness and mental aberrations being most common the outline which may be frequently vague or indistinct. Ingestion of high carbohydrate foods is often most significant finding.

	Test	Test Shown By:
Laboratory Tests	Comment:	Unfortunately, a satisfactory laboratory method of determining lactic acid levels has not yet been devised.
Clinical Tests	Endocardiograph	Split sounds, fibrillation and other deviations which are usually corrected within a few minutes after administration of B Complex.

Administration	**Dosage:** 1 to 4 per day is usual dosage. In beriberi syndrome (tachycardia, edema). amounts may be much higher and should be governed by the diuretic effect produced in these cases, kept at increased level as long as diuresis is produced.
	Effect: Ordinarily results on adequate dosage are very rapid, symptomatically being evident within a few days, within a few minutes where the Endocardiograph is being used to measure its effects.
	Side Effect: These are very rare. If, when they do occur, it seems a specific indication for Cataplex G, see part No. 3 under General Considerations for discussion.

Synergists:	Activity Contributed:
a. Organic Minerals	Source of potassium necessary in many synaptic and enzymatic reactions to which Vitamin B Complex contributes.
b. Calcium Lactate	Acts to combat acidosis, a condition frequently found concomitant with Vitamin B complex deficiency states.
c. Cataplex G	Source of enzyme precursors which act complimentary with those supplied by Cataplex B

CATAPLEX B

GENERAL CONSIDERATIONS

The energy that a cell needs to maintain itself and perform its various functions is supplied by the oxidation of the food within the cell. In this respect, Vitamin B complex performs an important role by catalyzing the various chain reactions through its co-enzymes. This to a very large extent is related to carbohydrate metabolism and as such we must consider not only the amount of Vitamin B complex which is provided by the diet, but also the requirements for that vitamin which may be created by the ingestion of excess amounts of high carbohydrate foods, particularly sugars. Thus, the requirements for Cataplex B vary according to the amounts of carbohydrates ingested. By this reason it may prove futile to administer Cataplex B without a corresponding reducing the overalimentation causing the initial problem. However, when both Cataplex B is given and carbohydrate intake is brought into range, results are usually satisfactory.

The nutritional effects of Cataplex B may be listed as follows:
1. Lactic acid metabolizing factor (oxidation of lactic and pyruvic acids).
2. Promotes motor nerve conductivity.
3. Essential in co-enzyme systems (acetylcholine reaction)
4. Opposes vaso-dilation due to lack of arteriole-capillary tone.

In the clinical application of Cataplex B, the following information is useful:

- **Cataplex B**, containing the B4 factor, has an effect of restoring function to localized areas in myo-neural disorders.

- In heart failure the urinary output may be low due to an inability of the heart to pump the blood in sufficient pressure to the kidneys. In these cases, **Cataplex B,** by increasing the work capacity of the heart, may raise the pressure sufficiently to produce a physiological diuresis.

- In all cases where the diastolic rest period is shortened (See Endocardiograph literature), **Cataplex B** should be preceded by **Cataplex G** until this is normal. Due to its vaso-dilating effects **Cataplex G** assures correction of deficiencies which may be aggravated by **Cataplex B** given prior to this correction.

CLINICALLY ASSOCIATED CONDITIONS

The following list shows but a few of the many possible clinically associated conditions in which **Cataplex B** might contribute important biochemical factors. **Cataplex B** should be considered as an important adjunct in most if not all degenerative and debilitating diseases and as such used in a much wider range of clinical situations than will be outlined.

NERVOUS AND PSYCHOGENIC
    Functional
        Asthenia
        Nervous Strain
    Metabolic
        Alcoholism
        Legs, Weakness of
        Neuromuscular Disorders
    Mentality
        Brain, Dysfunction of
METABOLIC DISORDERS
    Growth and Repair
        Deafness
    Intermediate Processes
        Diabetes Mellitus
    Collagen Diseases
        Rheumatoid Arthritis
    Acid-Base Balance
        Acidosis
    Water Balance
        Ascites
        Dropsy
        Edema
    Body Weight
        Appetite Decreased
EXOGENIC DISORDERS
    Inflammation
        Gingivitis
        Sciatica
VASCULAR DISORDERS
    Circulatory Diseases
        Tinnitus Aurium
GENETIC
    Female Disorders
        Amenorrhea
SPECIFIC DEFICIENCY DISEASES
    Nutritional Diseases
        Pellegra

CATAPLEX C

Label: Vitamin C – Contains 100 U.S.P. units of Vitamin C per tablet with naturally associated factors from alfalfa, mushroom, green buckwheat leaf, and bone marrow. Carrier Material: Fresh bone flour with milk solids as tablet binder. 1 to 4 tablets per day or as directed. 6 tablets per day furnish the full adult minimum daily Vitamin C requirement (600 U.S.P. units) if no other dietary Vitamin C is consumed. For best results tablets should be chewed or dissolved in the mouth.

Tissue or Function Supported	Promoting resistance

CLINICAL CONSIDERATIONS
Prominent Clinical Signs And Symptoms

Symptom
1) Infectious disease (Lowered resistance to bacterial invasion)
2) Adrenal insufficiency (Disturbance in potassium-sodium-chloride levels)
3) Inflammation (Gastritis, nephritis, etc.)
4) Healing
5) Scurvy (Spongy, bleeding gums, hemorrhage, etc.)

Possible Etiological Background
Perhaps of all the vitamin factors Vitamin C is the most concerned with oxygenation mechanisms, and this, in turn may account for its protein protective function. The increase in the oxygen carrying capacity of the blood when Vitamin C is supplied in deficiency states is evidence of this hypothesis. In addition, the natural Vitamin C complex contains the enzyme tyrosinase, a copper containing factor, copper being also active in formation of hemoglobin, an oxygenation factor of known activity.

Symptom Characteristics: Most of the disturbance of tissue in Vitamin C deficiency concerns itself with protein metabolism, i.e., integrity of the phagocyte, inflammation, capillary fragility, etc.

Laboratory and Clinical Tests **Remarks:** Blood tests and urine excretion tests on the synthetic ascorbic acid, though possible, are not generally applied, and we believe that such findings are secondary to the complete enzymatic relation which is obviously present. Therefore, observation of protein disturbances, such as outlined above, and the good judgement of the physician remain the course of reasoning in the selection of such factors in treatment.

Administration	**Dosage:** There are no contraindications for its use in any quantity (except, possible allergy); hourly dosage should be considered in acute conditions..
	Effect: Phagocytosis may be immediately increased. This effect may be considerably enhanced by the use of Calcium Lactate..
	Side Effect: None known..

Synergists:
a. Calcium Lactate
b. Cataplex G

Activity Contributed:
Source of ionizable calcium
Indicated cell proliferating influence

GENERAL CONTRIBUTED

Vitamin C complex is known as "the prima donna vitamin" and this is understandable because it serves the widest variety of protective functions in the body and needs the least physiological explanation of its mechanism for clinical use. Vitamin C, therefore, apparently "blends" well with the varied metabolic reactions in the body and, as such, "side-effects" are practically unknown. At the same time, the possible rewards are very considerable-consider for example we have the often made statements that an infection can only become overwhelming in the face of severe Vitamin C deficiency. The adrenal glands are also rich storage depots for Vitamin C and in their hyperactivity this reserve is depleted. All of which leads us to conclude that Vitamin C complex plays an important role in the defensive mechanisms of the body, and, by the same line of reason, its need is increased when these defenses are at an expense, as for example, during fever, toxemia and acute infections.

CATAPLEX C

CLINICALLY ASSOCIATED CONDITIONS

GASTROINTESTINAL-URINARY
  <u>Kidney and Bladder</u>
    Cystitis
    Nephritis
NERVOUS AND PSYCHOGENIC
  <u>Vasomotor</u>
    Blood Pressure Changes
METABOLIC DISORDERS
  <u>Growth and Repair</u>
    Caries
    Gums, receding of
  <u>Intermediate processes</u>
    Oxygen metabolism
  <u>Blood</u>
    Epistaxis
    Leukopenia
  <u>Respiratory</u>
    Bronchitis
    Emphysema

EXOGENIC DISORDERS
  <u>Infections</u>
    (Various kinds)
  <u>Inflammation</u>
    Mastitis
    Sinusitis
    Tonsillitis
    Gingivitis, etc.
VASCULAR DISORDERS
  <u>Circulatory</u>
    Bed Sores
    Leg Ulcers
  <u>Heart Disorders</u>
    Myocarditis
SKIN CONDITIONS
  Dermatitis
  Purpura

CATAPLEX D

Label: Concentrates of vitamin factors from fish liver oils. Carrier Materials: Milk solids, calcium phytate and calcium lactate. The calcium is used as a carrier for the Vitamin D and 1 tablet supplies one-tenth of the daily requirement of calcium. Each tablet contains 400 IU of Vitamin D with naturally occurring associated factors. Each tablet contains the full adult minimum daily requirement of Vitamin D. 1 to 2 tablets per day or as directed.

Tissue or Function Supported	Calcium Metabolism

CLINICAL CONSIDERATIONS
Prominent Clinical Signs And Symptoms

Symptom	Possible Etiological Background
1. Hyperirritability (Insomnia, restlessness, tachycardia, cramps) 2. Tetany (Muscle spasms) 3. Bone Disorders (Osteoporosis) 4. Lung Conditions (Bronchitis) 5. Lowered Resistance (Worse in winter due to lack of sunshine) 6. Indoor Living (Avoidance of exposure to sun) 7. Hypotension 8. Epistaxis (Nosebleed, also hemorrhage, some types) 9. Delayed Healing (Bed sores, ulcers, etc.)	As evidenced by the long history of beneficial effects of cod liver oil in a variety of diseases, as well as a world-wide recognized supplement for children, Vitamin D stands high on the list of therapeutically acceptable nutritional factors. Its specificity is associated with disturbances in calcium metabolism which in itself is one of the most complex of biological problems. The similarity of its effects to that of the parathyroid hormone call attention to its physiologic significance.

Symptom Characteristics: Two factors are generally considered: first, absorption and maintenance of calcium and blood levels; second, resistance of organism (probably secondary to first consideration). Consider benefits in tuberculosis.

Laboratory Tests	Test: Serum Calcium Plasma Protein	Need Shown By: Normal 10-11 mg. adults; 9-10 children. Calcium varies directly with protein content of blood and usually inversely with phosphorus.
Clinical Tests	Sulkowitch Reagent (*) See comments on page, 72	Decreased excretion indicating serum calcium less than 8.5 mg. per. 100 ml.

	Dosage: 3-6 per day for three weeks, one per day thereafter as indicated.
Administration	**Effect:** The synthetic varieties of Vitamin D have been found to be toxic. This is not true of the natural Vitamin D Complex, which, like cod liver oil, may be given a wide range of use without fear of toxicity in the dosage recommended.
	Side Effect: None known when used as directed.

Synergists:	Activity Contributed:
a. Cataplex F	Calcium Diffusor
b. Chlorophyll Complex (perles)	Prothrombin Factor (important in blood coagulation problems)
c. Calcium Lactate	Source Ionizable Calcium

CATAPLEX D

GENERAL CONSIDERATIONS

The nutritional effects of Vitamin D Complex may be listed as follows:

a. Acts to raise blood calcium level.
b. Acts to promote absorption of calcium.
c. Cooperates with Vitamin F Complex in calcium metabolism.

The similarity of the effects of Vitamin D to the parathyroid hormone are striking. In fact this hormone has been called the "winter hormone" because it is suggested that it performs where the patient does not get enough sunshine during the winter months to carry on the function) of Vitamin D. Clinically, Vitamin D has been found to be practically equivalent to parathormone in its ability to maintain blood calcium levels, an important consideration in the healing processes, and a factor in the resistance of the patient as evidenced by the accepted therapy in tuberculosis and other debilitating diseases by exposure to sunlight.

Some typical calcium deficiency symptoms where Vitamin D may be useful are as follows:

Insomnia	Hyperirritability
Restlessness	("nerve tension")
Cramps	Tetany
(Leg, stomach and menstrual)	("charley-horse")

CLINICALLY ASSOCIATED CONDITIONS

NERVOUS AND PSYCHOGENIC
   <u>Functional</u>
      Asthenia
      Hyperirritability
      Insomnia
      Nervous Strain
   <u>Vaso-Motor</u>
      Hypotension
METABOLIC DISORDERS
   <u>Growth and Repair</u>
      Bones, Healing of
      Osteoporosis
   <u>Intermediate Processes</u>
      Calcium Metabolism

<u>Collagen Diseases</u>
   Arthritis, Hypertrophic
<u>Blood</u>
   Epistaxis
EXOGENIC DISORDERS
   <u>Circulatory Diseases</u>
      Bed Sores
      Leg ulcers
GENETIC DISORDERS
   <u>Female Disorders</u>
      Dysmenorrhea
      Menstruation Symptoms

Clinical Test for Tetany: A blood pressure cuff and diastolic level determined. Holding the pressure just above the diastolic level (about 5 mm.) for a minute or two will produce a definite discomfort in the tetany prone patient. This is usually accompanied by a drawing up of the fingers (claw-like) and is indicative of hypocalcemia or alkalosis.

CATAPLEX E2

(VITAMIN E_2 C-Y 1732)

Label: A phospholipic synergist of alpha-tocopherol from beef chromatin. For experimental use as an adjuvant in Vitamin E deficiency states. A new product (1949) not as yet recognized as essential in human nutrition. Suggested dosage: 1 to 3 tablets per day, or as directed.

Tissue or Function Supported: A tissue oxygen conserving factor, acting primarily as a relaxant and antispasmodic.

CLINICAL CONSIDERATIONS
Prominent Clinical Signs And Symptoms

Symptoms:

1. Angina Pectoris (Chest pain usually radiating down left arm, brought on by exertion).
2. Indigestion Symptoms ("Nervous" type associated with nervous tension and cramps or spasms).
3. Hypertension (Where transitory elevations are brought about by mental instability or environment).
4. Cardiac Neurosis (Symptoms associated with the heart where primary "nervousness" is the problem).
5. Neurological Integrity (As occurring in biliary stasis, colitis, diarrhea, asthma, insomnia, palsy, etc.).

Possible Etiological Background

Apparently the effect of **Vitamin E_2** is synergistic with **Vitamin G Complex** and **Organic Minerals** in promoting the acetylcholine reaction necessary for synapse at the myoneural junction, possibly participating by establishment of the integrity of the oxidative mechanisms, thus assisting in the maintenance of neural control.

Symptom Characteristics: Spasticity, hyperirritability, and hypertonicity are the most characteristic findings. Cholinergic aspects of the autonomic system, myoneural junction disorders and neural control of gastrointestinal mechanisms (sphincters) are of particular importance.

	Test:	Need Shown By:
Laboratory Tests	X-Ray	Delayed emptying time of stomach
Clinical Tests	a. Palpation b. Pulse Rate c. Endocardiograph	Abdominal and muscular tension. Tachycardia Diminished diastolic rest interval

Administration	**Dosage:** 1 to 6 per day, regulated by symptomatic level of relief.
	Effect: Usually immediate, i.e., noticeable by the patient within the first day or two of treatment in indicated cases.
	Side Effect: None known when used as directed.

Synergists:	**Activity Contributed:**
a. Vitamin G Complex	Cholinesterase precursors
b. Organic Minerals	Organic potassium source
c. Orchex	Physiological tranquilize

GENERAL CONSIDERATIONS

The following information should be considered:

1. **Vitamin E_2**, along with **Vitamin G Complex**, has proved to be clinically effective to angina pectoris.
2. A wider application of use of **Vitamin E_2** will include certain types of stomach disorders where there is pain, but a specific diagnosis is lacking-so-called "pseudo-ulcers" or "nervous indigestion". **Vitamin E_2** has the effect of relieving the tension and pain associated with this clinical problem.
3. **Vitamin E_2** may be used in conjunction with any therapy where a tranquilizing effect is desired.

CATAPLEX E2

CLINICALLY ASSOCIATED CONDITIONS

GASTROINTESTINAL-URINARY
- <u>Liver and Gallbladder</u>
  - Biliary Stasis
  - Gallbladder Disease

NERVOUS AND PSYCHOGENIC
- <u>Functional</u>
  - Colitis, ulcerative
  - Hyperirritability
  - Insomnia
  - Ulcers, Gastric
- <u>Metabolic</u>
  - Neuromuscular Disorders
  - Tranquilizing Effects

METABOLIC DISORDERS
- <u>Body Weight</u>
  - Appetite Excessive

VASCULAR DISORDERS
- <u>Circulatory Diseases</u>
  - Intermittent Claudication
- <u>Heart Disorders</u>
  - Angina Pectoris
  - Myocarditis

SKIN DISORDERS
- Pruritis

FEMALE DISORDERS
- Dysmenorrhea
- Menopausal Symptoms

ASSOCIATED PRODUCTS:
Cardio-Plus: (See **Cardio-Plus** Product Bulletin, Page, 35)

CATAPLEX E

Label: Concentrates of Vitamin Factors from the juice of green peas (whole plant) and natural mixed tocopherols (Vitamin E) obtained from vegetable oils, 1 mg. Chlorophyll, and 35 mg. of Ribonucleic acid. Carrier Material: liver powder, wheat germ, and lettuce. The daily requirement of Vitamin E and its necessity for human nutrition have not been agreed upon by the consensus of medical opinion. 1 to 4 tablets per day, or as directed.

Tissue or Function Supported	Cell activity, as related to Vitamin E deficiency states.

CLINICAL CONSIDERATIONS
Prominent Clinical Signs And Symptoms

Symptom	Possible Etiological Background
1. Connective Tissue Disorders (Muscular weakness and atrophy, weakness of tendons, ligaments and fascia).	By promoting tissue repair rate, increases tissue response to stress requirements.
2. Intracellular Effects (Reported beneficial in virus infections such as herpes simplex, herpes zoster, colds, and others).	Intracellular metabolism, probably concerned with oxidative mechanisms.
3. Skin Conditions (Oil dermatitis, eczema, acne and others)	Increase of cellular activity, probably influencing epithelial proliferation rate.
4. Neurological Involvements (Hyperirritability, neuromuscular disorders)	Probably oxidative mechanisms.

Symptom Characteristics:	Generally involve the skin, muscles, ligaments and tendons, less frequently viral and neurological manifestations.	
Laboratory Tests	Test: None known	
Clinical Tests	a. Stretch Tests	Motility of parts (tendons, fascia)
	b. Palpation	Hernia, muscular atrophy, etc.
	c. Reflex Tests	Hyperirritability

Administration	**Dosage:** 3 per day in viral infections, hernia, skin conditions, initial dosage for day or two should be increased from 6 to 12.
	Effect: in hernia may be dramatic if in early stages and obturation has not occurred; often effective in viral and skin involvements.
	Side Effect: None known when used as directed.

GENERAL CONSIDERATIONS

The following nutritional effects are to be considered:

a. Promotes tissue repair rate
b. Acts to increase cellular activity.
c. Increases tissue response to stress.
d. Acts as nerve relaxant.

The non-specificity of symptoms of Vitamin E deficiency make it difficult to outline a clinical situation which fits these effects, however, it is believed that a much wider application of use exists than has been outlined.

CATAPLEX E

CLINICALLY ASSOCIATED CONDITIONS

NERVOUS AND PSYCHOGENIC
- Functional
  - Hyperirritability
- Metabolic
  - Neuromuscular Disorders
  - Tranquilizing Effects
  - Tremors, Muscular

METABOLIC DISORDERS
- Growth and Repair
  - Deafness
- Collagen
  - Arcus Senilis
  - Disc Lesions
  - Hernia
  - Ligaments, Deformity of

EXOGENIC DISORDERS
- Traumatic
  - Strictures Dermatitis

VASCULAR DISORDERS
- Circulatory Diseases
  - Hemorrhoids
- Heart Disorders
  - Myocarditis

SKIN DISORDERS
- Acne Vulgaris
- Eczema
- Psoriasis
- Skin Irritations

GENETIC
- Female
  - Amenorrhea
  - Uterine Congestion
  - Sterility
- Male
  - Sterility

CATAPLEX F

Label: Derived from unsaturated fatty acids; Arachidonic, Linolenic, Linoleic from Flax and Beef lipoids. Each tablet contains 1 milligram **Iodine-**protein complex. Carrier Materials: Milk solids, wheat and oat flour, (antioxidant). The daily requirements of Vitamin F and its necessity for human nutrition have not yet been agreed upon by the consensus of medical opinion. 1 to 4 tablets per day, or as directed.

Tissue or Function Supported   Calcium diffusing factor, promoting ionizable forms.

CLINICAL CONSIDERATIONS
Prominent Clinical Signs And Symptoms

Symptom	Possible Etiological Background
1. Increased metabolism (symptom of hypothyroidism, tachycardia, tremors, weight no., etc.)	Increased metabolic activity.
2. Skin Conditions (Sunburned lips, fever blisters, dry skin, acne, etc.)	Calcium diffusing effect.
3. Hair Integrity (Failing hair, graying, coarseness, thinning, etc.)	Skin and hair integrity shown to be factor in test animals.
4. Prostate Disease (Night urination, dribbling, back pain, etc.)	Probable influence through normalizing iodine metabolism through the thyroid.
5. Autonomic Unbalance (pyloric spasms, digestive complaints, "nervous" stomach, etc.)	Calcium metabolism through the autonomic nervous system.

	Test:	Need Shown by:
Laboratory Tests	a. Protein-Bound Iodine	Normal range: 3.0 to 8.0 mcg. Per 100 cc of serum. Increased concentrations found in hyperthyroidism.
	b. Total Protein	Normal range: 6.0 to 8.0 gm. Per 100 cc serum. Decreased value may indicate deficit in ionized calcium. (See Calcium Lactate Bulletin, page, 29 under Laboratory tests).
Clinical Tests	a. Pulse Rate	Tachycardia
	b. Prostate Examination	Enlargement
	c. Observation	Loss of integrity of skin and hair
	d. Endocardiograph	Diminished 2nd sound, mitral area

Administration	**Dosage:** The following schedule is recommended in prostatic hypertrophy and is applicable to most cases. 6 per day for 3 days, 4 per day for 2 weeks and one or two per day thereafter.
	Effect: The more acute the situation, the more rapid response; fever blisters, sunburned lips, skin conditions showing most rapid clinical evidence of effects. In prostate disease, response may depend upon history of venereal disease..
	Side Effect: None known.

Synergists	Activity Contributed
1. Calcium Lactate	Source of ionizable calcium
2. Cataplex F Perles	Iodine synergists
3. Thytrophin	Local environment of cells

GENERAL CONSIDERATIONS

The nutritional effects of Cataplex F may be listed as follows:

    a   Calcium diffuser   b.   Cooperates with Vitamin D

CATAPLEX F

GENERAL CONSIDERATIONS

The nutritional effects of Cataplex F may be listed as follows:

- c. Vitamin B6 synergist
- d. Skin integrity aid
- e. Antioxidant
- f. Beneficial in prostate disease

The following principals may apply:

1. **Cataplex F** has an important relation to iodine metabolism and its use is especially indicated in increased metabolic rates, as in hyperthyroidism.

2. **Cataplex F** has been found useful in certain types of skin disorders, especially where excess Vitamin D is involved, as in sunburned lips often seen in farmers and field workers.

3. **Cataplex F** is helpful in calcium metabolism problems and is indicated wherever Calcium Lactate is used because of its ability to diffuse calcium thereby making it available for tissue use. This is important in the treatment of brittle fingernails, canker sores, falling hair and fever blisters.

4. Because of its effects in calcium metabolism, **Cataplex F** is a valuable aid in the treatment of disorders of the autonomic nervous system (see page 91, Vitamin News).

5. **Cataplex F** has proved beneficial in prostate disease. For complete information – See Lee Foundation. Report No.1, "Vitamin F, in the Treatment of Prostatic Hypertrophy."

CLINICALLY ASSOCIATED CONDITIONS

GASTROINTESTINAL-URINARY
Liver and Gallbladder
- Gallbladder disease
- Indigestion, acute

Kidney and Bladder
- Cystitis
- Nephritis

NERVOUS AND PSYCHOGENIC
Functional
- Autonomic unbalance
- Dysphagia
- Salivary disorders
- Tachycardia

Metabolic
- Tremors, muscular

Vasomotor
- Dizziness
- Heat prostration

METABOLIC DISORDERS
Growth and Repair
- Deafness
- Nails, integrity of

Intermediate Processes
- Calcium metabolism

Respiratory
- Bronchitis
- Emphysema
- Coughs, chronic

EXOGENIC DISORDERS
Virus Infections
- Herpes Simplex

Toxic
- Poison Ivy and Oak

VASCULAR DISORDERS
Circulatory
- Tinnitus Aurium
- Heart Disorders
- Angina Pectoris
- Myocarditis

SKIN CONDITIONS
- Acne vulgaris
- Alopecia
- Dermatitis
- Skin irritations

GENETIC
Male Disorders
- Prostate disease

SPECIFIC DEFICIENCY DISEASES
Glandular
- Goiter

ASSOCIATED PRODUCTS

USF Ointment- Where Vitamin F factors are desired for topical application (See Page, 179)

CATAPLEX F PERLES

Label: Essential unsaturated fatty acids (Arachidonic, Linoleic, Linolenic) from Flax and Beef Lipoids with Soybean Lecithin – no daily requirement of "Vitamin F" and its necessity for human nutrition has not been established by the consensus of medical opinion. 1 to 3 Perles per day or as directed.

Tissue or Function Supported   Supplies vitamin forms of unsaturated fatty acids.

CLINICAL CONSIDERATIONS
Prominent Clinical Signs And Symptoms

<u>Symptoms:</u>

1. Hypothyroid symptoms (Wrinkles, thick dry skin, bradycardia, inability to tolerate stress, etc.)
2. Menstruation symptoms (Scanty menses, amenorrhea)
3. Menopausal symptoms (Hot flashes, lowered stress tolerance, irritability)
4. Vitamin D toxicity (Sensitivity to sunlight, sunburned lips)
5. Prostatitis
6. Falling hair
7. Hypercholesterolemia

<u>Possible Etiological Background</u>

The metabolism of iodine, with its consequential effects on thyroid activity are believed to be related to deficiency of vitamin forms of unsaturated fatty acids. In the main this involves hypothyroidism with subclinical manifestations of myxedema. The course of the deficiency follows lowered oxidation reactions with subsequent fibrotic tendencies and accumulations of sclerotic-type lesions involving the skin and its sub-strata layers. It is, perhaps, through the correction of these differences that Vitamin F has become known as "the cosmetic vitamin".

Symptom Characteristics:	These follow patterns usually encountered in hypothyroidism.	
Laboratory Tests	Test: Protein Bound Iodine	Need Shown by: Less than 3
Clinical Tests	Physical Examination	Signs and Symptoms of hypothyroidism.

Administration	**Dosage:** Usually 2 to 3 weeks are required before expecting noticeable improvement in symptomatic pattern. This effect is often dependent upon simultaneous administration of **Soybean Lecithin**.
	Effect: 3 to 6 per day. Bile Salts (**Cholacol**) may be necessary to promote absorption.
	Side Effect: None specifically accounted for, but rationalization would tend to point to hyperthyroidism if encountered. Of course, the fat nature of the product may cause disturbance secondarily in gallbladder disease calling for use of **Cholacol**.

<u>Synergists:</u>   <u>Activity Contributed:</u>

a. Thytrophin   Local Environment at of Calls
b. Super-EFF   Call Protective Phospholipids
c. Soybean Lecithin   Organic Phosphorus Source
d. Pituitrophin   Trophic Effect of Pituitary

GENERAL CONSIDERATIONS

When metabolic demands are increased (as in menopause, menstruation, pregnancy and senility) and the thyroid gland is unable to meet these demands, unpleasant reactions may occur until normal thyroid activity is obtained. Such reactions as increased irritability and inability to tolerate stress situations-working "under pressure" for example, are characteristic. These hypertonic responses may be due to lowering of the oxygenation activities and are, we believe, associated with hypothyroidism.

CATAPLEX F PERLES

GENERAL CONSIDERATIONS

In these cases, the blood iodine (PBI) will usually be found to be lowered (less than 3). Unsaturated fatty acids are known to increase the blood iodine and the effect here is thus indicative of normalizing thyroid function, i.e., relieving the hypothyroid state. The rationale here simply involves the biochemical nature of unsaturated fatty acids in that-being rated by their iodine numbers-they possess available bonds for iodine acceptance.

Where this rationalization has been clinically applied, very favorable clinical results have been obtained in a high percentage of cases.

The nutritional effects of **Cataplex F Perles** may be listed as follows-

CLINICALLY ASSOCIATED CONDITIONS

METABOLIC DISORDERS
   <u>Collagen</u>
      Arcus Senilis
      Arthritis, Hypertrophic
      Arteriosclerosis
EXOGENIC DISORDERS
   <u>Virus</u>
      Warts

FEMALE DISORDERS
   Menopausal Symptoms
   Menstruation Symptoms
   Uterine Congestion
SPECIFIC DEFICIENCY DISEASES
   Goiter
   Sterility

CATAPLEX G

Label: Content of Vitamin factors for which standards have been established: Riboflavin – 1 mg Niacin – 12 mg (One-third daily requirement per wafer, for adults). With synergists and extracts from yeast, sprouted grain and calf brain. Carrier Material: Phytin, 1 to 4 wafers per day or as directed.

Tissue or Function Supported In addition to being a source of lipotrophic factors, being specific thereby for liver tissue, it is also a source of factors which have been shown to be of benefit in neuro-muscular disorders, probably by supplying precursors for the formation of cholinesterase.

CLINICAL CONSIDERATIONS
Prominent Clinical Signs And Symptoms

Symptom	Possible Etiological Background
1. Night Sweats	Autonomic nervous system reaction, cholinergic response.
2. Paresthesia (Burning sensations on soles central nervous system origin of feet, crawling sensations)	Synaptic involvement, probably.
3. Erythema (Redness of palms of hands and soles of feet)	Associated with liver disease.
4. Paralysis (Loss of muscular control, numbness, angina-like spasms, ptosis, etc.)	Synapse at myoneural junction, usually involving potassium, necessary for cholinesterase reaction to occur.
5. Ascites (Also veinous congestion, visible veins on chest and abdomen, hemorrhoids, etc.)	Edema, secondary to liver failure.
6. Eye symptoms (Blurred vision, accommodation, sensation of "sand")	Muscle spasms and irritation.
7. Mental Symptoms (Melancholia, apprehension, loss of appetite (nervous)	Pellagra-type symptoms.
8. Digestive Complaints ("Nervous" indigestion, gastritis)	Cell proliferation failure causing achlorhydria, irritation; also synaptic relations governing peristalsis (parietal cells).

Symptom Characteristics: Neurological origin and symptoms of liver dysfunction.

Laboratory Tests Discussion: Most valuable laboratory finding is hypoproteinemia. It has been found that changes in serum cholinesterase parallel those of serum albumin, both substances being proteins formed by the liver. "Clinical Biochemistry" – Cantarow and Trumper.

Clinical Tests	Test:	Need Shown By:
	a. Phonocardiograph	Reading showing shortened diastolic rest period (tic-tac rhythm).
	b. Observation	Redness on palms of hands, veins showing on chest and abdomen.

Administration	**Dosage:** With sufficient dosage, up to 6 per day, effect is usually noted by patient within 24 hours when
	Specific symptoms are being observed. Best results are obtained by long, continued use. Organic Mineral Tablets, as a source of potassium, may be indispensable..
	Effect: 6 per day in initial stages, later 1 to 3 per day
	Side Effect: None known.

Synergists:	Activity Contributed:
1. Organic Minerals	Myoneural synaptic reactions occur in presence of potassium.
2. Choline and Betacol	Where liver disease is concerned.

CATAPLEX G

GENERAL CONSIDERATIONS

See Organic Mineral Bulletin, (See Page, 129) for further information.
The general nutritional effects may be listed as follow:

- a. Enzymatic tranquilizer
- b. Cell proliferating factor
- c. Acts as coronary relaxant
- d. Liberation of free choline to tissues (cholinesterase)
- e. Acts to normalize liver function
- f. Benefits autonomic nervous system
- g. Vaso-dilation effect
- h. Beneficial effect in digestive processes

Note:
1. When the synapse at the myoneural junction is effected by either a deficiency of enzymes (mediator substances) or a deficiency of potassium, it is apt to be delayed or not occur at all. The result may be paralysis, dystrophy or ptosis.
2. Unless degeneration has gone too far, the administration of **Cataplex G** (cholinesterase precursors) and **Organic Minerals** (as a source of potassium), often quickly restores the functional response. This failure of synapse may be suspected in localized areas of stress in various conditions, such as angina pectoris, coronary insufficiency, stomach spasms and complaints of "nervousness".
3. **Cataplex G** apparently has an influence on intracellular metabolism and may be considered a cell-proliferating factor judging by clinical results in some types of viral involvements and healing processes.
4. Beneficial in digestive processes requiring healing (gastritis) and in processes involving the pancreas and parietal cells of the stomach, also a tranquilizing effect in hyper-peristalic activity.

CLINICALLY ASSOCIATED CONDITIONS

GASTROINTESTINAL-URINARY
   <u>Liver and Gallbladder</u>
      Biliary Stasis
      Digestion Faulty
      Indigestion, Acute
      Liver Disease
   <u>Kidney and Bladder</u>
      Albuminuria
      Nephritis
NERVOUS AND PSYCHOGENIC
   <u>Functional</u>
      Autonomic unbalance
      Colitis
      Dysphagia
      Insomnia
      Hyperirritability
      Photophobia
      Nervous Strain
      Tachycardia
      Ulcers, Gastric
   <u>Metabolic</u>
      Alcoholism
      Numbness
   <u>Mentality</u>
      Backwardness, Children
      Brain, Dsyfunction of
   <u>Vaso-Motor</u>
      Blood Pressure Changes
      Hypersensitivity

METABOLIC DISORDERS
   <u>Growth and Repair</u>
      Aging Processes
      Deafness
      Eye Conditions
      Healing, Promotion of
   <u>Intermediate Processes</u>
      Cramps
      Protein Metabolism
   <u>Collagen Diseases</u>
      Cataracts
   <u>Acid Base Disorders</u>
      Acid, Cravings for
      Alkalosis
   <u>Water Balance</u>
      Ascites
      Dropsy
      Edema of Ankles
   <u>Blood</u>
      Anemia
   <u>Allergies</u>
      Antihistamine Effect
      Hives
   <u>Body Weight</u>
      Appetite Excessive
EXOGENIC DISORDERS
   <u>Infections</u>
      Vincent's Infection

CATAPLEX G

CLINICALLY ASSOCIATED CONDITIONS

EXOGENIC DISORDERS
- <u>Virus</u>
  - Earache
  - Warts
- <u>Toxic Disorders</u>
  - Delirium
- <u>Inflammation</u>
  - Mastitis
  - Diarrhea
  - Gingivitis
- <u>Traumatic</u>
  - Stroke, Recovery

VASCULAR DISORDERS
- <u>Circulatory Diseases</u>
  - Cold Hands and Feet
  - Intermittent Claudication
  - Leg Ulcers
  - Tinnitus Aurium
- <u>Heart Disorders</u>
  - Angina Pectoris

SKIN CONDITIONS
- Psoriasis
- Telangiectasia

GENETIC DISORDERS
- <u>Female</u>
  - Abortion
  - Dysmenorrhea
  - Endocervicitis

SPECIFIC DEFICIENCY
- <u>Glandular</u>
  - Gynecomastia
- <u>Nutritional</u>
  - Cheilosis
  - Glossitis
  - Conjunctivitis
  - Pellagra

ASSOCIATED PRODUCTS:

Drenamin: This product contains Vitamin G, useful where Vitamin G is desired as an adrenal hormone precursor. (See Page, 93)

Cardio-Plus: Also contains Vitamin G Complex, useful where Vitamin G is desired in connection with Heart Disorders. (See Page, 35)

CATAPLEX G

CHLOROPHYLL COMPLEX

Label: Fat-Soluble Chlorophyll Complex from Alfalfa, Buckwheat, and Soybeans. 385 Mgms per Perle.

Tissue or Function Supported Source of fat-soluble vitamin factors (particularly Vitamin K) and sex hormone precursors (Vitamin E complex factors).

CLINICAL CONSIDERATIONS
Prominent Clinical Signs And Symptoms

Symptoms:	Possible Etiological Background:
1. Vascular Changes (Telangiectasia, purpura, petechiae, etc.)	Capillary integrity, associated with prothrombin factor (Vitamin K).
2. Hypertension	Possible toxemia, also kidney involvement.
3. Acne (Associated with mense)	Deficiency of hormone precursors.
4. Healing (Ulcers, skin conditions, gastritis, etc.)	Healing action of chlorophyll.
5. Kidney Dysfunction (Also bladder irritation)	Protein metabolism, prothrombin factor (Vitamin K).
6. Toxemia (Associated with arthritis, arteriosclerosis, coronary sclerosis, etc.)	Probably guanidine-neutralizing effect its presence being a suspected factor in these diseases.
7. Hemorrhage (Excessive mense, nosebleed)	Prothrombin factor (Vitamin K)
8. Colitis (Gastritis, stomach ulcers)	Healing action of chlorophyll.

Symptom Characteristics: Usually concerned with blood clotting, vascular changes, or toxemia.

Laboratory And Clinical Tests: Prolongation of the blood clotting time beyond the usual 6 to 8 minute period is indicative of need.

Administration	
	Dosage: 1 to 6 per day or as directed. Bile Salts (**Cholocal**) may be necessary to promote absorption of fat-soluble factors.
	Effect: Blood clotting time may be changed in a few hours. The tonic effect and other noticeable changes may require several weeks.
	Side Effect: None known.

Synergists:	Activity Contributed:
Cataplex G	Cell-proliferating influence.
Cataplex A-C-P	Epithelial and connective tissue integrity.
Ferrofood	Compliments blood factors.
Chlorophyll Complex (perles)	Augments effects of fat soluble chlorophyll complexes.

GENERAL CONSIDERATIONS

In the use of **Chlorophyll Complex (perles)** both local and systemic effects must be taken into consideration, as follows:

1. The local effect of chlorophyll on the intestinal mucosa is to combat inflammation and promote healing, as would be indicated by a wide range of gastrointestinal disorders from diarrhea to stomach ulcers, colitis, gastritis, etc.

2. The systemic effect is to act as a detoxifying factor with a tonic effect, useful in most debilitated states associated with chronic disease.

3. Chlorophyll is an antagonist of guanidine.

CHLOROPHYLL COMPLEX

GENERAL CONSIDERATIONS

Clinical Application is from following stages:

1) Effect upon endocrine system as sex hormone precursors
2) Effect as prothrombin factor, Vitamin K, important in cardiovascular and circulatory problems
3) Effect in lowering blood pressure.
4) Effect in hemoglobin formation
5) Favorable effect in hypercholesterolemia
6) Favorable effect in arteriosclerosis
7) Source of fat-soluble vitamins (A, E, F, and K)

CLINICALLY ASSOCIATED CONDITIONS

GASTROINTESTINAL-URINARY
- Stomach and Intestine
  - Colitis
- Kidney and Bladder
  - Albuminuria
  - Kidney Stones
  - Nephritis

NERVOUS AND PSYCHOGENIC
- Functional
  - Colitis, Ulcerative
  - Ulcers, Gastric
- Vasomotor
  - Blood Pressure Changes

METABOLIC DISORDERS
- Growth and Repair
  - Aging Processes
  - Healing, Promotion of
  - Mouth-Tongue Disorders
  - Teething
- Intermediate Processes
  - Cholesterol
- Collagen Diseases
  - Arthritis, Rheumatoid

Blood
- Anemia
- Epistaxis

EXOGENIC DISORDERS
- Infections
  - Vincent's Infection
- Toxic
  - Burns, Systemic
- Inflammation
  - Mastitis
  - Diarrhea
  - Gingivitis

VASCULAR DISORDERS
- Circulatory
  - Bed Sores
  - Leg Ulcers
  - Tinnitus Aurium

SKIN CONDITIONS
- Acne
- Purpura
- Telangiectasis

ASSOCIATED PRODUCTS:

Chlorophyll (Aqueous) Capsules: Water-soluble, rapidly absorbed chlorophyll, for oral administration or topical use, but does not contain the fat-soluble vitamin factors A, E, F, and K.   (See Page, 193)

Chlorophyll Ointment: Topical application. (See Page, 71)

Additional Reading Material:

Vitamin News, page, 163

V-P Nutritional Abstracts (Chlorophyll)

Reprint "Chlorophyll for Healing" Science News letter

CHLOROPHYL OINTMENT

(CHLOROPHYLL, FAT SOLUBLE OINTMENT)

Label: Fat soluble Chlorophyll Complex Ointment from Lucerne, Buckwheat and Soybean

Tissue or Function Supported	Stimulant for tissue regeneration and healing.

CLINICAL CONSIDERATIONS
Prominent Clinical Signs And Symptoms

Symptoms:
1. Ulcers (Leg ulcers)
2. Dermatitis (Where lesions occur from scratching)
3. "Dry Socket" (Pain after tooth extraction)
4. Vaginitis (Inflammation in vaginal vault)
5. Inflammation (Bunions, corns, sore gums, etc.)
6. Bed sores (Pressure sores)

Possible Etiological Background:
Chlorophyll has an enviable reputation as a stimulant for tissue regeneration and healing. Aided by a grant from the American Medical Association, Drs. L.W. Smith and A.E. Levingston studied the healing influence of seventeen medicinal preparations on experimentally induced wounds and burns in 1,372 tests plus 878 controls. Only chlorophyll in these tests showed any consistent statistically significant effect in accelerating the healing of wounds and burns.
(Am. J. Surg., 62:358-369, 1943)

Symptom Characteristics:	Inflammation, lesions, and localized areas where tissue integrity is deficient.
Laboratory and Clinical Tests	None known.

Administration	**Dosage:** Topical application. **Note:** Should be lightly applied, heavy application does not increase its effectiveness, according to our reports.
	Effect: Treatment should be judged in relation to time of ordinary healing, i.e., at least one or two weeks before judging results. In case of "dry socket", result may be immediate.
	Side Effect: None known.

.Synergists:	Activity Contributed:
a. Carbamide (as wet poultice)	Healing effect
b. Vitamin F Ointment (May be mixed)	Calcium diffusing influence

GENERAL CONSIDERATIONS

Chlorophyll preparations are reputed to be very effective in controlling pain in skin abrasions, friction burns, burns in general, and after tooth extraction. This effect is very possibly due to the fact that chlorophyll destroys guanidine on contact, guanidine being a toxin released by burns, trauma, or muscle fatigue. Guanidine precipitates calcium from blood serum and is suspected to be a cause of calcification of coronary arteries, diffusing in from the muscle.

CHLOROPHYL OINTMENT

CHOLACOL II

Label: Each tablet contains: 8 mgs. Purified Bile Salts (Beef), 20 mgs. Collinsonia (root), 850 mgs. Montmorillonite. For use where a detoxifying, adsorbent action is desired, with a mild effect of bile salts. Suggested dosage: 4 tablets 15 minutes before each meal, or as directed.

Tissue or Function Supported Precipitates toxins and other substances in the intestinal tract and thus facilitates their removal, acting in this manner as an intestinal detoxicant.

CLINICAL CONSIDERATIONS
Prominent Clinical Signs And Symptoms

<u>Symptoms:</u>
1. Diarrhea
2. Allergy (food allergy)
3. Nausea
4. Constipation (some types)
5. Inability to gain weight
6. Indigestion (hyperacidity)
7. Flatulence (lower bowel gas)
8. Excessive appetite (due to faulty absorption)
9. Skin lesions (some types of psoriasis)
10. Costiveness (dry, hard stool)
11. Alkaline stool

<u>Possible Etiological Background:</u>
Symptoms listed are related to the effects produced by putrefaction, fermentation or rancidity or other products of intestinal toxemia, including both small intestine and colon. **Cholacol II**, by reason of its adsorptive power precipitates or filters these deleterious products and promotes their removal. Thus, faulty absorption due to over-eating or weakened digestion causing foci of morbid processes is combated and the intestinal environment tends to become cleared.

Symptom Characteristics: As described above, these will be reflected in disturbances in the intestinal environment, usually of a toxic nature. Note that specific gastrointestinal symptoms may be lacking, the toxic end-products of intestinal toxemia being the primary consideration. These may relate to allergies (asthma, for example), arthritis, skin conditions, etc. Some form of flatulence, vertigo, nausea, hypertension or tachycardia is usually evident.

Laboratory Tests <u>Test:</u> <u>Need Shown By:</u>
Bromthymol Blue (Stool) Test   Acid reaction

Clinical Tests A Therapeutic Test of two or three days use is usually sufficient to show etiological background of gastric hyperacidity or intestinal toxemia, response being immediately evident by clinical results.

Administration

Dosage: Activity is dependent on mechanical (physical) adsorptive properties, therefore results are proportional to dosage employed and amount of toxemia present. 4 tablets before each meal is usually adequate. In diarrhea, 4 tablets with each bowel movement is usually effective in 24 hours where intestinal toxemia is the problem (diarrhea of neurological or psychic origin does not respond). Schedule should be alternated according to clinical response, i.e., reduced or discontinued when symptoms clear, also, series of two to three weeks on and off its use may be advisable. The consideration in all cases is that this product does not provide substantial nutritional support but is useful rather because of its physical properties (see note at end of this bulletin)..

Effect: On adequate dosage, lower bowel gas, hyperacidity, and diarrhea are usually promptly relieved. Allergies, constipation, skin conditions (involving systemic considerations) require longer period for response-three to six weeks.

Side Effect: A hasty unfavorable appraisal of the general effects of this product because of occasional side-effects encountered is unwarranted and such side-effects need careful analysis because they are generally due to gastritis, an inflammatory condition of the tract which is neurologically stimulated when **Cholacol II** is introduced, a condition requiring **Comfrey, Pepsin & E$_3$** for its treatment. On the other hand, this same mechanical activity acts to stimulate a tract which is sluggish (but not irritated) and in this respect the product is very beneficial. Simply stated, this means that **Cholacol II** should not be used where food roughage (such as endive, raw foods, etc.) are cause for complaints, in other words, where a bland diet is indicated. In the main, however, these side-effects are in the minority and beneficial results are to be expected.

CHOLACOL II

Synergists:
a. Zypan
b. Zymex
c. Comfrey, Pepsin & E_3
d. Organic Minerals

Activity Contributed
Digestive Catalyst
Intestinal Detoxicant
Hydrophilic Colloids
(*) See below

GENERAL CONSIDERATIONS

Cholacol II has a slight cholagogue effect, however, it is designed to be used as an intestinal cleanser and detoxifier because of its exceptional adsorbent qualities.

(*) Clinically this clay acts differently than purified forms in many other products in that it has a particular affinity for the potassium ion and in this respect is helpful in adrenal insufficiency where potassium is not properly eliminated. By the same line of reason, however, it may aggravate an already existent potassium deficiency state, usually evidenced by tachycardia or aggravation of constipation. This calls for the use of **Organic Mineral** tablets. It also raises the acidity of the stool and thereby aids in overcoming intestinal stasis.

CLINICALLY ASSOCIATED CONDITIONS

GASTROINTESTINAL-URINARY
  Stomach and Intestine
    Alimentary Canal Flora
    Mucous Colitis
    Flatulence
NERVOUS AND PSYCHOGENIC
  Vasomotor
    Hypotension
METABOLIC DISORDERS
  Intermediate Processes
    Cholesterol Metabolism
  Allergies
    Antihistamine Effects
    Allergies
    Sneezing Attacks
  Body Weight
    Appetite Excessive

EXOGENIC DISORDERS
  Inflammation
    Diarrhea
SKIN DISORDERS
    Acne Vulgaris
GLANDULAR
    Adrenal Insufficiency

CHOLACOL

Label: (Bile Salts with Collinsonia) Each tablet contains: 2 grs. Purified Bile Salts (Beef), 5 grs. Collinsonia (root). For the promotion of liver function where impaired by bile salt deficiency. Dosage: 1 to 3 tablets per day, or as directed.

Tissue or Function Supported Fat absorption (emulsification) and cholagogue.

CLINICAL CONSIDERATIONS
Prominent Clinical Signs And Symptoms

Symptoms:

1. Acholic stool (Light or gray colored)
2. Constipation
3. Faulty absorption of fat-soluble vitamins (A, E, F, K) (Excessive appetite prolongation of blood clotting time indicative of K deficiency)
4. Cholecystecomy
5. Indigestion symptoms (Intolerance of fats, nausea)

Possible Etiological Background:

As with other gastric secretions, for example, hydrochloric acid-not only is the amount produced important, but also the time of release from stored compartments into the intestinal environment. The administration of bile salts apparently acts to initiate this effect, thus the supplementation is enhanced by physiological reserves.

Symptom Characteristics: Two factors are to be considered: 1) Acholic or clay-colored stools, and, 2) Neurological failure (bile fails to release due to spastic states). The deficiencies of fat-soluble vitamins are difficult to trace to this source, but nevertheless should be constantly kept in mind.

Laboratory Tests	Test:	Need Shown By:
	Urine Bile and Bilirubin	Presence indicates obstruction in biliary tract and Cholacol **(bile salts) should not be administered.**
	Contra-**Indication:**	**Betafood** is indicated instead.

Clinical Tests Screen Test: **Note:** A screen-test for the more specific test above is to shake urine in Test tube. A frothy appearance indicates possible presence of bile.

Administration	
	Dosage: In constipation a step ladder dosage may be required, 3 first day, 6 second, 9 third, later reduced to effective control levels.
	Effect: Usually effective on sufficient dosage.
	Side Effect: See "Laboratory Tests" above. Cholagogues (bile salts) may be cause of distress in biliary stasis because bile flow being inhibited or obstructed for various reasons, the stimulatory action places further stress upon an already overburdened part. As mentioned above, **Betafood** is the product of choice in these cases because while it acts to thin the bile, it has no stimulatory action and therefore relieves the pressure rather than adding to it.

Synergists:	**Activity Contributed:**
a. Betafood	Bile thinning influence
b. Zypan	Digestive catalyst
c. Di-Sodium Phosphate	Liver stimulant

Note: For source of fat-soluble vitamins where absorption is being impaired, use **Chlorophyll Complex (perles)** particularly in Vitamin K deficiency states.

CHOLACOL

GENERAL CONSIDERATIONS

Nutritional effects of **Cholacol** may be listed as follows:

A. Stimulates bile flow
B. Combats constipation
C. Promotes absorption of fats and fat-soluble vitamins
D. Its contained Collinsonia combats hemorrhoids and varicose veins (reputedly) known to be aggravated when bile salts alone are used in susceptible cases.

Rationalization for clinical use is as follows:

1. Diminished bile flow, usually indicated by light-colored (or clay-colored) stool, shows need for bile salts (except where blockage has occurred, usually indicated by jaundice).
2. Constipation, indigestion symptoms, flatulence and other gastrointestinal symptoms may indicate need for **Cholacol**.
3. Clay-colored (acholic) stools indicate presence of fat in stool, faulty fat digestion and need for **Cholacol**.
4. Prolongation of the blood clotting time (prothrombin time) may show failure to absorb Vitamin K; Vitamins A, E and F may also be concerned according to their deficiency symptoms.
5. Indicated in almost all liver insufficiency states.
6. Indicated in almost all cholecystectomies (gallbladder removal).
7. Clinical reports favor use in excessive appetite, apparently due to low blood fat reacting on appetite centers in brain which **Cholacol** tends to correct.

Note: **Cholacol II** differs from **Cholacol** in that the former contains the adsorbent mineral, montmorillonite in abundance, but less bile salts and collinsonia. **Cholacol II** is, therefore, the product of choice where the primary effect desired is adsorption and precipitation of toxins for intestinal detoxification; while **Cholacol** is the product of choice where the stimulatory action of bile salts is desired.

CLINICALLY ASSOCIATED CONDITIONS

GASTROINTESTINAL-URINARY
   <u>Liver and Gallbladder</u>
      Constipation
      Liver Disease
METABOLIC DISORDERS
   <u>Body Weight</u>
      Obesity

EXOGENIC DISORDES
   <u>Traumatic</u>
      Sedimentation Rate
SKIN CONDITIONS
   Psoriasis

CHOLINE

Label: 400 mgs. Choline Bitartrate per tablet. A nutritional factor useful in intestinal colic, hypertension and tachycardia where due to its deficiency. Suggested schedule: 1 to 2 tablets with each meal, or as directed.

Tissue or Function Supported: Lipotropic factor.

CLINICAL CONSIDERATIONS
Prominent Clinical Signs And Symptoms

Symptoms:

1. Gallbladder Symptoms (Nausea, intolerance to fats, chronic indigestion, jaundice, constipation, etc.)
2. Liver Disease (Fatty degeneration, venous congestion, diminished urination, hemorrhoids, constipation)
3. Capillary Stasis (Pallor pasty complexion, diminished blood volume, purpura, etc.)
4. Hypertension Symptoms (Morning headache, chronic fatigue, tachycardia, etc.)
5. Fatty Degeneration (Artherosclerosis, fatty liver, also fatty heart and kidney)
6. Colic and Hyperperistalsis (Intestinal colic, frequent bowel movements, gas pains, sphincter spasms)
7. Tachycardia (With associated symptoms as listed above)

Possible Etiological Background:

Acts as physiological detergent and thus promotes bile flow by reducing surface tension of fat particles, augmenting the action of bile salts in this respect. It is also possible to account for its lipotropic activity by this means. We have observed that the reduced surface tension apparently extends to systemic considerations, acting to augment capillary circulation as well as lymphatic drainage. A neurological effect is also observable, apparently acting through the autonomic nervous system (cholinergic effect), since it has been shown to be beneficial in biliary stasis i.e., gallbladder dysfunction associated with colic. Intestinal peristalsis and sphincter control (sphincter of Oddi) also are apparently under this influence. Symptomatic relief of conditions involving increased cerebrospinal fluid pressure have also been observed leading to the supposition that its detergent effects can be extended to this level as well.

Symptom Characteristics: Two aspects are considered: 1) Circulatory deficiency, 2) Neurological control as described above. General considerations include fat and cholesterol metabolism as may occur in liver, gallbladder and arteriosclerotic patients.

Laboratory and Clinical Tests See Product Bulletin on **Betacol**, page 11.

Administration

Dosage: 2 tablets with each meal is apparently adequate in most cases..

Effect: Generally shows improvements within one week as described above, except in most chronic cases. Hypertension and circulatory disorders may require extended therapy and increased dosage before symptomatic evidence is obvious.

Side Effect: None known in dosage recommended.

Synergists:	Activity Contributed:
a. Betacol	Basic liver supplement
b. Betafood	Bile-thinning factor
c. Di-Sodium Phosphate	Liver stimulating factor
d. Zypan	Digestive catalyst

GENERAL CONSIDERATIONS

The nutritional effects of **Choline** may be listed as follows:

1. **Choline**, acting as a physiological detergent or "wetting agent", compliments the action of bile by promoting dispersion of fat particles. This "wetting action", so to speak, also acts to promote capillary circulation according to clinical evidence we have observed, accepting a pale, pasty skin as evidence of poor capillary circulation, which **Choline** tends to correct.

CHOLINE

GENERAL CONSIDERATIONS

2. The attributed detergent effect may also be one of the factors concerned with the well-known effect of **Choline** in promoting the dispersion of fatty deposits in the liver.

3. **Choline** apparently possesses an antispasmodic effect which is evidenced in biliary stasis by promoting release of sphincters controlling bile flow.

4. Lymph, tissue fluids and cerebrospinal fluids are apparently also under the influence of the above mechanisms, headaches resulting from spinal-block anesthesia and other related conditions having been reported relieved by **Choline**, symptomatically at least.

CLINICALLY ASSOCIATED CONDITIONS

GASTROINTESTINAL-URINARY
    Liver and Gallbladder
        Biliary Stasis
        Gallbladder Disease
        Liver Disease
NERVOUS AND PSYCHOGENIC
    Functional
        Dysphagia
    Metabolic
        Neuromuscular Disorders
        Numbness
    Mentality
        Brain, Dysfunction of
    Vasomotor
        Blood Pressure Changes
        Dizziness

METABOLIC DISORDERS
    Intermediate Processes
        Reactions to Foods
    Collagen
        Arteriosclerosis
EXOGENIC DISORDERS
    Traumatic
        Sedimentation Rate
VASCULAR DISORDERS
    Circulatory Diseases
        Varicose Veins
SKIN DISORDERS
    Psoriasis
    Telangiectasia
FEMALE DISORDERS
    Uterine Congestion

COLLINSONIA ROOT

Label: Collinsonia (Root) 380 mgs. per capsule. Of reputed value in Varicose Vein conditions and Hemorrhoids. Dosage: 4 capsules per day, or as directed. Sold for experimental use only.

Tissue or Function Supported	Possible benefit in liver conditions, acting as vascular astringent.

CLINICAL CONSIDERATIONS
Prominent Clinical Signs And Symptoms

Symptoms:

1. Symptoms of liver disease (Venous congestion such as: visible veins on chest and abdomen as well as hemorrhoids and varicose veins)

2. Pregnancy schedule (Prophylaxis in hemorrhoids and varicose veins)

3. Circulatory symptoms (Due to varicosities such as: leg pains, leg ulcers, leg cramps)

Possible Etiological Background:

While the mechanism of the effects of this product remain obscure, clinical reports of its effectiveness are ample and the nature of this information is such that the etiological background of benefit in liver disease shows as the most likely possibility.

Note: See Homeopathic list at end of this bulletin.

Symptom Characteristics: Circulatory changes involving gross deformities such as varicosities and hemorrhoids are most outstanding, although less severe abnormalities should not obviate the reason for therapeutic intention as experience shows it serves well prophylactically.

	Test:	Need Shown By:
Laboratory and Clinical Tests	Physical Examination	Veinous congestion

Administration	**Dosage:** Usual suggestion is four capsules daily. This may safely be increased if necessary. Best obtained when full glass of water is consumed taken preferably between meals or at. Bedtime.
	Effect: Good results have been reported in relieving the pains caused by varicosities, apparently having an effect upon the deep seated veins from which the pain arises. With conventional therapy, Collinsonia Capsules offer a valuable adjunct in the treatment of the conditions described.
	Side Effect: None known.

Synergists:	**Activity Contributed:**
a. Cyruta Plus	Vascular Integrity
b. Phosfood	Blood viscosity effect
c. Cataplex B	Lactic Acid Metabolizing influence
d. Cataplex G	Vasodilating action
e. Chlorophyll Complex (perles)	Prothrombin factors

GENERAL CONSIDERATIONS

1. Indicated in any condition where the vascular system has lost its tone and the blood vessels have been enlarged, such as hemorrhoids and varicose veins.

2. May also be sued prophylactically in these conditions, a good example being in pregnancy where it does much to relieve the varicosities and hemorrhoids which so frequently attend this state.

3. As an adjunct in liver diseases, particularly where evidence of venous congestion exists.

COLLINSONIA ROOT

GENERAL CONSIDERATIONS

The Homeopathic Material Medica (ninth edition) by William Boericke, MD., page 226 report in part as follows COLLINSONIA CANADENIS (Stone-Root):

Pelvic and portal congestion, resulting in hemorrhoids and constipation, especially in females. Depressed arterial tension, general atony of muscular fiber. Chronic nasal, gastric and pharyngeal catarrh, due to portal circulation. Dropsy from cardiac disease. Pruritis in pregnancy, with piles. Constipation of children from intestinal atony. Said to be of special value when given before operations for rectal disease. Sense of weight and constriction. Venous congestion.

Head: Dull frontal headaches; from suppressed hemorrhoids. Chronic catarrh. Yellow-coated tongue. Bitter taste.

Rectum: Sensation of sharp sticks in rectum. Sense of constriction. Vascular engorgement of rectum. Dry feces. Most obstinate constipation, with protruding hemorrhoids.

Female: Dysmenorrhea; pruritis of vulva; prolapse of woomb; pain on sitting down; cold feeling in thighs after menstruation. Sensation of swelling of labia and of clitoris.

Respiratory: Cough from excess use of voice, "Ministers sore throat"; hoarseness.

Heart: Palpitation, rapid but weak; oppression, faintness, and dyspnea.

Modalities: Worse, from slightest mental emotion or excitement; cold. Better, heat.

CLINICALLY ASSOCIATED CONDITIONS

METABOLIC DISORDERS
    Legs, weakness of
    Dropsy
CIRCULATORY DISORDERS
    Hemorrhoids
    Varicose Veins
SKIN CONDITIONS
    Purpura

CONGAPLEX

(ANTI-CORYZA CAPSULES)

Label: A concentrate of nutritional (alkaline) mineral factors from alfalfa leaf and sea lettuce (dulse). For the correction of physiological unbalances due to lack of leafy vegetable components in the diet.—As a food supplement, one capsule per day is suggested. For a quick alkalinizing effect, one capsule every 15 minutes until six have been taken. (Often very helpful in warding off a cold).

Tissue or Function Supported	For the correction of physiological unbalances due to lack of alkaline minerals.

CLINICAL CONSIDERATIONS
Prominent Clinical Signs And Symptoms

Symptoms:	Possible Etiological Background:
1. Common Colds 2. Acidosis (Anoxia, hyperirritability, tachycardia)	The symptoms of the common cold may be amenable to nutritional support, apparently their need being increased with the infection.

Administration	**Dosage:** 1 to 4 per day, as required.
	Effect: Usually effective in relief of symptoms associated with the common cold when due to this cause.
	Side Effect: None known

Synergists:	Activity Contributed:
a. Organic Minerals	Source of potassium
b. Min-Tran	Source of calcium lactate and sea kelp
c. Carbamide	Blood buffer salt source
d. Vitamin C Complex	Vitamin C source

GENERAL CONSIDERATIONS

The etiological background of the common cold has yet to be definitely established. Various possibilities have been investigated, including virus, allergy and acidosis. There is, no doubt, some basis for each of these factors, and in reality, a strong possibility exists that the reaction of a cold is a combination of the three in most cases.

POTASSIUM: In both the virus and allergic reaction range, we are dealing with intercellular components, specifically concerned with protein metabolism. In this respect, we must consider the important role of potassium in such reactions. Both alfalfa leaf and sea lettuce are rich sources of potassium, and, when processed by methods which maintain their biological activities, ac, we believe, as specific intercellular factors.

CALCIUM LACTATE: Another factor to consider is the similarity of respiratory disturbances to the reactions in acidosis, increased pulse rate, hyperirritability, etc. The effect of calcium in combating the effects of fever is well known to those who have had clinical experience with the ionizable forms as would be the example with Calcium Lactate.

CARBAMIDE: This is another factor which needs to be considered. Carbamide is a desensitizing factor (denatures protein) and is recognized as a diuretic agent. The relationship to the kidney function in colds is obvious.

VITAMIN C COMPLEX: This provides a protein protective action which is also important, since the factors we are considering are being viewed from the protein metabolism factors. Clinical experience with Vitamin C shows that its ability to abort the common cold is often outstanding.

CONGAPLEX

CYROFOOD

Label: Contains concentrates from alfalfa, carrot, veal bone, beef and fish liver lipoids, yeast, wheat germ, rice and peanut bran, liver, mushroom, green peas (whole plant) with milk solids and oat flour. This product is sold for use as a part of the nutritional pattern of a human diet. It has no drug use known to us in the dosage recommended. 4 to 12 tablets daily.

Tissue or Function Supported Multiple essential food concentrate containing nutritive factors of above mentioned foods, dehydrated to maintain biological potency.

CLINICAL CONSIDERATIONS
Prominent Clinical Signs And Symptoms

Symptoms:

1) Chronic fatigue (Failure to meet ordinary requirements of daily activities).
2) Hypertension or Hypotension (Deviations in blood pressure for no discernible cause).
3) Chronic Diseases (Particularly degenerative disease).
4) Lowered Resistance (Susceptibility to infections, colds, flu, etc.).
5) Glandular Insufficiency (Endocrinopathies in general including liver disorders).
6) Nutritional Response (Failure to respond to specific nutritional schedule).
7) Prophylaxis (Widespread conditions of malnutrition).

Possible Etiological Background

Philip Norman, M.D., prominent nutritional consultant, has stated that dietary excesses aggravate dietary deficiency states. By the same line of reasoning, **Cyrofood Tablets** which is a combination of selected essential food concentrates, as described on the above label, acts as a nutritional "governor" to regulate diverse physiological mechanisms in situations where only one or two may be given specific nutritional support on a recommended program. Also, **Cyrofood Tablets** by covering the broadest possible spectrum of nutritional factors is one of the most useful multiple food products for prophylactic purposes, because it is an established basic nutritional concept to get ALL of the factors concerned in deficiency states. We must also consider that **Cyrofood Tablets** are a valued source of trace minerals and that in these products the minerals are organically combined with their naturally associated enzyme and protein complexes.

Symptom Characteristics: In addition to complaints by the patient of specific indications of malnutrition, there in also usually wide variety of so-called "vague symptoms" which may be related to malnutrition in general, such as insomnia, paresthesia, traveling sensations, tightness in head, blotchy complexion, weakness, etc.

Clinical and Laboratory Tests Discussion: One of the greatest needs of practitioners in the healing arts today is the development of an adequate method of measuring of nutritional deficiency states. So far attempts in this direction have been feeble indeed, and, as a result, we must rely upon clinical results to show as the effectiveness of nutritional entities. Cyrofood Tablets and Powder have been appraised by thousands of doctors on this basis and for over 30 years have remained among their most valued nutritional products.

Administration

Dosage: **Cyrofood Tablets** are our most economical supplements. Cyrofood Powder is in a convenient form to add to cereals, salads, or to mix with peanut butter or mayonnaise as spreads or dressings. **Cyrofood Tablets** are a convenient form of essential foods, and are economical, particularly where large family groups are concerned.

Effect: These are almost too inconsequential to mention, but we must consider that activation of the detoxification mechanisms may produce seemingly adverse reactions. In most cases this is simply a matter of interpreting the reaction and continued usage merits a confident appraisal.

Side Effect: None known when used as directed.

Synergists:	**Activity Contributed:**
Organic Minerals	Organic Potassium Source
Calcium Lactate	Diffusible Calcium Source
Chlorophyll Complex (perles)	Chlorophyll Source

CYROFOOD

GENERAL CONSIDERATIONS

Cyrofood Tablets, especially combined natural food concentrates, differ from synthetic vitamin formulas in that they may safely given in the most extremes of delicately balanced physiological mechanisms without fear of overdosage or of producing adverse reactions, as for example in infants or enfeebled, aged individuals.

While The controversy between synthetic and natural vitamins has, and probably will continue to be an issue with clinicians for some time to come, the evidence pointing to toxic effects of various ingredients (chemicals) included in synthetic formulas is very considerable and impressive to the cautious doctor. On the other hand, the low potency-broad spectrum formula of natural ingredients in **Cyrofood**, a nutritional complex, affords the clinician a product of choice.

The potential benefits in either case must be decided by clinical observation upon known patients, using their objective symptoms and detectable responses as a method of judgement. In this respect, we believe **Cyrofood** will adequately provide conclusive evidence and to its inherent benefits to any fair-minded and astute clinical observer.

CLINICALLY ASSOCIATED CONDITIONS

As malnutrition is, we believe, in the etiological background of most common diseases, especially the degenerative varieties, we feel that the essential multiple food concentrate **Cyrofood** is indicated in all such disorders, not necessarily as a "specific" but to fortify the usual complex nutritional deficiency pattern which is usually present.

CYRUTA

(CYRUTA C-Y 1729)

Label: Dehydrated extract of buckwheat seed and green leaf. Each wafer contains 90 mgs. Inositol. 1 to 4 wafers per day or as directed.

Tissue or Function Supported Cholesterol metabolism.

CLINICAL CONSIDERATIONS
Prominent Clinical Signs And Symptoms

<u>Symptoms:</u>

1. Hypertension (Morning headaches, pain in back of head, throbbing sensations, vertigo and chronic fatigue).
2. Arteriosclerosis (Vertigo, tinnitus, loss of memory, repetitiousness).
3. Circulatory Disorders (Capillary fragility, purpura, telangiectasia, bruises from slight trauma).
4. Healing Processes (Inflammatory conditions, rheumatoid arthritis, for example).

<u>Possible Etiological Background:</u>

By acting to mobilize calcium for blood coagulation and connective tissue sue, and also to metabolize cholesterol from tissue deposits, **Cyruta** is useful in all problems dealing with capillary fragility and promotion of arterial elasticity, problems found primarily in the geriatric groups afflicted with arteriosclerotic changes, hypertension and arthritic tendencies.

Symptom Characteristics: Involve circulatory mechanisms and healing processes.

	Test:	Need Shown By:
Laboratory Tests	Blood Cholesterol	Hypercholesterolemia
Clinical Tests	a. Blood Pressure	Hypertension
	b. Observation	Evidence of venous congestion, capillary fragility, purpura

Administration	**Dosage:** 2 per day maintained over a long period of time is satisfactory in most cases of hypertension, increased dosage required in purpura and other such lesions.
	Effect: Prophylactic results in hypertension have been very satisfactory. A 20% drop in systolic level is not unusual in initial stages, progressively lowering under long term use. Importance of protracted treatment should be stressed.
	Side Effect: Reactions in the hypotensive patient may occur, but these are rare, and hypotension alone should not because for dismissing possibilities of use in this type patient, particularly if circulatory lesions are involved. In the coronary or potential coronary patient, a different situation is encountered: the mobilization of tissue deposits of calcium and cholesterol into the general circulation may temporarily raise the blood levels, particularly of cholesterol. IF the bile route is able to handle this situation no adverse results will be experienced. Therefore, in all patients in which coronary insufficiency is suspected, **A & F with Betafood** should be administered for at least 10 days before **Cyruta** is added to the schedule. (**A & F with Betafood** lowers the viscosity of the bile, promoting better elimination of cholesterol, one of the bile constituents).

<u>Synergists:</u>	<u>Activity Contributed</u>:
a. Soybean Lecithin	Cholesterol antagonist
b. Phosfood Liquid	Lowers viscosity of blood

GENERAL CONSIDERATIONS

The nutritional effects may be listed as follows:

    a. Promotes formation of calcium for blood and connective tissue use.

    b. Factor in cholesterol metabolism

CYRUTA

GENERAL CONSIDERATIONS

Rationalization for clinical application is as follows:

1. As one of the most important members of the Vitamin C complex group, Cyruta, which has been clinically proven, has a broad spectrum of use. As such, Cyruta should be considered wherever Vitamin C Complex is indicated.

2. The establishment of the protein integrity of the tissues concerned is probably the basic mechanism whereby this product obtains its effects. In this respect, the protective action on phagocytes is to be considered, making it an important factor in promoting resistance.

CLINICALLY ASSOCIATED CONDITIONS

NERVOUS AND PSYCHOGENIC
    <u>Functional</u>
        Headaches
    <u>Metabolic</u>
        Torticollis
    <u>Vasomotor</u>
        Blood Pressure Changes
METABOLIC
    <u>Intermediate Processes</u>
        Cholesterol Metabolism
    <u>Collagen</u>
        Arcus Senilis
        Arteriosclerosis
        Arthritis

EXOGENIC
    <u>Traumatic</u>
        Strictures
VASCULAR
    <u>Circulatory</u>
        Buerger's Disease
        Tinnitus Aurium

CYRUTA-PLUS

Label: Dehydrated buckwheat juice, whole plant, exclusive of seed extract. 1 to 4 tablets per day, or as directed by physician.

Tissue or Function Supported   Capillaries

CLINICAL CONSIDERATIONS
Prominent Clinical Signs And Symptoms

Symptoms:	Possible Etiological Background
1. Migraine headaches	Capillary damage may permit proteins from blood serum to leak into the cerebrospinal fluid.
2. Gingivitis	Promotion of fibrin in blood clotting and healing processes.
3. Ulcerative colitis	Etiology may be similar to gingivitis in the capillary lesions, see Dr. Norman's book on *"Ulcerative Colitis"*.
4. Radiation injuries.	Will be helped by Vitamin P group in overcoming tissue damage as reported by the atomic energy commission.

Symptom Characteristics: Follow the general pattern of blood clotting (fibrin) and healing mechanisms, particularly in relation to capillary integrity.

Laboratory and Clinical Tests   None known.

Administration

Dosage: 1 to 4 tablets per day or as directed.

Effect: Capillary strengthening, repair burst, inflamed, or ruptured capillaries, tone capillary walls.

Side Effect: None known when used as directed.

Synergists:	Activity Contributed:
a. Chlorophyll Complex (perles)	Source of fat-soluble vitamins, particularly Vitamin K.
b. Phosfood Liquid	Lowers blood viscosity.

GENERAL CONSIDERATIONS

Cyruta Plus is a source of the Vitamin P factors of the Vitamin C complex. Prothrombin is made in the liver with Vitamin K required for its formation. Evidence of Vitamin K deficiency are venous congestion and the formation of telangiectases. Should these evidences occur, Chlorophyll Complex (Fat soluble factors from the green leaf) which carries the Vitamin K group would be indicated.

CLINICALLY ASSOCIATED CONDITIONS

NERVOUS AND PSYCHOGENIC
   <u>Functional</u>
      Headaches
      Migraine Headaches
   <u>Metabolic</u>
      Torticollis
   <u>Vasomotor</u>
      Blood Pressure Changes

METABOLIC
   <u>Intermediate Processes</u>
      Cholesterol Metabolism
      <u>Collagen</u>
      Arcus Senilis
      Arteriosclerosis
      Arthritis

EXOGENIC
   <u>Traumatic</u>
      Strictures
VASCULAR
   <u>Circulatory</u>
      Buerger's Disease
      Tinnitus Aurium

CYRUTA-PLUS

DERMATROPHIN

(EPITHELIAL CYTOTROPHIN)

Label: Cytotrophic Extract of Epithelial Tissue—An extract intended to supply the specific determinants of the above mentioned tissue and to aid in improving the local nutritional environment. For experimental use in cooperation with conventional Therapeutic methods. Mfg. under U.S. Patent No. 2,374,219. One to three tablets per day, or as directed. (One per day should be maximum dosage for first week).

Tissue or Function Supported	Skin

CLINICAL CONSIDERATIONS
Prominent Clinical Signs And Symptoms

Symptoms:	Possible Etiological Background:
1. Alopecia 2. Acne (Scar formation) 3. Dry cracks in skin (Hands and feet) 4. Electrical burns (X-Ray burns)	Improvement of local environment of skin tissues and other protomorphogen effects are accountable for in the circumstances given, being specific for skin epithelium as far as present clinical results are concerned.

Symptom Characteristics: The dermal layers are thickest on the scalp, nape of neck and hands and feet, areas where clinical results have been most favorably reported, indicating its influence where this tissue is concerned.

Laboratory and Clinical Tests   None known.

Administration	**Dosage:**	See label above for dosage and uses with the Page Food Plan (Refer to the back of the book).
	Effect:	Immediate clinical observation of results are not ordinarily to be expected since structural changes are usually involved, as would apply to arthritis, for example. Rapid results may be obtained in more functional types of disorders such as insomnia, restlessness, hyperirritability, etc.
	Side Effect:	These seldom occur and when they do may be considered as an indication for **Calcium Lactate**, the ionizable form of calcium more directly concerned with the relief of calcium deficiency symptoms.

Synergists:	Activity Contributed
a. Vitamin A-C-P Complex	Epithelial and Connective Tissue Integrity
b. Vitamin G Complex	Cell Proliferating Influence
c. Chlorophyll Complex	Detoxification and Healing Factor
d. Cyruta A	(In case of X-Ray burns)
e. Pituitary Cytotrophin	(In case of alopecia)

GENERAL CONSIDERATIONS

Rationalization for clinical use is as follows:

1. Aids in combating cicatrization and promotion of healing in traumatic lesions.

2. May be used as a general supplement in practically all skin conditions.

Note: In the case of psoriasis, clinical evidence of results have not been established.

DERMATROPHIN

CLINICALLY ASSOCIATED CONDITIONS

EXOGENIC DISORDERS
   <u>Toxic</u>
      X-Ray burns
VASCULAR DISORDERS
   <u>Circulatory Diseases</u>
      Bed Sores
      Leg Ulcers
SKIN DISORDERS
   Alopecia
   Dermatitis
   Eczema
   Skin Irritations

DISODIUM PHOSPHATE

Label: Di-Sodium Phosphate (for food use) Contents: 8 ounces

Tissue or Function Supported Liver and gallbladder (blood buffer salt factor)

CLINICAL CONSIDERATIONS
Prominent Clinical Signs And Symptoms

Symptoms:

1) Constipation (costiveness)
2) Biliousness (Marked by grayish, dull, pallor of skin, waxy or oiliness)
3) Acholic stools (Clay-colored stools due to presence of undigested fats)
4) Acidosis symptoms (Tachycardia, breathlessness, hyperirritability)
5) Adrenal insufficiency (hypotension, neurasthenia, chronic fatigue, etc.)

Possible Etiological Background:

Di-basic sodium phosphate, best known as a blood buffer salt, has properties which have been shown to be clinically effective in treatment of gallbladder and liver disorders. While the mechanism whereby this is accomplished is rather obscure, we do know that the product acidifies the urine while at the same time it combats acidosis indicating a breakdown to its components, sodium and phosphorus, apparently the sodium being retained and the phosphorus excreted.

Symptom Characteristics: Clinically associated with sluggish liver and gallbladder activity.

	Tests:	Need Shown By:
Laboratory Tests	None known.	
Clinical Tests	Litmus Paper	Blue reaction.

Note: Dry paper gently in heat. If paper remains blue it is due to fixed alkali, the positive reaction; if it turns red again, it is due to volatile alkali (ammonium) and test is not positive.

Administration	**Dosage:** For constipation, 1 tsp. In glass of warm water before breakfast (because of its low ionization point, will not dissolve in cold water); to promote fat digestion, ½ tsp. In 1 or 2 ounces of warm water before meals.
	Effect: In both constipation and fat digestion, effect is usually prompt. Acholic stools often relieved within a week or two.
	Side Effect: A patient with alkalosis may not be able to tolerate the use of this product, indicating the need for **Cal-Amo**. Long term use in increased dosage should be avoided for the same reason, 2 or 3 teaspoonfuls per week seems reasonable after initial deficiency of blood buffer salts have been restored. This should be administered entirely on a symptomatic basis, i.e., for relief of constipation. Other means should be sought for the correction of this condition. (See Synergists listed below).

Synergists:	**Activity Contributed:**
a. Betacol	Liver Metabolizing Influence
b. Organic Minerals	Source Organic Potassium
c. Zypan	Digestive Catalyst
d. Betafood	Bile Thinning Factor

CLINICALLY ASSOCIATED CONDITIONS

GASTROINTESTINAL-URINARY
    Liver and Gallbladder
        Biliary Stasis
        Constipation

Gallbladder Disease
Jaundice
Liver Disease

DISODIUM PHOSPHATE

CLINICALLY ASSOCIATED CONDITIONS

METABOLIC DISORDERS
    <u>Body Weight</u>
        Appetite Decreased
DERMAL DISORDERS
    <u>Skin Disorders</u>
        Acne Vulgaris
        Psoriasis

DRENAMIN

Label: Each Tablet contains 3 mgs of Vitamin C, .33 mg. Riboflavin, 4 mg Niacin, and specific lipoproteins of the chromatin of Beef Adrenals, with naturally associated factors from Alfalfa, Mushroom, Green Buckwheat Leaf, Yeast, Sprouted Grain, Calf Brain and Bone Marrow. Carrier Materials: Fresh Bone Flour and Phytin. 3 to 12 tablets per day or as directed.

Tissue or Function Supported Intended to supply the specific tissue determinants of the adrenal glands with organic synergists found useful in promoting adrenal function, mainly Vitamin C and G complexes.

CLINICAL CONSIDERATIONS
Prominent Clinical Signs And Symptoms

Symptoms:	Possible Etiological Background:
1. Nervous Complaint (Chronic fatigue, "nervousness", tachycardia and other symptoms)	Insufficiency of adreno-sympathetic system.
2. Respiratory Disorders (Asthma, sinusitis, colds, pneumonia, coughs, etc.)	Resistance factor, disturbance in histamine-adrenaline metabolism due to adrenal insufficiency.
3. Vaso-Motor Disturbances (Hypo-/hpertension, circulatory symptoms)	Adreno-Sympathetic reaction.
4. Blood Sugar Disturbances (Hypo-/hypertension)	Trophic relation with pancreas and liver.
5. Allergic Reactions (Hives, dermatitis, sneezing attacks, frequent colds)	Histamine-adrenaline imbalance.
6. Reactions to Potassium Foods (Molasses, veal, vegetable juices, olives, etc.)	Elevated serum potassium, found in advanced hypoadrenia.
7. Abnormal Craving for Salt (Table salt)	Reaction indicating need of sodium to compensate for excess potassium.
8. Lowered Resistance (Coughs, weakness residual effects of illness)	Probably concerned with defense and other mechanisms, the stress syndrome.

Symptom Characteristics: Usually involve the vaso-motor mechanisms, respiratory tract or allergic reactions, fatigue being a common finding. Illnesses which may be traced to pneumonia or severe shock (mental or physical) often are due to the adrenal failure syndrome.

Laboratory Tests	Test:	Need Shown By:
	a. 17-Ketosteroid Test	Below or above 12-15 mg 24 hours
	b. Sodium-Potassium Serum Ratio	See Chart in "Applied Physiology of the Adrenal Glands"
Clinical Tests	Test:	Need Shown By:
	a. Postural Blood Pressure Test	Failure to show rise of systolic pressure on rising (standing position).
	b. Potassium Tolerance Test	Inability to tolerate potassium-rich foods (advanced states only).
	c. Observation	Weight loss, bronzing of skin.
	d. Phonocardiograph	Fibrillation (with hypotension). Tachycardia (with hypertension). High second sounds over mitral area.

	Dosage: 3 per day for 3 days, 6 to 9 per day thereafter, each patient manages dosage according to degree of fatigue.
Administration	**Effect:** Changes in Postural Blood Pressure are often noted within 20 minutes. Chronic conditions require long term schedule.
	Side Effect: None known specifically, however, note that fatigue may not be immediately relieved in some cases. In fact, there may be a temporary "let-down" feeling which is a specific indication of adrenal response and indicative of a need for use of synergists as listed below.

DRENAMIN

Synergists:	Activity Contributed:
1. Organic Minerals	Organic Potassium Source
2. Sodium Citrate	Source of sodium

Note: Management of the adrenal patient depends upon an understanding of the physiological mechanisms involved. See "Applied Physiology of the Adrenal Glands" (free on request) for complete discussion of the clinical aspects.

GENERAL CONSIDERATIONS

The adrenal glands enter into a variety of physiological effects and are known to be concerned with the following mechanisms:

- a. Resistance
- b. Detoxification
- c. Mineralization
- d. Histamine-adrenalin regulation
- e. Glucose-glycogen metabolism
- f. Vaso-motor regulation (Sodium-Potassium-Chloride)

The adrenal glands are particularly associated with the following types of diseases:

1. Respiratory diseases
2. Allergic reactions
3. Inflammatory diseases
4. (Particularly Rheumatoid Arthritis)
5. Neuresthenic diseases
6. (Neurocirculatory asthenia)
7. Blood pressure aberrations

The adrenals--"the stress glands"—have been shown to be the first of the endocrine axis to fail under various conditions of stress, such as burns, poisons and other toxic manifestations—as well as being susceptible to failure from protracted stress and strain of "ordinary" everyday activities. Conclusive evidence was offered by McCarrison to show that the adrenals were also the first to fail under the stress of malnutrition. Interestingly, our experience shows the adrenals to be the first to respond to nutritional therapy.

CLINICALLY ASSOCIATED CONDITIONS

GASTRO-INTESTINAL-URINARY
   Kidney and Bladder
      Uremia
NERVOUS AND PSYCHOGENIC
   Functional
      Asthenia
      Dysphagia
      Migraine Headaches
      Sweat Gland Activity
   Metabolic
      Legs, Weakness of
   Vaso-Motor
      Dizziness
      Heat Prostration
      Hypotension

METABOLIC DISORDERS
   Intermediate Processes
      Carbohydrate Metabolism
      Cholesterol Metabolism
      Salt Metabolism
   Acid-Base Balance
      Acidosis
      Alkalosis
   Water Balance
      Edema
   Blood
      Leukopenia
   Respiratory
      Bronchitis
      Emphysema
   Allergies
      Asthma

EXOGENIC DISORDERS
   Infections
      Pneumonia
   Virus Infections
      Colds, Flu, Grippe
      Herpes Zoster
   Toxic
      Burns, Systemic
      Eclampsia
      Halitosis
      X-Ray Burns
   Inflammation
      Sinusitis
SKIN CONDITIONS
   Pruritis
FEMALE DISORDERS
   Menopausal Symptoms
GLANDULAR
   Adrenal Insufficiency

DRENATROPHIN

(ADRENAL CYTOTROPHIN)

Label: Cytotrophic Extract of Beef Adrenals—A tissue extract intended to supply the specific determinant factors of the above mentioned organ and to aid in improving the local nutritional environment for that organ. For experimental use in cooperation with conventional Therapeutic methods. One to three tablets per day, or as directed. (One per day should be maximum dosage for first week.)

Tissue or Function Supported   Intended to supply the specific tissue determinants of the adrenal glands.

CLINICAL CONSIDERATIONS
Prominent Clinical Signs And Symptoms

Symptoms:

1. Respiratory Tract (Asthma, bronchitis, sinusitis)
2. Allergic Reactions (Skin conditions, rash, dermatitis, etc.)
3. Joint Inflammation (Rheumatoid arthritis)
4. Neurasthenia (Exhaustive states, diminished stamina)
5. Vasomotor Reactions (Blood pressure changes)
6. Lowered Resistance (Colds, flu, pneumonia)

Possible Etiological Background:

Apparently the regulation of the acid-alkaline balance through the blood buffer salts (sodium, potassium and chloride) is under control of the adrenal glands, and in dysfunction this blood buffer system is inadequate, resulting in respiratory embarrassment (anoxia), inflammatory conditions and exhaustion. The adrenals also regulate adrenalin metabolism which opposes histamine in its effects, accounting for the allergic susceptibility of these patients. Sodium retention-potassium deficit is associated with hyperadrenia (hypertension); potassium retention-sodium deficit is associated with hypoadrenia (hypotension)

Symptom Characteristics: Blood pressure changes, respiratory involvements and skin conditions are usual pattern of objective symptoms; subjective symptoms involve autonomic unbalance and stamina, energy regulation in general.

	Test:	Need Shown By:
Laboratory Tests	a. 17-Keotsteroid Test	Normal 12-15 mg. 24 hour specimen
	b. Sodium-Potassium Ratio	See chart in "Applied Physiology of Adrenal Glands"
	Test:	Need Shown By:
Clinical Tests	a. Postural Blood Pressure Test	In hypoadrenia systolic fails to show rise in standing position.
	b. While Line Test	Dermographic "white line" appears after stroking with blunt instrument
	c. Endocardiograph	Fibrillation (with hypotension), high second sounds over mitral-pulmonary valves.
Administration	**Dosage:** 1 to 3 per day, one per day maximum for first week, later regulated according to patient's reported degree of fatigue.	
	Effect: Characteristically there is an immediate improvement where indicated, followed by "let-down" period, probably calling for pituitary support at this stage if encountered.	
	Side Effect: Understanding of reactions is outlined in "Applied Physiology of the Adrenal Glands" which should be used as a guide in governing physiological support.	
Synergists:	**Activity Contributed:**	
a. Ostogen	A source of biologically active uncooked veal bone calcium-protein-enzyme complex which supplies phosphatase and other bone factors.	
b. Catalyn	To supply additional synergistic vitamin and trace mineral complexes which may not be adequately provided in the dietary.	

DRENATROPHIN

GENERAL CONSIDERATIONS

The adrenal glands enter into a variety of physiological effects and are known to be concerned with the following mechanisms:

- a. Resistance
- b. Detoxification
- c. Mineralization
- d. Histamine-adrenalin regulation
- e. Glucose-glycogen metabolism
- f. Vasomotor regulation (Sodium-Potassium-Chlorides)

The adrenal glands are particularly associated with the following types of diseases:

1. Respiratory diseases
2. Allergic reactions
3. Inflammatory diseases (Particularly Rheumatoid Arthritis)
4. Neurasthenic diseases (Neurocirculatory asthenia)
5. Blood pressure aberrations

The adrenals—"the stress glands"—have been shown to be the first of the endocrine axis to fail under various conditions of stress, such as burns, poisons, and other toxic manifestations—as well as being susceptible to failure from protracted stress and strain of "ordinary" everyday activities. Conclusive evidence was offered by McCarrison to show that the adrenals were also among the first to fail under the stress of malnutrition.

CLINICALLY ASSOCIATED CONDITIONS

GASTROINTESTINAL-URINARY
   <u>Kidney and Bladder</u>
      Uremia
NERVOUS AND PSYCHOGENIC
   <u>Functional</u>
      Asthenia
      Dysphagia
      Migraine Headaches
      Sweat Gland Activity
   <u>Metabolic</u>
      Legs, Weakness of
   <u>Vasomotor</u>
      Dizziness
      Heat Prostration
      Hypotension
METABOLIC DISORDERS
   <u>Intermediate Processes</u>
      Carbohydrate Metabolism
      Cholesterol Metabolism
      Salt Metabolism
   <u>Acid-Base Balance</u>
      Acidosis
      Alkalosis
   <u>Water Balance</u>
      Edema
   <u>Blood</u>
      Leukopenia
   <u>Respiratory</u>
      Bronchitis
      Emphysema
   <u>Allergies</u>
      Asthma
EXOGENIC DISORDERS
   <u>Infections</u>
      Pneumonia
   <u>Virus Infections</u>
      Colds, Flu, Grippe
      Herpes Zoster
   <u>Toxic</u>
      Burns, Systemic
      Eclampsia
      Halitosis
      X-Ray Burns
   <u>Inflammation</u>
      Sinusitis
SKIN CONDITIONS
      Pruritis
FEMALE DISORDERS
      Menopausal Symptoms
GLANDULAR
      Adrenal Insufficiency

FERROFOOD

Label: Each capsule contains 10 mgs. Of Iron, organically combined as Iron Phytate, Cytotrophic Extract of Spleen 38 mgs., B_{12} 1.75 mcgm, specific unsaturated fatty acids from beef and fish liver lipoids, with extracts of alfalfa, beef liver and fresh raw veal bone (including bone marrow). Two capsules of this product contains the average adult minimum daily requirement of iron. This product is sold for use as a part of the nutritional pattern of a human body. It has no drug use known to us in the dosage recommended. Suggested schedule: 1 to 3 capsules per day or as directed.

Tissue or Function Supported	Hematopoietic system.

CLINICAL CONSIDERATIONS
Prominent Clinical Signs And Symptoms

Symptoms:

1. Anemia (Classical features: pallor of skin, mucous membrane, nails; tachycardia, anoxia, weakness, hyperirritability, restlessness)
2. Predisposing Factors: (Hypochlorhydria [low salt diets and common in pregnancy], faulty diet, mental stress, overwork, environment)
3. Frequently occurring in: (Nephritis, pregnancy, febrile diseases, hemorrhage, toxemia, amenorrhea, neuralgia, loss of libido)
4. Other Considerations: (Rheumatoid arthritis, bed sores, vertigo, dysphagia, drowsiness, fatigue, headaches, gingivitis, glossitis, tinnitus, hypotension)
5. Gastrointestinal Conditions: (Vomiting, diarrhea, colitis, indigestion, constipation, gallbladder disorders)

Possible Etiological Background

The etiological background of anemia includes many factors in addition to iron and B12. Lecithin, chlorophyll, unsaturated fatty acids, spleen, bone marrow and others have been reported as having a productive influence in anemias. Insufficiency of gastric secretions, particularly hydrochloric acid, is commonly involved in chronic anemias. The integrity of the R.B.C." and its physiology would also include such regulatory mechanisms as acid-base balance, fluid balance and protein metabolism as well as, circulatory disturbances, the metabolic rate and integrity of the reticuloendothelial system. The prominence of anemia in nephritis and nephrosis leads to the conclusion that the kidney is an important organ in the anemia syndrome, probably by direct action of preventing hemolysis brought about by toxins or by other enzymatic influences not as yet completely understood. Vitamin T, as found in sesame butter, has recently been reported as an antianemia factor.

Symptom Characteristics: Blood tests are the only positive means of diagnosis. However, it is well to keep in mind the high incidence of anemia in the general population and it therefore seems likely that a physiological antianemia formula (**Ferrofood**) may be recommended in many more cases than is practical to diagnose by specific blood tests, although these are always desirable.

	Test:	Need Shown By:
Laboratory Tests	Blood Count	Evidence of anemia
Clinical Tests	Tallqvist's Hemoglobin Scale	Color chart readings

Note: Antianemia supplementation may be particularly important in the recuperative phases of infectious diseases, particularly where there has been fever such as commonly occurs in cold, flu, pneumonia, etc. Also to be considered is the use of **Ferrofood** for blood donors following transfusions and contributions to blood banks.

Administration	**Dosage:** 1 to 3 per day. Initial dosage may be increased in severe cases.
	Effect: On sufficient dosage, observable results may be experienced by the patient in as little as one or two days.
	Side Effect: Unlike many inorganic iron products in general use, Ferrofood does not tend to be constipating. Side effects are rare.

FERROFOOD

Synergists:	**Activity Contributed:**
a. Zypan	Digestive catalyst QIC1 source
b. Chlorophyll Complex (perles)	Influence in anemia reported
c. Soybean Lecithin	Influence in anemia reported
d. Sesame Butter (Commissary)	The sesame products are sources of Vitamin T, important in platelet formation and anemia.

GENERAL CONSIDERATIONS

1. **Ferrofood** is an antianemia complex product containing unsaturated fatty acids, spleen extracts, Vitamin B_{12} in addition to organically combined iron, differing from usual hemotinics by supplying a variety of substances designed to combat anemia.

2. **Ferrofood** may be used as a dietary addition, not only in frank anemia, but also where tonic and blood building effects are desired, as would be the case, for example in emaciation and recuperation.

CLINICALLY ASSOCIATED CONDITIONS

GASTROINTESTINAL-URINARY
    <u>Kidney and Bladder</u>
        Albuminuria
        Cystitis
        Nephritis
NERVOUS AND PSYCHOGENIC
    <u>Functional</u>
        Asthenia
    <u>Metabolic</u>
        Numbness
    <u>Vasomotor</u>
        Hypotension

METABOLIC DISORDERS
    <u>Intermediate Processes</u>
        Oxygen Metabolism
        Drowsiness
    <u>Blood</u>
        Anemia, Pernicious
        Anemia, Secondary
EXOGENIC DISORDERS
    <u>Toxic</u>
        X-Ray burns
GENETIC
    <u>Female</u>
        Amenorrhea
        Pregnancy Schedule

ASSOCIATED PRODUCTS:

Spleen PMG: (See Page, 163)

FOR-TIL B12

Label: Each capsule contains 420 mgms. of Tillandsia extract fortified with 3 micro-grams of natural Vitamin B_{12} (with intrinsic factor). Use: To supply the Vitamin E Chlorophyll complex of green plant. Suggested Dosage: 1-4 capsules per day or as directed.

Tissue or Function Supported   Nutritional Alternative

CLINICAL CONSIDERATIONS
Prominent Clinical Signs And Symptoms

Symptoms:
Associated with chronic disease conditions such as:
- Lowered stamina
- Impotency
- Premature senility
- Arteriosclerosis
- Emaciation
- Chronic fatigue
- Anemia
- Mental aberrations (Such as repetitiousness, forgetfulness, irritability, insomnia, etc.)

Possible Etiological Background:
Both Vitamin B_{12} and the chlorophyll-Vitamin E complex factors present are known for their general beneficial effects in a wide variety of disorders where sufficient evidence of a specific diagnosis may be lacking, but rather the condition exists as a series of rather vague complaints of debilitation and a nutritional alterative becomes desirable-in addition, of course, to specific therapies indicated.

Symptom Characteristics: Associated with the aging processes in general and with those attendant in most chronic diseases.

Laboratory and Clinical Tests   None known

Administration
Dosage: 1 to 4 per day is usual dosage. Sufficient time should be given, at least three weeks before expecting maximum clinical benefits..

Side Effect: None known.

Synergists: | **Activity Contributed:**
a. Chlorophyll Complex (perles) — Prothrombin factor (K)
b. Pituitrophin — Trophic effects of pituitary gland

GENERAL CONSIDERATIONS

Nutritional effects and rationalization for clinical application as follows:
1. Intended as a food adjunct in the nutritional program of the convalescent, undernourished or geriatric patient.
2. Benefits in glandular insufficiency states by reason of its contained B_{12}, E, Chlorophyll complex.
3. Loss of sex interest may be benefited by sex hormone precursors.
4. Clinical problems of senescence, senility and debilitation marked by repetitiousness, confusion and depression.
5. Hyperirritability of undetermined origin.

CLINICALLY ASSOCIATED CONDITIONS

NERVOUS AND PSYCHOGENIC
   Functional
      Asthenia
   Mentality

Backwardness in Children
Vaso-Motor
   Hypotension

CLINICALLY ASSOCIATED CONDITIONS

METABOLIC DISORDERS
   <u>Growth and Repair</u>
      Aging Processes
   <u>Female Disorders</u>
      Amenorrhea
      Menopausal Symptoms

GASTREX

Label: Intended for the relief of gastritis. Contents: A natural colloidal silica, with trace minerals, Tillandisa, Okra, Extracts of Stomach and Duodenum, and Di-Sodium Phosphate. The active ingredients of this product are derived from food sources only. Suggested Dosage: 2 or 3 capsules before each meal.

Tissue or Function Supported Concentrated nutritional factors for the promotion of healing of gastrointestinal lesions.

CLINICAL CONSIDERATIONS
Prominent Clinical Signs And Symptoms

Symptoms:
1. Ulcer syndrome (Acid rebound; patient eats, five or six hours later has gastric pain which eating again relieves. Seasonal syndrome, attacks show recurrent pattern).
2. Gastritis (Colitis, diarrhea, flatulence)
3. Indigestion symptoms (Heartburn, "water-brash", sour eructations, etc.)

Possible Etiological Background:
A complex of ingredients which have proven beneficial in the treatment of gastrointestinal problems related to the gastric ulcer.

Symptom Characteristics: The characteristic gastric ulcer syndrome.

	Test:	Need Shown By:
Laboratory Tests	X-Ray Examination	Evidence of gastric ulcer.
Clinical Tests	a. Case History	Typical gastric ulcer syndrome.
	b. Palpation	Abdominal tenderness.

Administration

Dosage: As shown on label (above) or taken at time of discomfort.

Effect: Gastrex tends to normalize acid flow and prevent acid rebound as well as to promote healing of gastric lesions.

Side Effect: Where hyperperistalsis is present, dosage may be reduced until normalized by Okra, Pepsin E3 Capsules and Organic Minerals; Phosfood may be necessary to control nausea. There are not side-effects known to attribute directly to Gastrex.

Synergists:
a. Pituitrophin (See Side-Effects above)
b. Chlorophyll Complex (perles)

Activity Contributed:
Promotion of Healing Processes
Healing Effects of Chlorophyll

GENERAL CONSIDERATIONS

Intended for use as a source of colloidal silica with trace minerals as an aid in healing processes of stomach and intestinal lesions by providing specific factors known to be beneficial where gastritis exists.

Rationalization for clinical use:
1) Useful in gastric hyperacidity, particularly in the acid rebound type of case evidencing the symptoms of the ulcer syndrome: eat, pain, eat, relief, etc.
2) Complaints of pyrosis (heartburn), "water-brash", sour or watery eructations, burning sensations, etc. indicate its need.
3) Specifically indicated in ulceration and inflammation of the gastric mucosa, a valuable adjunct to any therapeutic means employed in this type of gastric disturbance.

GASTREX

GENERAL CONSIDERATIONS

4) In considering the gastric ulcer syndrome, the neurological aspects need to be given fullest possible support. These may differ with each case and a review of the factors concerned may be helpful. In this respect, it is suggested that the following product bulletins be reviewed:

Phosfood   **Cataplex F**
Calcium Lactate   **Organic Minerals**
Cataplex E2   **Cataplex G**

5) For further information regarding treatment of gastric ulcers, see "Gastric Ulcers", Therapeutic Foods Manual.

CLINICALLY ASSOCIATED CONDITIONS

GASTRO-INTESTINAL-URINARY
<u>Stomach and Intestines</u>
   Colitis, Mucous
<u>Liver and Gallbladder</u>
   Digestion Faulty

NERVOUS AND PSYCHOGENIC
<u>Functional</u>
   Ulcers, Gastric

HEPATROPHIN

Label: Cytotrophic Extract of Beef Liver—A tissue extract to supply the specific determinant factors of the above mentioned organ and to aid in improving the local nutritional environment for that organ. For experimental use in cooperation with conventional therapeutic methods. One to three tablets per day, or as directed. (One per day, should be maximum dosage for first week.)

Tissue or Function Supported Liver

CLINICAL CONSIDERATIONS
Prominent Clinical Signs And Symptoms

Symptoms:

1. Venous Congestion (Dilated veins showing over chest and abdomen)
2. Protein Metabolism (Decreased serum albumin)
3. Carbohydrate Metabolism (Deviations in blood sugar pattern)
4. Water Balance (Ascites, edema due to liver failure)
5. Kidney Disorders (Diminished urination, protein metabolism related to kidney disorders)
6. Toxemia (Leukocytosis, intestinal toxemia related to liver dysfunction)

Possible Etiological Background:

Lipotropic factors-or fat metabolizing factors-are but one phase of consideration in liver dysfunction…various hormones, carbohydrates, proteins, and tissue factors must be taken into consideration. Of these, perhaps the most important, is the determinant factor of the liver cells themselves otherwise known as **Hepatrophin**. The multiple role played by the liver in a wide variety of vital processes, emphasizes the importance of support of the integrity of the cells themselves by use of determinant factors which support their intrinsic integrity. While this rationalization is sound, the tracing of clinical results cannot be provided in such a positive manner since the liver is still "the organ of mystery" for the physiologist and evaluation of therapeutic measures is, therefore, difficult. **Symptom Characteristics:**

While disturbances in fat metabolism are fairly obvious, it is within the range of protein metabolism wherein the diagnostician must search of the answers to many liver problems. For instance, an ostensible kidney case may simply be a manifestation of liver failure to provide the protein necessary for the repair of that organ. Perhaps the most common finding in liver dysfunction is venous or portal circulation engorgement.

Laboratory Tests	Most Frequently Used Tests:	Indications Commonly Relied Upon:
	a. Urine for presence of bile	Venous congestion-dilated veins over chest and abdomen
	b. Icterus Index	Indigestion symptoms, acholic stool
	c. Van Den Bergh Reactions	Enlarged liver or spleen
	d. Cephalin-Cholesterol Flocculation	Jaundice or ascites
	e. Galactose Tolerance	Oliguria
	f. Decreased serum albumin	Leukocytosis
Clinical Tests	a. Observation of above findings	Hemorrhoids
	b. Palpation	Enlarged liver and spleen
	c. Blood pressure	Elevated diastole considered significant
	d. Phonocardiograph	Usually a feature in heart failure
	e. Case History	History of hepatitis
Administration	**Dosage:** One to three per day is usual dosage. Long term therapy should be stressed rather than acceleration of dosage.	
	Effect: Appreciable effects depend upon length of time of treatment, dietary management of patient and synergistic products used.	
	Side Effect: None known. (This is a distinct advantage because in use of cholagogues, lipatropic factors and laxatives side-effects are common. Therefore, **Hepatrophin** provides an excellent means of initiating patient into liver program without possibility of these reactions occurring).	

HEPATROPHIN

Synergists:	Activity Contributed:
a. Betacol	Liver metabolizing influence
b. Choline	Lipotropic factor
c. Betafood	Bile-thinning influence (carbohydrate and fat metabolism)

GENERAL CONSIDERATIONS

DISCUSSION: The etiological background of liver dysfunction should be brought into focus in two major categories, as follows:

    A. Where response to selected therapy is slow or failing.

    B. In most chronic, degenerative diseases.

While liver involvement is present in most chronic disease, the screening of patients requiring specific liver support presents a problem which must be answered. The following suggests a screening process useful in determining the most needful of these cases:

1. Evidence of venous congestion by signs of dilated veins showing over chest and abdomen, also hemorrhoids and varicose veins would come in this category.

2. Kidney pathology. Since kidney pathology may rest largely on deviations in protein metabolism, over which the liver has primary control, all kidney cases require liver support on this basis. Clinical results bear out this statement.

3. Most chronic diseases involving the degenerative processes, and, specifically wasting diseases and disturbances in water balance, edema and ascites, require specific liver support. This would include most cases of congestive heart failure.

CLINICALLY ASSOCIATED CONDITIONS

GASTROINTESTINAL-URINARY
  <u>Liver and Gallbladder</u>
    Constipation
    Hepatitis
    Jaundice
    Liver Diseases
  <u>Kidney and Bladder</u>
    Albuminuria
    Nephritis
NERVOUS AND PSYCHOGENIC
  <u>Functional</u>
    Epilepsy
  <u>Metabolic</u>
    Alcoholism
  <u>Vasomotor</u>
    Dizziness
    Shock
METABOLIC DISORDERS
  <u>Growth and Repair</u>
    Aging Processes
  <u>Collagen Diseases</u>
    Arcus Senilis
    Arteriosclerosis
    Arthritis
    Bone, Pain in
    Cataracts

METABOLIC DISORDERS
  <u>Acid-Base Balance</u>
    Ketosis
  <u>Water Balance</u>
    Ascites
    Dropsy
    Edema
  <u>Blood</u>
    Anemia, Pernicious
    Epistaxis
  <u>Allergies</u>
  <u>Body Weight</u>
    Appetite Decreased
    Obesity
EXOGENIC DISORDERS
  <u>Toxic</u>
    Delirium
    Eclampsia
    Halitosis

INOSITOL

Label: 400 mgms. per tablet, natural Vitamin B8, a Lipotrophic factor useful in alleviating liver dystrophy where due to its deficiency. Dose: 1 to 4 tablets with each meal.

Tissue or Function Supported   Lipotrophic factor.

CLINICAL CONSIDERATIONS
Prominent Clinical Signs And Symptoms

Symptoms:	Possible Etiological Background:
1. Diabetes Mellitus 2. Muscular dystrophies 3. Parasympatheticotonia 4. Gallbladder disease 5. Liver disease 6. Hypothyroidism 7. Muscular pains	Because its effects are primarily as activators of the A.T.P. (adenosine triphosphate) mechanisms and these are difficult to trace clinically, prominent clinical signs and symptoms are lacking. However, the use of Inositol seems advisable in the conditions shown.

Symptom Characteristics: Phosphorylation (introducing phosphoric acid radical into an organic molecule) involves energy mechanisms with resultant oxygenation reactions and energy catalysts. For this reason, symptoms usually indicated are related to utilization of fats and sugars or involve the energy-consuming muscle system.

	Test:	Need Shown By:
Laboratory Tests	a. Creatinine (Pathologically)	Urinary excretion
	b. Alkaline Phosphatase	Increased in liver-biliary disorders
	Test:	Need Shown By:
Clinical Tests	(Blood Cholesterol)	(Elevated)

Note: The blood cholesterol is elevated in hypothyroidism, clinical evidence of which is usually available, and since in this condition oxygenation mechanisms are deficient, rationalization would direct one's attention to consideration of Inositol Tablets.

Administration	**Dosage:** There seems to be no limit to the amount of **Inositol** that may be administered, apparently being nontoxic in any amount that would ordinarily be given.
	Effect: By itself there may be little noticeable effect which may be determined by clinical observations, apparently in this respect requiring synergists as listed below. It should be stated, however, that where phosphorilization reactions are being considered, **Inositol** may be the "spark plug" upon which the success of the program depends.
	Side Effect: Fever blisters have been reported, apparently due to the activation of phosphoric acid mechanisms. Studies need to be made of its effects on blood phosphorus levels.

Note: **Inositol** has been called "the muscle sugar vitamin" and its synergists fall along this pattern. For complete discussion see "Neuro-Muscular Disorders", Therapeutic Foods Manual. Most important synergists are listed below:

Synergists:	Activity Contributed:
Myotrophin	Super-EFF
Organic Minerals	Cataplex E
Cataplex G	Arginex

GENERAL CONSIDERATIONS

Aside from its well-known function as a lipotrophic factor, **Inositol** has other postulated effects. These may be listed as follows:

a. Possible relation to phosphorilization by means of stabilization of adenosine triphosphate mechanisms (energy "sparkplug" of muscle cells).

b. By means of above, may be important factor in muscle metabolism and other energy producing mechanisms, particularly oxidation of fats, the probable means whereby it acts as a lipotrophic agent.

INOSITOL

GENERAL CONSIDERATIONS

The rationalization for clinical use is as follows:

1. Beneficial effects have been noted in diabetes mellitus, apparently by utilization of glycogen from the cell through the above described activity.
2. We may reason that its effect on phosphorus metabolism may be beneficial in lowered metabolic states, such as may occur in thyroid and pituitary disorders, emaciation, atrophy and other debilitated states.
3. Clinical application has shown it to have a very beneficial effect in synergizing the action of glutamic acid in mental conditions, where the combined use of **Inositol** and glutamic acid has produced much more favorable results then one would have been led to suspect from use of either alone.

CLINICALLY ASSOCIATED CONDITIONS

NERVOUS AND PSYCHOGENIC
   <u>Metabolic</u>
      Neuro-Muscular Disorders
      Numbness
      Torticollis
   <u>Mentality</u>
      Brain, Dysfunction of
      Backwardness in Children
   Vaso-Motor
      Hypotension
   <u>Lesions</u>
      Cerebral Palsy
      Multiple Sclerosis

METABOLIC DISORDERS
   <u>Intermediate Processes</u>
      Diabetes Mellitus
   <u>Collagen</u>
      Arcus Senilis
EXOGENIC DISORDERS
   <u>Toxic</u>
      Nightmares
VASCULAR DISORDERS
   <u>Circulatory Diseases</u>
      Buerger's Disease

IPLEX

(OCULOTROPHIN)

Label: Cytotrophin Extract of Beef Eye—An extract intended to supply the specific determinant factors of the above mentioned tissue, and to aid in improving the local nutritional environment. For experimental use in cooperation with conventional Therapeutic methods. Mfg. under U.S. Patent No. 2,374,219. One to three tablets per day, as directed. (One per day should be maximum dosage for first week.)

Tissue or Function Supported   Eye

CLINICAL CONSIDERATIONS
Prominent Clinical Signs And Symptoms

Symptoms:	Possible Etiological Background:
1) Complaints originating from the eyes, such as eye strain and fatigue, failing vision, headaches. 2) Strabismus (Spontaneous origin in children) 3) Accommodation defects (Far and Nearsightedness) 4) Aging processes (Usual tissue changes of eye associated with aging processes)	Supplies specific determinant factors and aids in improving local nutritional environment and as such has been found useful in nearly all uncomplicated eye conditions. However, fullest clinical response is obtained only when synergists, as indicated, are simultaneously administered. See "Synergists" below.

Symptom Characteristics: In the use of this product, we restrict its effects to the general integrity of the eye tissue itself, bearing in mind that most ordinary eye complaints are neurological and muscular in origin calling for neuromuscular support. Also specific vitamin deficiencies are frequently concerned, Vitamins A and G complexes, particularly.

Laboratory Tests
    Test: Need Shown By:
Rapidly failing vision, pain, persistent blurring of vision and other unusual symptoms may indicate serious disorders such as glaucoma, cataracts, iritis, detached retina and others, calling for an ophthalmologist in diagnosis.

Clinical Tests
    Test: Visual Charts   Need Shown By: To determine visual efficiency as well as to determine therapeutic progress.

Administration

Dosage: One per day should be maximum for first week, increased according to symptomatic response thereafter.

Effect: Favorable results are often noted by patient within a few weeks, or even days.

Side Effect: Should not be given during stage of inflammation or infection because of local release of histamine which may result in temporary pain or discomfort. In more serious eye conditions, when used in connection with conventional therapeutic methods, its use should be in very small dosage (1/4 tablet) until tolerance is determined.

Synergists:	Activity Contributed:
Cataplex G	Enzymatic Tranquilizer
Organic Minerals	Source Organic Potassium
Cataplex A-C-P	Epithelial and Connective Tissue Factor
Wheat Germ Oil Perles	Anti-oxidant
Calcium Lactate	Source of Ionizable Calcium

Note: Most eye conditions involving nervous strain are benefited by recommendations given in Therapeutic Foods Manual under "Neuromuscular Disorders"

GENERAL CONSIDERATIONS

IPLEX has been found useful in nearly all uncomplicated eye conditions, such as ordinary eye strain and usual tissue changes associated with failing vision and aging processes.

In most cases where eye complaints are the problem however, additional aggravating circumstances need to be considered. Of these the following are considered as being most common:

IPLEX

CONDITION:	INDICATED SYMPTOMATICALLY BY:	NUTRITIONAL SUPPORT:
Autonomic Unbalance	Photophobia, dysphagia, tachycardia	Organic Minerals Cataplex G
Anoxia	Breathlessness, cramps brought on by Exertion, bruising easily	Cataplex E2 Wheat Germ Oil
Acidosis	Irregular respiration, tachycardia	Sodium Citrate Drenamin
Vitamin A deficiency	Tear duct infection, granulation tissue, Epithelial cells, night blindness	Cataplex A-C-P
Vitamin G deficiency	"Bloodshot eyes", conjunctivitis, styes, feeling of "sand"	Cataplex G

Note: In glaucoma, AC Carbamide provides an acceptable physiological diuretic. See "Glaucoma" in Therapeutic Foods Manual for further information.

CLINICALLY ASSOCIATED CONDITIONS

NERVOUS AND PSYCHOGENIC
- <u>Functional</u>
  - Photophobia

METABOLIC DISORDERS
- <u>Growth and Repair</u>
  - Eye conditions
- <u>Collagen</u>
  - Arcus Senilis

LACTIC ACID YEAST

Label: (A Mycelium type yeast). Ingredients: Mycelium yeast, hops, malt, sugar, corn, rye, rice and tapioca flours. 4 wafers per day, or as directed.

Tissue or Function Supported	Intestinal environment by production of lactic acid.

CLINICAL CONSIDERATIONS
Prominent Clinical Signs And Symptoms

Symptoms:
1. Constipation (Costiveness, hard, dry stools characteristic)
2. Malassimilation (Weight loss)
3. Foul stools
4. Body and breath odors
5. Diarrhea

Possible Etiological Background

A favorable intestinal environment not only eliminates a source of intestinal toxins, but also, through bacterial action, provides production of bulk essential for peristalic movement. Failure to produce sufficient lactic acid for bacterial integrity may account for many gastrointestinal difficulties.

Symptom Characteristics: The need for this product should be extended beyond the ordinary indications of gastrointestinal complaints to include a wide variety of conditions in which malassimilation and toxemia are prevalent, including emaciation, inability to gain weight and recuperation. Lack of exercise is a frequent finding in cases showing need of this product.

	Test	Test Shown By:
Laboratory Tests	None known.	
Clinical Tests	pH of Stool (Bromthymol Blue Indicator)	Alkaline reaction
Administration	**Dosage:** Varies with each case. Initial dosage of 9 per day is suggested, later reduced to symptomatic levels, see "Side-Effects" below	
	Effect: Eventual benefits in constipation and related disorders are to be expected in the majority of cases. This is dependent upon adequate dosage "enough", and providing sufficient time for environmental changes to occur, usually 2 to 3 weeks.	
	Side Effect: In initial stages of use increased gas formation may be noted. This is because gas formed at certain pH-levels, a zone which may be passed through and lactic acid production is increased, ceasing when normal pH is obtained. Doubling the dosage hastens this phase of treatment and shortens the symptomatic manifestations-which, incidentally, is a positive sign for the patient's need of the product.	

Synergists:	Activity Contributed:
a. Zypan	Digestive Catalyst
b. Cholacol II	Intestinal Adsorbent.
c. Pancreatrophin	Local Enviroment of Cells.

GENERAL CONSIDERATIONS
1. Produces lactic acid by fomentation of sugars and starches, thereby inhibits the growth of toxic bacteria in the alimentary system.
2. Acts to correct persistent alkaline stools, the most common finding in chronic constipation.
3. A completely physiological method of treatment of constipation and may be used indefinitely where effective.
4. Because it improves digestion and assimilation it is especially indicated in emaciation and weight gain failure.
5. Lactic Acid Yeast is the only acidophilic organism which will ferment any carbohydrate into lactic acid. Other such organisms such as lactobacillus acidophilus require milk sugar (lactose) for the formation of lactic acid.

LACTIC ACID YEAST

GENERAL CONSIDERATIONS

Physiological review:
- A. The stomach contains acids whose function is to break down protein foods, with the aid of pepsin, into peptones and proteases which pass on into the small intestine.
- B. In the small intestine, which is alkaline by nature, the protein digestion is completed, with the aid of trypsin. This is done by completing the disintegration of the partially digested proteins in to the individual building blocks of amino acids.
- C. After this, the contents of the intestine must be acidified to kill the undesirable and toxic microorganisms which are contained in the food waste derivatives and which can exist only in an alkaline medium.
- D. This is where **Lactic Acid Yeast** enters the picture, to supply lactic acid (through the action of the lactic acid yeast organism) to acidify this intestinal mass in the large intestine and colon.

CLINICALLY ASSOCIATED CONDITIONS

GASTROINTESTINAL-URINARY
    <u>Stomach and Intestines</u>
        Alimentary Canal Flora
    <u>Liver and Gallbladder</u>
        Constipation

METABOLIC DISORDERS
    <u>Body Weight</u>
        Appetite Diminished
        Appetite Excessive*

(*) Lactic Acid Yeast taken before meals may reduce appetite-taken after meals it tends to increase the appetite.

MAMMARY PMG

Label: Cytotrophic Extract of Beef Mammary Gland-A tissue extract intended to supply the specific determinant factors of the above mentioned organ and to aid in improving the local nutritional environment for that organ. For experimental use in cooperation with conventional Therapeutic methods. Mfg. under U.S. Patent No. 2,374,219. One to three per day, or as directed. (One per day should be maximum dosage for first week).

Tissue or Function Supported   Mammary glands

CLINICAL CONSIDERATIONS
Prominent Clinical Signs And Symptoms

Symptoms:
Disorders related to female breasts such as:
1. Nipple pain
2. Lymph node enlargement
3. Underdevelopment
4. Mastitis
5. Menstrual pain
6. Nipple inflammation
7. Congestion
8. Lactation insufficiency

Possible Etiological Background:
As with ovarian function, the mammary integrity may depend upon the close interrelationship with other glands, see **Ovatrophin** bulletin for synergistic products. Etiological background includes epithelial integrity, see "Symptom Characteristics" below.

Symptom Characteristics: Aside from specifically referable findings, we have found that epithelial integrity is usually involved, desquamation of the endothelium providing the means of a circulatory barrier in the lymphatic and capillary network, apparently by this means. In these cases, **Cataplex A-C-P** is indispensable.

Clinical and Laboratory Tests   Physical examination, otherwise none known. (Biopsy)

Administration	
Dosage:	1 to 3 per day.
Effect:	Effectiveness depends upon etiological background and appropriate selection of synergists, see "Symptom Characteristics" above, also "General Considerations" following.
Side Effect:	None known.

Synergists:	Activity Contributed:
Cataplex A-C-P	Effect on Epithelial Integrity
Inositol	(Beneficial in lactation)
Chlorophyll Perles	Sex hormone Precursors (Tillandsia E3 Complex)
Pituitrophin	Trophic Influence on Endocrines

GENERAL CONSIDERATIONS

The broad physiological background of mammary influence and changes would include the broad field of menopausal, menstrual, and lactation activities as well as adrenal, thyroid, and pituitary influences. See "Signs and Symptoms" in the Manual of Clinical Trophology, and **Ovatrophin** bulletin in this book for discussion. *Practical Endocrinology*, by Harrower, (see index) also gives a discussion of possibilities in this respect. However, specific signs and symptoms are lacking and sufficient clinical evidence has not been accumulated which would afford making positive statements as to its effects in these related conditions.

CLINICALLY ASSOCIATED CONDITIONS

EXOGENIC DISORDERS
   <u>Inflammation</u>
      Mastitis

MAMMARY PMG

MANGANESE-B$_{12}$

(Manganese Phytate-B12)

Label: Each tablet contains: 300 Mgms. Manganese Phytate, 5 Mcgms. Vitamin B$_{12}$ for organic Cobalt. For use as a nutritional supplement in Manganese deficiency states. This product is sold for use as a part of the nutritional pattern of a human diet. It has no drug use known to us in the dosage recommended. Maximum Dosage: 3 tablets per day, or as directed.

Tissue or Function Supported Magnesium is a muscle builder, bone hardener and a ligament strengthener. Especially helpful for patients with flat feet and misalignment of the spine, particularly in terms of lower back pain and slipped discs.

Laboratory and Clinical Tests: none known

CLINICAL CONSIDERATIONS

This product is especially developed for the patient who needs **Trace Minerals B6**, but who cannot tolerate the high organic iodine content of the **Trace Minerals B6**.

Contrary indications
None known

ASSOCIATED PRODUCTS:

See "**Trace Minerals B6**" (Product Bulletin) for indications of low back pain, flat feet, and poor muscle tone of the entire muscular and ligament structure of the body. (See Page, 177).

MANGANESE-B$_{12}$

MIN-TRAN

Label: (A Food Mineral tranquilizer) Each tablet contains 5 grains of Calcium Lactate and 5 grains of Pacific Sea Kelp for the correction of restlessness due to nutritional deficiency of these minerals. Dosage: 2 or 3 tablets taken one half hour before meals and at bedtime or 6 to 12 tablets per day.

Tissue or Function Supported   Complex of alkaline minerals and ionizable calcium.

CLINICAL CONSIDERATIONS
Prominent Clinical Signs And Symptoms

<u>Symptoms:</u>
1. Tachycardia (Persistent)
2. Hyperthyroidism (Weight loss, tremors, etc.)
3. Cramps (Menstrual, muscle)
4. "Nervous" Tension (Associated with muscle tonus)
5. Low Back Pain (Associated with muscular fatigue)
6. Insomnia (Associated with restlessness)

<u>Possible Etiological Background:</u>
Increasing the metabolism via thyroid activity is associated with calcium loss, increased oxygenation and high blood iodine (with inability of the thyroid to accept iodine from the blood). Thus increasing the blood iodine (via kelp source) and the replacement of the calcium loss is basic. Apparently this situation exists at the functional level long before it develops pathologically judging from widespread response when this product is used as a mineral tranquilizer.

Note: that calcium deficiency is recognized as being one of our most common deficiencies. The relation of this to the thyroid gives us a clue as to its etiological background.

Symptom Characteristics: Related to the hypermetabolic state, the most reliable symptom of which is persistent tachycardia.

Laboratory Tests	Protein Bound Iodine Basal Metabolic Rate Inorganic Iodine Blood cholesterol	Increased Increased Lowered Lowered	Note that satisfactory diagnosis by laboratory methods may only be obtained if a consistency of findings results-(in most cases). These findings indicate hyperthyroidism
Clinical Tests	Therapeutic Test		12 Min-Tran per day evidenced when symptomatic relief of the above symptoms points to hyperthyroidism.
Administration	**Dosage:** 12 per day in initial stages, later reduced to amount required for relief of symptoms.		
	Effect: Usually immediate, within ½ hour in case of muscle or menstrual cramps on sufficient dosage, seldom longer than two or three days are required to judge its effectiveness in the relief of these symptoms.		
	Side Effect: As can be understood, since this product is indicated primarily in the hypermetabolic state, its lack of effect in hypometabolism may be diagnostic. This specifically calls for thyroid support, Thytrophin, Cataplex F Perles, and Soybean Lecithin.		

<u>Synergists:</u>
Organic Minerals
Sea Water (Commissary)

<u>Activity Contributed</u>:
Potassium Source
Trace Mineral Source

GENERAL CONSIDERATIONS

One of the most common clinical complaints heard today is "nervousness". While "nervousness" is unrecognized as technical terminology, its clinical recognition is well established as evidenced by the sale of millions of dollars of drug tranquilizers. These, at best, have their effects at the psychic levels and have no basis in physiological medicine. They cannot replace the mineral losses brought about by the factors which indicate their need. In the first place, the drug approach to this problem may likely have not been brought into existence had they avoided demineralization.

MIN-TRAN

GENERAL CONSIDERATIONS

We may thus assume that there are two factors involved in every stress situation culminating in the need for tranquilization:

1. The psychic factor which is stimulatory in its effect, and the results of this stimulation which places a "cost" upon the physiological mechanisms involved, namely, demineralization through glandular stimulation.

The first of the above factors may be environmental, economic or social in origin and may or may not be under clinical management possibilities. However, the second factor-the demineralization resulting from the first-definitely amenable to nutritional support.

FOR THESE REASONS WE RECOMMEND **Min-Tran**, the food mineral tranquilizer in all cases where tranquilizers are indicated. The clinical response from the use of **Min-Tran** in these circumstances has been highly satisfactory. It is, perhaps, one of our most widely indicated products.

Note: Orchex, recommended as the physiological psychic tranquilizer, is the physiological counterpart to **Min-Tran** and is recommended for this aspect of the tranquilization problem.

CLINICALLY ASSOCIATED CONDITIONS

GASTROINTESTINAL-URINARY
- Liver and Gallbladder
  - Biliary Stasis
  - Gallbladder Disease
- Kidney and Bladder
  - Albuminuria
  - Cystitis
  - Urinary Incompetence

NERVOUS AND PSYCHOGENIC
- Functional Disorders
  - Asthenia
  - Chorea
  - Dysphagia
  - Hyperirritability
  - Nervous Strain
  - Sweat Gland Activity
- Metabolic
  - Legs, Weakness of
  - Tremors, Muscular
- Vasomotor
  - Blood Pressure Changes
  - Heat Prostration
  - Hypotension
  - Shock

METABOLIC DISORDERS
- Growth and Repair
  - Bones, Healing of
  - Caries
  - Gums, Receding of
  - Healing, Promotion of
  - Nails, Integrity of
  - Osteoporosis
  - Teething

METABOLIC DISORDERS
- Intermediate Processes
  - Calcium Metabolism
  - Cramps
  - Protein Metabolism
  - Drowsiness
- Acid-Base Disorders
  - Acids, Craving for
  - Acidosis
  - Alkalosis
- Blood
  - Epistaxis
  - Leukopenia
- Respiratory
  - Bronchitis
  - Emphysema
  - Coughs, Chronic
- Allergies
  - Antihistamine Effect
  - Hives
- Body Weight
  - Obesity

EXOGENIC DISORDERS
- Vincent's Infection
- Brucellosis
- Febrile Diseases
- Lymph Node Infections
- Pneumonia
- Rheumatic Fever
- Virus Infections
  - Colds, Flu, Grippe
  - Earache
  - Herpes Simplex
  - Herpes Zoster
  - Lumbago
  - Warts

EXOGENIC DISORDERS
- Toxic Disorders
  - Burns, Systemic Effects
  - Eclampsia
  - Poison Ivy and Oak
- Inflammation
  - Mastitis
  - Gingivitis
  - Periodontoclasia
  - Denture Irritation
  - Sinusitis

VASCULAR DISORDERS
- Circulatory Diseases
  - Bed Sores
  - Leg ulcers

SKIN DISORDERS
- Dermatitis
- Purpura
- Skin Irritations

GENETIC DISORDERS
- Female Disorders
  - Abortion
  - Dysmenorrhea
  - Endocervicitis
  - Menopausal Symptoms
  - Menstruation Symptoms
  - Pregnancy Schedule

SPECIFIC DEFICIENCY
- Glandular
  - Adrenal Insufficiency
  - Goiter

MYOTROPHIN

HEART CYTOTROPHIN (CARDIOTROPHIN)

Label: Cardiotrophin, Cytotrophic Extract of Beef Heart—A tissue extract intended to supply the specific determinant factors of the above mentioned organ and to aid in improving the local nutritional environment for that organ. For experimental use in cooperation with conventional Therapeutic methods. (One to three tablets per day, or as directed. (One per day should be maximum dosage for first week.

Tissue or Function Supported Muscle tissue, particularly cardiac, supplying nutrients for the local nutritional environment of muscle cells.

CLINICAL CONSIDERATIONS
Prominent Clinical Signs And Symptoms

Symptoms:	Possible Etiological Background:
1. Loss of Muscle Integrity (Atrophy, weakness, tonus, prolapse, etc.) 2. Carbohydrate Metabolism (Failure of muscle cells to metabolize glucose-glycogen) 3. Cardiac Weakness (Decompensation or failure due to lack of muscle tonus, nutrition to cell) 4. Sedentary Occupations (Predisposing heart failure) 5. Circulatory Problems (Due to tonus of musculature of arterial coats)	**Cardiotrophin** apparently assists the entire muscular system by influencing the nutritional aspect of selective absorption range of the muscle cell membrane. This selective range includes glucose uptake and is related to the important energy mechanism (ATP). Exercise is the usual activator of this system, being particularly significant in the case of the diabetic and potential heart rate failure patient. As such, **Cardiotrophin** provides a valuable remedy for these patients, particularly where such activity would be inadvised or otherwise unobtainable.

Symptom Characteristics: Important relation to carbohydrate metabolism via ATP mechanisms, as well as muscle integrity per se must be considered.

Laboratory Tests	Test: Creatine (urine)	Need Shown By: Pathologically found in wasting muscular disease.
Clinical Tests	Endocardiograph	Diminished, elongated first sounds, proportionately elevated second sounds.
Administration	**Dosage:** One tablet per day for first week or until level of tolerance is determined (See Side-Effects, below). Later level of administration depends upon the symptomatic level of response, observing exercise tolerance as indicator.	
	Effect: A tonic effect is usual in indicated cases. Its specific effect upon heart integrity must be determined by Endocardiograph readings or other diagnostic means.	
	Side Effect: These rarely occur. Reactions such as tachycardia may be attributed to disturbance in potassium-glucose metabolism. (The transfer of glucose to the muscle cell is accompanied by utilization of serum potassium, the administration of insulin being one of the few therapeutic means of reducing serum potassium temporarily. Calcium is one of the counterbalancing factors for potassium, NaCl another when serum potassium is in excess. In most cases, however, indications are potassium deficiency and **Organic Minerals** is the product of choice in this event. **Cardiotrophin** taken over a period of time may progressively lower the blood sugar level and hypoglycemia may be aggravated. This same effect, of course, is beneficial in hyperglycemia.	

Synergists:	Activity Contributed:
Organic Minerals	Potassium source (see remarks above)
Calcium Lactate	Ionizable calcium source (see above)
Betafood	Sugar metabolizing influence (see above)

GENERAL CONSIDERATIONS

Clinical rationalization for use is suggested as follows:
1. As a potentiator of nutrition to the muscle cell, thus useful in muscular weakness, atrophy, etc. In this respect, myoneural junction disorder must also be considered. See "Myoneural Junction Disorders" in Clinical Trophology.

MYOTROPHIN

GENERAL CONSIDERATIONS

2. As a nutritional factor favoring the geriatric patient, its tonic effect being most evident in these patients.
3. As a nutritional factor in increasing the energy metabolism of the muscle cell via the ATP mechanisms, apparently in same relation as exercises, which to the limits of tolerance is beneficial both to the diabetic and congestive heart failure patient.
4. Because of its effects in carbohydrate metabolism, as a possible factor in conditioning the hyperkalemia patient, a finding in Addisons Disease, which may also result in heart block. See notes under Side-Reactions for details.

CLINICALLY ASSOCIATED CONDITIONS

METABOLIC DISORDERS
<u>Intermediate Processes</u>
Diabetes Mellitus

VASCULAR DISORDERS
<u>Heart Disorders</u>
Heart abnormalities

NEUROTROPHIN PMG

Label: Cytotrophic Extract of Beef Brain – A tissue extract intended to supply the specific determinant factors of the above mentioned organ, and to aid in improving the local nutritional environment for that organ. For experimental use in cooperation with conventional Therapeutic methods. Manufactured under U.S. Patent No. 2,374,219. One to three tablets per day, as directed. (One per day should be maximum dosage for first week).

Tissue or Function Supported   Brain tissue.

CLINICAL CONSIDERATIONS
Prominent Clinical Signs And Symptoms

Symptoms:
1. Slowness of thought
2. Loss of memory
3. Psychoneurotic manifestations
4. Uncontrolled mental activity (Nightmares, epilepsy, day dreaming, inability to concentrate, etc.)
5. History of trauma (Concussion, anoxia)
6. Diabetes (traumatic origin) (Diabetes following brain injury)

Possible Etiological Background:

The difficulty of evaluating Brain Cytotrophin from a clinical viewpoint stems from the etiological background wherein the function of the brain still lies in an obscure area of research.

Symptom Characteristics: No outstanding characteristics have become evident, however, as a supportive measure in most central nervous system involvement's, logic would dictate its clinical application as a prophylactic measure. It should also be noted that a great variety of diseases are associated with encephalitis and so the incidence of traumatic involvement of brain tissue may be much greater than ordinarily suspected, cerebral anoxia is another consideration in the same category.

	Test:	Need Shown By:
Laboratory Tests	Encephalograph Readings	Epileptic-type readings
Clinical Tests	Psychiatric Examination	Schizophrenia and other findings
Administration	**Dosage:** 1 or 2 tablets per day. Increased dosage has not shown proportionate benefits.	
	Effect: See "Etiological Background" above. Slowness of thought shows the most promising clinical observation.	
	Side Effect: None known.	

Notes: Synergists are very important, **Cataplex G** and **Organic Minerals** as activators of cholinesterase reactions are of primary consideration; **Orchex** in relation to oxygen metabolism; **Cataplex B**, lactic and pyruvic acid metabolism; and **Zymex** in relation to intestinal toxemia. (NOTE: Mono-Sodium-Gluconate, available under various trade names, is a source of natural glutamic acid. This product along with **Inositol Tablets** has produced many favorable clinical results in mental conditions). **Protefood** may be very important in all mental considerations.

GENERAL CONSIDERATIONS

The general indications for use are as follows:
    a. History of trauma to brain tissue (concussion, anoxia)
    b. Deviations from normal thinking processes
    c. Uncontrolled mental activity

The rationalization for clinical application is as follows:
1. Slowness of thought in persons otherwise normal in their thinking processes is the most common indication.
2. Diabetes which follows brain injury is another indication.
3. Some cases of schizophrenia and epilepsy have been reported as beneficially effected.

NEUROTROPHIN PMG

GENERAL CONSIDERATIONS

4. No observable results have been reported in Parkinson's Disease, multiple sclerosis or cerebral palsy, possibly because these involve degenerative changes or traumatic lesions beyond the point of repair by these methods.

CLINICALLY ASSOCIATED CONDITIONS

NERVOUS AND PSYCHOGENIC
    Functional
        Epilepsy
    Metabolic
        Tranquilizing Effect
    Mentality
        Backwardness in Children
        Brain, Concussion of
        Brain, Dysfunction of

EXOGENIC DISORDERS
    Toxic
        Delirium
        Nightmares
    Traumatic
        Stroke, Recovery from

NIACINAMIDE-B_6

Label: Niacinamide-50 mg; B_6—10 mg, with trace minerals from sugar cane concentrate. For use in correcting deficiency reactions of these vitamin factors such as the Pellagra Syndrome. Suggested dosage: 2 to 6 capsules per day, or as directed.

Tissue or Function Supported Deficiency states related to the Pellagra syndrome.

CLINICAL CONSIDERATIONS
Prominent Clinical Signs And Symptoms

Symptoms:	Possible Etiological Background:
1. Dermatitis (Bilateral lesions) 2. Psychic Manifestations (Melancholia, depression, neurasthenia) 3. Paresthesia (Burning, prickling sensation) 4. Sensitivity to sunlight 5. Loss of appetite (Severe) 6. Diarrhea	Niacinamide is an essential part of the enzyme system concerned with oxidation in the living cell; Vitamin B_6 augments this effect by playing an important function in the conversion of tryptophane to niacinamide and also in metabolizing unsaturated fatty acids to Vitamin F forms, and thus seems to be involved in fat metabolism. B_6 is also concerned with protein metabolism, its need has been shown to be increased in high protein diets.

Symptom Characteristics: Primarily involve neurological mechanisms, particularly concerned with enzymatic reactions.

Clinical and Laboratory Tests None known. However, recent experience with baby formulas where its deficiency created tetany-like reactions shows that B_6 deficiency is a possible differentiation factor where laboratory tests show that calcium deficiency is not the cause of this disorder.

Administration	
Dosage:	2 every hour for 4 or 5 hours may be necessary in initial stages, later reduced to symptomatic requirements. See "Synergists" listed below.
Effect:	Effective in producing a tranquilizing effect where indicated, particularly applicable to the hyperirritability characteristic of the menopausal state, probably by reason of adrenal involvement at this stage.
Side Effect:	None known.

Synergists:	Activity Contributed:
a. Organic Minerals	Potassium Source (resting potential)
b. Vitamin B Complex	Motor Nerve Conductivity Influence
c. Calcium Lactate	Ionizable Calcium Source

Note: 3 of each of the above, taken with 3 Niacinamide-B_6 capsules, usually is effective in producing a marked tranquilizing effect in the hypertonic patient within 20 minutes and may be used routinely where this effect is desired.

GENERAL CONSIDERATIONS
The nutritional effects may be listed as follows:
  a. B_6 has been reported as a fatty acid metabolizer (synthesis of Vitamin F forms in the liver).
  b. Antipellagra factors.
  c. Source of trace minerals from sugar cane.

Note: B6 is found in high amounts in the adrenals and as such may act as an adrenal hormone precursor.

CLINICALLY ASSOCIATED CONDITIONS

NERVOUS AND PSYCHOGENIC
   Functional
      Hyperirritability
      Nervous Strain

Metabolic
   Tranquilizing Effects
GENETIC
   Menopausal Symptoms
SPECIFIC DEFICIENCY DISEASES
   Pellagra

ASSOCIATED PRODUCTS:
Orchex: (See Page, 125)

NIACINAMIDE-B_6

OKRA, PEPSIN, E₃

(COMFREY, PEPSIN, E₃ CAPSULES)

Label: Each capsule contains 255 mgm. Of the root of Symphytum Officinale (Comfrey) carrying a vegetable mucin, 65 mgm. Pepsin (1:3000), 15 mgm. Of an extract of Tillandsia, 20 mgm. Of Vitamin E_3 (a saponifiable complex from wheat germ and beef chromatin), and 1/50 grain of Pineal Substance. Excipient: Carbamide. Dose: One capsule after each meal or as directed, swallowed with water. Use: As an aid to digestion.

Tissue or Function Supported Source of hydrophylic colloids and enzyme factors which aid digestive processes, acting to promote healing and relieve irritation.

CLINICAL CONSIDERATIONS
Prominent Clinical Signs And Symptoms

Symptoms:

1. Diarrhea (Caused by local irritation)
2. Constipation (Costiveness, lack of motility of feces)
3. Indigestion Symptoms (Ulcer syndrome, heartburn, fullness after meals, etc.)
4. "Intestinal Flu" (Gastro-intestinal symptoms associated with colds, flu, grippe, etc.)
5. Colitis (Ulcerative and mucous colitis, gastritis, etc.)
6. Gouty Diathesis (Uric acid metabolism)
7. Hemorrhoids (Aggravated by costiveness)

Possible Etiological Background:

Comfrey (otherwise known as Boneset) has a long history of use as an alterative, known for its healing properties, particularly where lesions may be due to gastritis. Costiveness (dry, hard stool) is usually benefited by the mucilagenous, hydrophylic colloids which provide motility to the feces. Diarrhea, usually caused by local irritation, is also usually benefited. Allantoin is considered to be the active ingredient, which is related in some way to uric acid metabolism. The biochemical aspects are discussed in a booklet published by the Lee Foundation on Comfrey, titled "A Narrative of and Investigation Concerning an Ancient Medicinal Remedy and its Modern Utilities" by Chas. J. Macalister, M.D.

Symptom Characteristics: Intestinal irritation (usually accompanied by either constipation or diarrhea) is the most outstanding characteristic. Hypochlorhydria is most constant finding, calling for Zypan as an adjunct.

	Test:	Need Shown By:
Laboratory Tests	a. Urinalysis	Indicanuria
	b. Blood Uric Acid	Normal 1 to 3 mg./100 mg. whole blood
Clinical Tests	Abdominal palpation	Rigidity, evidence of hypermobility, tenderness, indicating gastritis
Administration	**Dosage:** 3 per day is usual dosage (with meals). This may be increased to one capsule every half-hour in acute conditions such as gastrointestinal involvements of colds and flu, diarrhea and gastric ulcers.	
	Effect: Immediate benefits reported in most gastrointestinal disorders on sufficient dosage. Effect in constipation is secondary to correction of basic cause.	
	Side Effect: None known.	

Synergists:	**Activity Contributed:**
a. Zypan	Digestive catalyst
b. Di-Sodium Phosphate	Liver stimulant
c. A F with Betafood	Bile thinning factor
d. Anti-Gastrin	Useful in ulcer syndrome

GENERAL CONSIDERATIONS

The nutritional effects of Comfrey, Pepsin, E_3 may be listed as follows:

    a. Acts to reduce irritation in the intestinal tract.

    b. Aids in the digestion of proteins

    c. Reputed aid in healing processes.

OKRA, PEPSIN, E$_3$

GENERAL CONSIDERATIONS

The clinical rationalization is as follows:

1. A valuable adjunct in the treatment of gastrointestinal disorders involving local inflammation and irritation. This generally presents itself clinically as diarrhea.

2. Its effects in promoting healing may be attributed to its reputed effect of promoting phagocytosis and raising the blood calcium levels. (NOTE: Common name is Boneset, also reflected in scientific name "Symphytum" which means "putting together"). Allantoin, well known for its healing properties, is a natural constituent of Comfrey and has been found to be clinically beneficial in gout, probably by reason of the biochemical similarity between this substance and uric acid, the "vehicle" being changed, uric acid excretion is facilitated.

3. It possesses mucilaginous properties which promote motility to the stool where hard, dry stools are the cause of difficult bowel movements resulting in hemorrhoids and constipation.

4. When the contents are removed from the capsule and mixed with water and applied locally as a wet poultice, the effect is very beneficial for example in ingrown toenails, festers, ulcers and similar lesions.

5. This product is particularly beneficial for the aged, where Zypan as a source of other digestive aids, often proves indispensable to the comfort and feeling of well-being of this type patient.

CLINICALLY ASSOCIATED CONDITIONS

GASTROINTESTINAL-URINARY
   Stomach and Intestine
      Achlorhydria
      Alimentary Canal Flora
      Colitis, Mucous
   Liver and Gallbladder
      Constipation
      Digestion Faulty
NERVOUS AND PSYCHOGENIC
   Functional
      Colitis, Ulcerative
      Ulcers, Gastric
METABOLIC
   Growth and Repair
      Healing, Promotion of

METABOLIC
   Collagen Diseases
      Gout
   Blood
      Anemia, Pernicious
   Allergies
      Sneezing Attacks
EXOGENIC
   Virus
      Colds, Flu, Grippe
      Herpes Zoster
   Inflammation
      Diarrhea
SKIN CONDITIONS
      Acne Vulgaris

ORCHEX

Label: Enzymatic Extract of Bovine Orchic Gland. Each capsule contains Orchic Hyaluronidase from approximately 2 grams of fresh glandular material, 25 mgms of Niacinamide and 5 mgms. of Pyridoxine Hydrochloride (Vitamin B6) with trace minerals from sugar cane concentrate added for synergistic action. For experimental use in determining its value in correcting states of metabolic unbalance due to malnutrition. One to three capsules per day as directed.

Tissue or Function Supported   Physiological tranquilizing effect.

CLINICAL CONSIDERATIONS
Prominent Clinical Signs And Symptoms

Symptoms:

1. Hyperirritability (Nervous tension, lowered tolerance to stress)
2. Melancholia (Depression, loss of psychic tone)
3. Hypertension (Aggravated by psychic manifestations)
4. Capillary Engorgement (Bruising on slight trauma, "black and blue spots")
5. Pellagra Symptoms (Loss of appetite, mental depression, skin lesions)
6. Neuresthenia (Adrenal insufficiency)
7. Menopausal Symptoms (Nervousness, insecurity, mental aberrations, etc.)
8. Alterative (Lack of feeling of well-being)

Possible Etiological Background:

The probable mechanism of the tranquilizing effects observed clinically by the use of this product are through the oxygenation mechanisms, perhaps being specific for nerve cells, including brain cell activity. Vitamin B_6, also included in this preparation, is known to be a factor in fatty acid metabolism, acting also in this respect as an antioxidant, we believe. Included also are trace minerals and niacinamide, important enzyme system activators. In addition Orchex contains hyaluronidase-otherwise known as "the spreading factor"- which serves usefully in hypertension. Orchex is therefore admirably suited for physiological replacement where drug therapy is being used with the intention of producing a tranquilizing effect.

Symptom Characteristics: Psychic in nature, melancholia, depression, loss of basal tone of feeling for life being most common findings.

	Test:	Need Shown By:
Laboratory Tests	None known.	
Clinical Tests	Test: a. Transient Tachycardia b. Blood Pressure c. Psychiatric Examination	Need Shown By: Aggravated by emotional strain Transient variety, aggravated by emotional strain. Anxiety states

Administration	**Dosage:** 3 to 6 per day. Increased amounts do not seem to materially increase benefit.
	Effect: A pleasant increase in the feeling of well-being is usually experienced within a few days, blood pressure drop is proportional to the psychic benefits. In the latter case, long term dosage is recommended.
	Side Effect: None known.

Synergists: **Activity Contributed:**
a. Cataplex G   Enzyme activator (anti-spasmodic factor)
b. Calcium Lactate   Blood calcium factor
c. Organic Minerals   Potassium source (parasympatheticotonia)

GENERAL CONSIDERATIONS

The nutritional effects of Orchex may be listed as follows:
a. Oxygenation: Apparently through this mechanism it produces a beneficial effect in normalizing nerve activity.
b. "Spreading Factor": Source of hyaluronidase, a factor of benefit in circulatory relations.
c. Fatty acid metabolism: Synthesis of Vitamin F forms in the liver, a Vitamin B_6 synergistic effect.

GENERAL CONSIDERATIONS

d. A tranquilizing effect is experienced in the pellagra syndrome (characterized by anorexia, depression, gastritis and dermatitis).

e. Clinically, has been reported of benefit in the mental aberrations of the menopausal patient (depression, hyperirritability, etc.)

f. Useful in the neuroasthenic state of the adrenal patient according to clinical reports.

g. The nervous tension associated with hypertension is apparently benefited as well as systemic effects of the enzymatic effects of hyaluronidase being possible from long term use.

h. Capillary engorgement, a condition possible in oxygen deficiency states, may be benefited, oxygen being necessary to constrict capillaries which have become congested and engorged from traumatization.

Note: Vitamin B_6 is found in adrenal tissue, and we may assume adds support to the function of these glands. This may be of particular importance to the menopausal patient judging from clinical benefits noted when sued in this state. Some investigators claim that the adrenals—at least to some degree—take over functions of the ovaries at this period and for this reason the adrenals have been referred to as "the ovaries of the aged".

CLINICALLY ASSOCIATED CONDITIONS

NERVOUS AND PSYCHOGENIC
    Functional
        Hyperirritability
        Nervous Strain
    Metabolic
        Tranquilizing Effect
    Vaso-Motor
        Blood Pressure Changes
        Hypersensitivity
METABOLIC DISORDERS
    Intermediate Processes
        Oxygen Metabolism
    Body Weight
        Appetite Excessive

EXOGENIC DISORDERS
    Toxic
        Nightmares
        Delirium
VASCULAR DISORDERS
    Heart Abnormalities
        Anginal Pectoris
GENETIC
    Female
        Menopause Symptoms
        Uterine Congestion
GLANDULAR
    Adrenal Insufficiency

ORCHIC PMG

(ORCHIC CYTOTROPHIN)

Label: Cytotrophic Extract of Beef Orchic Substance-A tissue extract intended to supply the specific determinant factors of the above mentioned organ and to aid in improving the local nutritional environment for that organ. For experimental use in cooperation with conventional Therapeutic methods. One to three tablets per day, or as directed. (One per day should be maximum dosage for first week).

Tissue or Function Supported	Testes

CLINICAL CONSIDERATIONS
Prominent Clinical Signs And Symptoms

Symptoms:
1. Orchitis (Idiopathic)
2. Spermatogenesis (Infertility due to diminished sperm count)
3. Male Climacteric (As alterative)
4. Testicular Atrophy (Frequently accompanying liver cirrhosis, seen in alcoholism)
5. Cryptorchism (undescended testes)
6. Gynecomastia

Possible Etiological Background:

The intimate relationship between vitamins and hormones is illustrated in the frequent occurrence of atrophy of the testes and gynecomastia in liver disease, especially cirrhosis…some have claimed that the absorption of Vitamin E is inhibited by diminished bile secretion and that the untoward results are due to avitaminosis. This lends emphasis to the importance of administering nutritional support to these cases, supplying not only the probable vitamin concerned, but also the cell determinants for that organ. Note that the testes are very sensitive to changes in food intake and that prolonged fasting or malnutrition produces testis involution among undernourished boys.

Symptom Characteristics:	Aside from obvious localized involvements, secondary to sex characteristics are to be considered.	
Laboratory Tests	Tests: Sperm Count 17-Ketosteroid	Need Shown By: Normal 180-360 million spermia 10-15 mg. (Callow's Method), normal.
Clinical Tests	Palpation-physical examination, observation, etc.	
Administration	**Dosage:** 1 to 3 per day.	
	Effect: An interval of at least 6 weeks should be given before determining effects.	
	Side Effect: None known.	

Synergists:
a. Vitamin E Complex
b. Chlorophyll Complex (perles)
c. Pituitary Cytotrophin

Activity Contributed
Tissue response to stress
Sex hormone precursors (Tillandsia E_3-Complex)
Trophic influence on endocrines

GENERAL CONSIDERATIONS

It is interesting that the first studies of hypogonadism were investigations of a Russian religious sect, the Skoptsi, who practiced castration in young children. These studies showed that the testes were not only concerned with reproduction, but, in addition, exert important effects upon somatic growth, fat distribution and psychic development. As the years went by, numerous physiological experiments became fashionable for a decade or two- the famous "monkey gland operation for rejuvenation", for example. A study of the early publications reveals that in this field, as in so many other branches of endocrinology, convenient bioassay methods played a decisive role. All of which reemphasizes the importance of rigorous objectivity in evaluation of these phenomenon. The **Cytotrophic Extract of Orchic** as such, although relatively new in this field, promises to be productive of evidence of a satisfactory nature, but should be viewed with the same objectivity. Clinical reports, to date, have encouraged further investigation of this hypothesis.

CLINICALLY ASSOCIATED CONDITIONS

(See "Clinical Considerations" above)

ORCHIC PMG

ORGANIC BOUND MINERALS
(ORGANIC MINERALS)

Label: Contains colloidal minerals of sea lettuce (dulse) and alfalfa. The necessity in human nutrition for the minerals contained herein have not been agreed upon by the consensus of medical opinion. 1 to 3 tablets per day or as directed.

Tissue or Function Supported As a source of organic potassium it supplies this important intercellular component. (Only small amounts of potassium are found in the blood compared with the cells. Potassium is known to support the autonomic nervous system and is concerned with the function of the adrenal glands.

CLINICAL CONSIDERATIONS
Prominent Clinical Signs And Symptoms

Symptoms:	Possible Etiological Background
1. Suffocation symptoms (Frequent signing, breathlessness, dislike for closed rooms, high altitudes discomfort, irregular respiration).	Decreased control of respiratory mechanisms, autonomic unbalance, also symptoms of acidosis.
2. Hyperirritability symptoms (Tachycardia, photophobia, insomnia, voice affected during stress dysphagia, "cold-sweat" type perspiration, goose flesh easily formed).	Autonomic unbalance, sympathetic dominance, probably due to lack of parasympathetic counter-balancing effect.
3. Dehydration symptoms (Dryness of mouth, skin, mucous membranes, dry hard stool, diminished urination and perspiration).	Dehydration symptoms of acidosis, likely to occur in alkaline mineral deficits.
4. Neurasthenia (Carrying alert, quick movements, avoidance of emotional situations which provoke symptoms, increased metabolism suggestive of hyperthyroidism).	Decreased resting potential of cells.
5. Spasticity (Esophageal cramps, sphincter spasms-pyloric, etc., spastic constipation, etc.).	Autonomic unbalance.

Symptom Characteristics: The most common complaint is "nervousness". This general symptom is usually traceable to organs receiving the greater number of nerve impulses, such as the eyes, throat, and heart. Thus, the patient will usually have symptoms of sensitivity to bright light, a tightness or "lump" in the throat (voice affected with excitement) and an awareness of a fast, pounding beat that fails to calm down after excitation or after retiring. The manifestation of symptoms is almost always within the neurological pattern.

	Test:	Need Shown By:
Laboratory Tests	Sodium-Potassium Ratio	See "Applied Physiology of the Adrenal Glands" for graph of ratio.
Clinical Tests	Postural Blood Pressure	Failure to show rise in standing position.

Administration	**Dosage:** 1 to 3 tablets per day until symptoms are abated, then 1 to 4 tablets per week may be all that is required. Tablets may be given any time as needed. Greatest need, however, may be following meals, due to carbohydrates depressing blood potassium.
	Effect: Relief of symptoms may often be within 20 minutes upon administration of organic potassium. The patient may feel more tired and sleepy for one or two days following use. This is because the stress the body has been laboring under has been removed. In a few days the recuperation has been completed and normal responses are to be expected.
	Side Effect: The sodium-potassium levels are influenced by the adrenals and most reactions that might occur when **Organic Minerals** are administered may be traced to adrenal dysfunction. In this event, **Organic Minerals** should be withheld and **Drenamin** used until normal. It may be that the adrenals will not respond to either of the above courses because of a degenerated gland, in which case, it may be well to investigate the possibility of Addisons Disease. Note that an overdosage of these tablets can bring about a temporary condition of over sensitiveness of the entire parasympathetic system. A few doses of **Phosfood Liquid** relieves this.form of calcium more directly concerned with the relief of calcium deficiency symptoms.

ORGANIC BOUND MINERALS

Synergists:	Activity Contributed:
a. Ostogen	A source of biologically active uncooked veal bone calcium-protein-enzyme complex which supplies phosphatase and other bone factors.
b. Catalyn	To supply additional synergistic vitamin and trace mineral complexes which may not be adequately provided in the dietary.

GENERAL CONSIDERATIONS

The metabolism of potassium is one of the most important considerations in the entire biochemical array. However, since its activity is largely within

the cell itself, studies made upon the blood have been largely unproductive. An excess of cellular potassium is unknown. The symptoms manifest by

its deficiency or excess are closely related to the refractory period (or resting potential) of the nerve cell (Bernstein theory, see Best and Taylor, *Physiological Basis of Medicine*).

The nutritional effects of potassium may be listed as follows:

    a. Increases resting potential of cell (according to Bernstein Theory)

    b. Necessary for vagus support

    c. Combats acidosis

    d. Necessary for sugar utilization

    e. Cooperates with cholinesterase (myoneural junction synapse)

    f. Acts as physiological stimulant for adrenals

IMPORTANT: Since potassium metabolism is under the control of the adrenal glands, an understanding of the Adrenal's relationship is necessary for rationalization of its use. This is discussed in the article "Applied Physiology of the Adrenal Glands."

CLINICALLY ASSOCIATED CONDITIONS

EXOGENIC DISORDERS
    Infection
        Rheumatic Fever
    Inflammation
        Sciatica
    Traumatic
        Sedimentation Rate
GENETIC
    Female
        Dysmenorrhea
        Uterine Congestion
GASTROINTESTINAL-URINARY
    Liver and Gallbladder
        Constipation
        Indigestion, Acute
METABOLIC DISORDERS
    Acid-Base Balance
        Acidosis
        Ketosis
        Urine, pH of Blood

METABOLIC DISORDERS
    Blood
        Leukopenia
    Allergies
        Antihistamine Effects
METABOLIC DISORDERS
    Growth and Repair
        Caries
        Eye conditions
        Teething
        Tumors, Fibroid
        Intermediate Processes
        Cramps
        Carbohydrate Metabolism
        Diabetes Mellitus
    Collagen Diseases
        Arteriosclerosis
        Gout

ORGANIC BOUND MINERALS

CLINICALLY ASSOCIATED CONDITIONS

NERVOUS AND PSYCHOGENIC
- Functional
  - Autonomic Unbalance
  - Chorea
  - Dysphagia
  - Hyperirritability
  - Nervous strain
  - Photophobia
  - Sweat Gland Activity
  - Tachycardia

NERVOUS AND PSYCHOGENIC
- Metabolic
  - Neuromuscular Disorders
  - Numbness
  - Tranquilizing Effects
  - Torticollis
- Mentality
  - Backwards in Children
  - Brain, Dysfunction of
- Lesions
  - Palsy

SPECIFIC DEFICIENCY
- Glandular
  - Goiter

VASCULAR DISORDERS
- Heart
  - Angina Pectoris
  - Myocarditis

ASSOCIATED PRODUCTS: Min-Tran: The concentration of potassium in **Min-Tran** is much less than in Organic Minerals, however, appreciable amounts of potassium are present. **Min-Tran** contains, in addition, **Calcium Lactate** and iodine as well as other alkaline minerals, and is not as likely to produce reactions in hypoadrenia where potassium is in excess since potassium and calcium act to balance one another in the body chemistry. (See Page, 115)

OSTROPHIN PMG

Label: Each tablet contains 225 mg extract from fresh veal bone, and 45 mg of cold sterilized veal bone meal organically combined with 4 mg manganese. Carrier Materials: calcium lactate, carrot powder. Mfg. Under U.S. Pat. No., 2,374,219. Use: To provide raw bone nutritional factors.

Tissue or Function Supported Source of rare amino acids and contains enzyme phosphatase which is found only in raw (uncooked) foods in the diet.

CLINICAL CONSIDERATIONS
Prominent Clinical Signs And Symptoms

Symptoms:
1. Bone and Joint Symptoms (Arthritis, joint pains, ligamentous problems, pain in bones, etc.)
2. Connective Tissues (Supportive tissue as irritated gums, loose teeth, receding gums)
3. Calcium Utilization (Osteoporosis, rheumatoid arthritis, osteomyelitis, etc.)
4. Circulation Symptoms (Headaches, varicose veins, hemorrhoids, veinous congestion)

Possible Etiological Backgrounds:
Apparently Ostrophin promotes the calcium and protein metabolizing systems of the body through its rare amino acids and enzyme content, a faulty metabolism brought on, we believe, by lack of raw food factors in the diet as evidenced by deficiency of raw foods in the diet bringing on kindred clinical pictures as demonstrated by Pottenger.

Symptom Characteristics: In a wide range of connective tissue diseases, this product may be considered as a useful adjunct. Generally, calcium utilization problems and loss of integrity of the ligamentous structures are concerned.

	Test:	Need Shown By:
Laboratory Tests	X-Ray	Bone porosity, "spurs", etc.
Clinical Tests	Observation Bleeding, spongy gums, joint motility, venous congestion, etc.	

Administration	**Dosage:** 1 to 4 per day.
	Effect: May be rapid in case of loss of integrity of the tooth socket, gum tissue lesions and some types of pain in the bones; arthritic lesions, bone repair and other similar problems may require long-term use..
	Side Effect: None known.

Synergists: | **Activity Contributed:**
a. Calcium Lactate | Source of ionizable calcium
b. Bio-Dent | Raw bone factors

GENERAL CONSIDERATIONS

1. Utilization of calcium, phosphorus and protein is promoted by Ostrophin and its use is indicated where such supplementation is being used but response is lacking. This is particularly applicable where patient is lacking raw foods in the diet.
2. Phosphatase is found in highest amounts in growing bone and its use is valuable as an adjunct wherever evidence of need for repair of bone is encountered.
3. This product has been found useful in sore, receding or spongy gums as well as joint pains, loose teeth and other conditions where one would expect its rare amino acid content is the active factor.

CLINICALLY ASSOCIATED CONDITIONS

NERVOUS AND PSYCHOGENIC
   Functional
      Headaches
      Migraine Headaches
   Metabolic
      Torticollis

Lesions
   Cerebral Palsy
   Multiple Sclerosis
   Palsy

OSTROPHIN PMG

CLINICALLY ASSOCIATED CONDITIONS

METABOLIC DISORDERS
    <u>Growth and Repair</u>
        Bones, Healing of
        Gums, Receding of
    <u>Intermediate Processes</u>
        Calcium Metabolism
    <u>Collagen Diseases</u>
        Bursitis
        Cataracts
        Disc lesions
        Dupuytren's Contracture
        Hernia

    <u>Collagen Diseases</u>
        Ligaments, Deformity of
        Peyronie's Disease
    <u>Blood</u>
        Anemia
    LXOGENIC DISORDERS
    <u>Circulatory Diseases</u>
        Buerger's Disease
        Hemorrhoids
        Intermittent Claudication
        Varicose Veins

OVATROPHIN PMG

(Ovary Cytotrophin)

Label : Extract of Beef Ovaries—A tissue extract intended to supply the specific determinant factors of the above mentioned organ and to aid in improving the local nutritional environment for that organ. For experimental use in cooperation with conventional Therapeutic methods. Mfg. under U.S. Patent No. 2,374,219. One to three tablets per day, or as directed. (One per day should be maximum dosage for first week.)

Tissue orFunction Supported Ovary

CLINICAL CONSIDERATIONS
Prominent Clinical Signs and Symptoms

<u>Symptoms:</u> <u>Possible Etiological Background:</u>

Note: Pages, 534 to 556, *Practical Endocrinology*, by Harrower, give a comprehensive review of ovarian dysfunction. The clinical picture described in these pages is too long to tell in detail here but the possibilities covered may be listed briefly as follows:

1. Amenorrhea
2. Delayed Puberty
3. Dysmenorrhea
4. Dysovarism
5. Frigidity
6. Infantilism
7. Menopause
8. Metrorrhagia
9. Menorrhagia
10. Ovarian Irritability
11. Ovarian Poisoning
12. Premature Senility

Symptom Characteristics: Aside from the classically recognized possibilities of ovarian dysfunction, we have observed the most common characteristic to be deviations in calcium metabolism, and of being a particular variety apparently concerned with intercellular calcium metabolism in which blood calcium levels may or may not be disturbed. In these cases, calcium administration may either prove disappointing or actually produce reactions. **Ovex**, as well as **Ovary Cytotrophin** is indicated.

	Tests:	Need Shown By:
Laboratory Test	a. Urinary 17-Ketosteroids	Slightly diminished, level further depressed in old age.
	Tests	Need Shown By
Clinical Tests	a. X-Ray of bone	Osteoporosis (most frequent in aged)
	b. Vaginal Smear	Shows degree of estrogen deficiency

Administration	**Dosage:** One per day should be maximum for first week, later increased to 2 or 3 per day.
	Effect: Response is generally satisfactory where specific symptoms are being observed. Synergistic support may be very important, see "General Considerations" following, for suggested schedule; also, "Signs and Symptoms" in the Manual of Clinical Trophology for specific indications.
	Side Effects: Side effects occurring are usually nonspecific, i.e., not directly referable to the ovaries themselves, but rather either due to trophic effects of ovarian hormones on the thyroid or pituitary adrenals—or to metabolic insufficiencies usually manifest as disturbances in calcium metabolism. **Anti-Pyrexin**, **Calcium Lactate** and **Pituitary Cytotrophin** are the usual recourses, otherwise see references listed above for specific indications.

Synergists: See "General Considerations" following page

GENERAL CONSIDERATIONS

Improvement of functional ability of ovaries via protomorphogen activity thus normalizing hormonal control is rationalization for clinical application. Simultaneously with ovarian support, we should consider the close interrelationship with other endocrine glands, namely: the thyroid, adrenals, and pituitary glands, and the important function of the uterus as well.

OVATROPHIN PMG

GENERAL CONSIDERATIONS

In clinical application, therapy directed towards these related glands may provide the successful difference which ovarian support alone may lack. It is this interrelationship which provides the clinician with his most difficult problems in these cases. For this reason, we are offering the following schedule for use in determining the most likely related products in these situations:

GONADAL MANIFESTATION	CONCOMITANT FINDINGS	PRODUCT RECOMMENDATIONS
1. Amenorrhea	Anemia, neurasthemia, developmental deficits	Ferrofood, Pituitrophin, Ovex
2. Dysmenorrhea	Hyperthyroid tendencies, hyperpituitarism, calcium deficiency states	Trace Minerals B12, Calcium Lactate, Pituitrophin
3. Metrorrhagia	Adrenal insufficiency, ovarian insufficiency	Drenamin, Calcium Lactate, Ovex, Chlorophyll Complex Perles
4. Menopausal Symptoms	Pituitary hyperactivity, adrenal insufficiency, hyperthyroidism	Calcium Lactate, Trace Minerals B12, Pituitrophin, Soybean Lecithin

When the foregoing is attended by freak thyroid or adrenal symptoms, as follows:

Thyroid involvements
1. Hypothyroidism – **Vitamin F Perles, Pituitary Cytotrophin, Thyroid Cytotrophin***
2. Hyperthyroidism – **Calcium Lactate, Organic Iodine, Pituitary Cytotrophin, Thyroid Cytotrophin***

*Thyroid Cytotrophin indicated in both states. Hypothyroidism is attended with bradycardia, hyperthyroidism with tachycardia

Adrenal involvements
1. Hypoadrenia -- **Calcium Lactate, Lecithin, B12, Adrenamin***
2. Hyperadrenia – **Organic Iodine, Calcium Lactate, Adrenamin***

*Adrenemin indicated in both states. Hypoadrenia is attended with hypotension, neurasthenia, hyperadrenia is attended with hypertension, masculation.

Note: The above suggestions are simply an outline of possible therapeutic courses which may be followed. Changes in the clinical picture should be observed and the schedule altered according to indications. **Ovary Cytotrophin** is recommended in all cases as the basic nutritional support.

CLINICALLY ASSOCIATED CONDITIONS

Female Disorders

Amenorrhea	Leukorrhea	Uterine Congestion
Dysmenorrhea	Menstruation Symptoms	Vaginitis

ASSOCIATED PRODUCTS:

Ovex	Contains the enzymatic principles and is independent of ovary function, and, as such it may be used either with or without
Ovary Cytotrophin	Which contains the protomorphogen principles influencing the local nutritional environment of the cells (See Pages, 135-138)

OVEX OR OVEX P

Label: Aqueous Extract of bovine or porcine ovarian tissue. Each tablet represents approximately 3 grams of fresh material. For experimental use in determining its value in metabolic unbalance due to malnutrition. 1 to 3 tablets per day or as directed.

Tissue or Function Supported   Ovary

CLINICAL CONSIDERATIONS
Prominent Clinical Signs And Symptoms

<u>Symptoms:</u>   <u>Possible Etiological Background</u>

Note: Pages 534 to 556, *Practical Endocrinology*, by Harrower, give a comprehensive review of ovarian dysfunction. The clinical picture described in these pages is too long to repeat in detail here, but the possibilities covered may be listed briefly as follows:

Amenorrhea	Frigidity	Metrorrhagia
Delayed Puberty	Infantilism	Ovarian Irritability
Dysmenorrhea	Menopause	Ovarian Poisoning
Dysovarism	Menorrhagia	Premature Senility

Symptom Characteristics: Aside from the classically recognized possibilities of ovarian dysfunction, we have observed the most common characteristic to be deviations of calcium metabolism, and of being a particular variety apparently concerned with intercellular calcium metabolism in which blood calcium levels may or may not be disturbed. In these cases, calcium administration may either prove disappointing or actually produce reactions. **Ovatrophin**, as well as **Ovex**, is indicated.

	Test:	Need Shown By:
Laboratory Tests	Urinary 17 Ketosteroids	Slightly diminished, level further depressed in old age
Clinical Tests	a. X-Ray of Bone b. Vaginal Smear	a. Osteoporosis (most frequent in aged) b. Shows degree of estrogen deficiency
Administration	**Dosage:** 2 or 3 per day.	
	Effect: Response is generally satisfactory where specific symptoms are being observed. Synergistic support may be very important, see "General Considerations" following, for suggested schedule; also, "Signs and Symptoms" in Manual of Clinical Trophology for specific indications.	
	Side Effect: Side-effects occurring are usually nonspecific, i.e., not directly referable to the ovaries themselves, but rather either due to trophic effects of ovarian hormones on the thyroid or pituitary or adrenals-or to metabolic insufficiencies usually manifest as disturbances in calcium metabolism. **Antronex, Calcium Lactate** and **Pituitrophin** are the usual recourses.	

<u>Synergists:</u>   <u>Activity Contributed:</u>

See "General Considerations" following

GENERAL CONSIDERATIONS

Simultaneously with ovarian support, we should consider the close interrelationship with other endocrine glands, namely: the thyroid, adrenals and pituitary glands, and the important function of the uterus as well. In clinical application, therapy directed towards these related glands, may provide the successful difference which ovarian support alone may lack.

It is this interrelationship which provides the clinician with his most difficult problems in these cases. For this reason, we are offering the following schedule for use in determining the most likely related products in these situations.

<u>GONADAL MANIFESTATION</u>	<u>CONCOMITANT FINDINGS</u>	<u>PRODUCT RECOMMENDATIONS</u>
1. Amenorrhea	Anemia, neurasthemia, developmental deficits	Ferrofood, Pituitrophin, Ovex
2. Dysmenorrhea	Hyperthyroid tendencies, hyperpituitarism, calcium deficiency states	Trace Minerals B12, Calcium Lactate, Pituitrophin,

OVEX OR OVEX P

GONADAL MANIFESTATION	CONCOMITANT FINDINGS	PRODUCT RECOMMENDATIONS
3. Metrorrhagia	Adrenal insufficiency, ovarian hyperthyroidism	Drenamin, Calcium Lactate, Ovex, Chlorophyll Complex Perles
4. Menopausal Symptoms	Pituitary hyperactivity, adrenal insufficiency, hyperthyroidism	Calcium Lactate, Trace Minerals B12, Pituitrophin, Soybean Lecithin

When the foregoing is attended by frank thyroid or adrenal symptoms, as follows:

   A. Thyroid involvements
      1. Hypothyroidism--Cataplex F Perles, Pituitrophin, Thytrophin*
      2. Hyperthyroidism—Calcium Lactate, Organic Iodine, Thytrophin*

*Thytrophin is indicated in both states. Hypothyroidism-as attended with Bradycardis, hyperthyroidism with tachycardia.

   B. Adrenal Involvements
      1. Hypoadrenia—Calcium Lactate, Lecithin, B12, Drenamin*
      2. Hyperadrenia—Organic Iodine, Calcium Lactate, Drenamin*

*Drenamin indicated In both states. Hypoadrenia is attended with hypotension, neurasthenia; hyperadrenis In attended with hypertension, masculation.

Note: The above suggestions are simply an outline of possible therapeutic courses which may be followed. Changes in the clinical picture should be observed and the schedule altered according to indications. Ovatrophin is recommended in all cases as the basic nutritional support.

CLINICALLY ASSOCIATED CONDITIONS

FEMALE DISORDERS
   Amenorrhea
   Dysmenorrhea
   Leukorrhea
   Menstruation Symptoms
   Uterine Congestion
   Vaginitis

PANCREATROPHIN PMG

Label: Cytotrophic Extract of Beef Pancreas. A tissue extract intended to supply the specific determinant factors of the above mentioned organ and to aid in improving the local nutritional environment for that organ. For experimental use in cooperation with conventional Therapeutic methods. This product is sold for use as part of the nutritional pattern of a human diet. It has no drug use known to us in the dosage recommended. (Excipient: Dehydrated Buckwheat Juice) Three to six tablets per day, or as directed. (Three per day should be maximum dosage for first week)

Tissue or Function Supported Local nutritional environment of pancreas cells.

CLINICAL CONSIDERATIONS
Prominent Clinical Signs And Symptoms

Symptoms:
1. Hyperglycemia (Diabetic tendency)
2. Emaciation (Wasting diseases)
3. Upper back pain (Pain in area of clavicles)
4. Acholic stool (Undigested foods, light or clay colored)
5. Healing reactions (Diabetic ulcers, etc.)

Possible Etiological Background:
Since the discovery of insulin, this function of the pancreas has tended to overshadow the important role of this organ in other aspects of intermediate metabolism, specifically its role in protein digestion.

Recall that trypsin, a product of the pancreatic juice, is a potent proteolytic enzyme, and the possibility exists for this enzyme to be excessive and become systemic in distribution. Emaciation and other wasting situations may, according to our observations result from this.

Symptom Characteristics: Relate mostly to carbohydrate or protein metabolism. The latter manifest as a muscular dystrophy or atrophy.

Laboratory Tests	Test:	Need Shown By:
	Blood sugar	Elevated
	Enzyme Tests	(These have largely been unsatisfactory)

Clinical Tests Discussion: One of the most commonly omitted diagnoses is that of pancreas dysfunction in the absence of diabetes, yet this organ provides the main bulwark between digestion and the assimilation of foods. The difficulty arises from adequate methods of diagnosis.

Administration	**Dosage:** 3 per day in usual dosage. Some reports indicate benefits from increasing dosage to as high as 12 per day. This should be regulated upon symptomatic basis.
	Effect: Upper back pain (see above) when from this cause is usually relieved within a few hours. Blood sugar levels and protein metabolism are to be judged over a period of weeks. Digestion may be variably improved, differing with each case.
	Side Effect: None known.

Synergists: | **Activity Contributed:**
a. Sea Water (Commissary) | Source of trace minerals particularly zinc which is necessary for pancreas function
b. Zypan | Source hydrochloric acid and pancreatic factors

GENERAL CONSIDERATIONS

Insufficiency of the pancreas may be considered one of the most commonly omitted diagnose, in the patient suffering from chronic fatigue, emaciation, lowered resistance and a variety of general symptoms not directly associated with sufficiency of the gastric secretions.

Substance in fact to the above statement is provided by Harrower on page 482 of his book, *Practical Endocrinology*, which reads, in part, as follows:

"The frequency with which diabetics suffer from concomitant infections is well known…small pimples often become serious boils…and may spread with amazing rapidity. Infections that may ordinarily be considered trivial frequently becoming quite serious in the diabetic.

PANCREATROPHIN PMG

GENERAL CONSIDERATIONS

In the experimental work on animals it has been found that the removal of the pancreas in one step is almost invariably fatal. The significant fact is that these animals do not heal. This may be obviated by the implantation, in the abdominal wall, of a small piece of pancreatic tissue, preferably from the tail of the pancreas…even a small graft is enough to preserve the immunizing response to infection. This seems to afford the best kind of evidence of a relation between the internal secretion of the pancreas and the power to overcome bacterial infection."

Note: with the notable exception of diabetes, the clinical associated conditions are rather obscure, protein and carbohydrate metabolism (with their meaning, ramifications) being primary consideration. We therefore do not list specific entries in this case.

PAROTID PMG

(PAROTID CYTOTROPHIN)

Label: Cytotrophic Extract of Beef Parotid—A tissue extract intended to supply the specific determinant factors of the above mentioned organ and to aid in improving the local nutritional environment for that organ. For experimental use in cooperation with conventional Therapeutic methods. Manufactured under U.S. Patent No. 2,374,219. One to three tablets per day, or as directed. (One per day should be maximum dosage for first week.)

Tissue or Function Supported Determinant factors of parotid gland.

CLINICAL CONSIDERATIONS
Prominent Clinical Signs And Symptoms

Symptoms:

1. Developmental characteristics (Undescended testicles, under-developed children)
2. Thyroid derangements (Goiter, hypothyroidism, thyrotoxicosis)
3. Salivary disorders (Diminished salivation, enlargement of salivary glands, "stones," etc.)
4. Specific disease history (Orchitis, mumps)
5. Iodism (Sensitivity to iodine administration)

Possible Etiological Background:

The vestigial organ, the thyroglossal duct, calls attention to the relation between the thyroid and the parotid glands, suggesting that the assimilation of thyroxine or its metabolism may be related to parotid determinants. The large chromosome cells in both the parotid and orchic glands suggest the relationship, evident as concomitant inflammations in infectious diseases.

Symptom Characteristics: While application remains on an empirical basis, direction of attention is in connection with thyroid problems, possible traumatic interruption of normal function via history of mumps or orchitis being a strong clinical consideration, particularly when difficulties stem from this origin (sterility)

Laboratory and Clinical Tests See "Organic Iodine" Bulletin (Also palpation of glands, history of mumps, underdevelopment, thyroid, etc.)

Administration	
Dosage:	1 to 3 per day, taken with meals.
Effect:	Beneficial particularly in underdeveloped children along with other nutritional factors.
Side Effects:	None known

Synergists:	Activity Contributed:
1. Pituitary Cytotrophin	Trophic Influence on Endocrines
2. Thyroid Cytotrophin	Local Nutritional Environment of Cells
3. Pancreas Cytotrophin	Proteolytic Enzyme Relation
4. Vitamin F Complex	Calcium Diffusing Influence
5. Vitamin G Complex	Cell Proliferating Influence
6. Vitamin A-C-P Complex	Epithelial and Connective Tissue Integrity

GENERAL CONSIDERATIONS

The parotid protomorphogen, like the pituitary, may have a wide spread range of clinical application. We have had reports of uses in various conditions, apparently involving the thyroid gland and its functions.

We may rationalize this as follows:

1. Parotitis (mumps) shows a close relationship between the tissues of the parotid gland and testes, sterility resulting in many cases. Histologically both tissues are of very large chromosomes.
2. Embryologically we have evidence of a relation between the thyroid and the parotid via the vestigial thyroglossal duct, a structure which now may be observed with a possible understanding of its former importance. It is interesting, in this respect, to note that the thyroid hormone is the most compatible with oral administration.

PAROTID PMG

GENERAL CONSIDERATIONS

3. The theory to be applied here is that the possibility exists that the salivary secretions mark the thyroid for reabsorption or at least enter into its metabolic mechanisms.
4. Clinical experience with **Parotid Cytotrophin** seems to substantiate this hypothetical basis, therefore, our recommendation for its experimental use in thyroid involvements.

CLINICALLY ASSOCIATED CONDITIONS

NERVOUS AND PSYCHOGENIC
<u>Functional</u>
    Salivary Disorders
<u>Mentality</u>
    Backwardness in children

METABOLIC DISORDERS
<u>Growth and Repair</u>
    Mouth-Tongue Disorders
<u>Blood</u>
    Anemia

GLANDULAR
    Goiter

PHOSFOOD LIQUID

Label: For the correction of a nutritional deficiency of phosphates. Each 10 drops contain approximately 130 mg of Ortho-Phosphoric Acid and 21 mg of Phytin (cereal source) of which 5.6 mg is Inositol. Suggested dosage: 10 drops in ½ to 1 glass of water after each meal or as directed.

Tissue or Function Supported — As a source of ortho-phosphoric acid, it supplies phosphorus and is thus related to calcium metabolism. As such, it supports nerve function and aids in controlling calcium levels.

CLINICAL CONSIDERATIONS
Prominent Clinical Signs And Symptoms

Symptom	Possible Etiological Background
1. Stiffness (Feeling of muscle and joint stiffness, particularly in the morning)	Calcium carbonate deposits in soft tissues; viscosity of synovial fluid.
2. Nausea (Vomiting type of indigestion, pyloric spasms, "butter-fly stomach")	Neurological response through autonomic nervous system.
3. Myositis (Cramp sensation when one position is held for a length of time, "writers' cramp", stiff legs, etc.)	May be related to circulatory disturbance via blood viscosity.
4. Lowered metabolism (Slow starters, Bradycardia, sensitivity to cold weather)	Hypothyroid type symptoms. Accelerator control of glands.
5. Edema (Some types, observe concomitant symptoms)	Where there is a phosphorus deficiency, normalization of cell salts releases water from the tissues.
6. Arteriosclerosis (Hypertension, "pipe-stem" arteries of advanced case)	Combats calcium carbonate deposits; also lowering of blood viscosity improves circulation, especially to coronary arteries.
7. Symptoms occurring at night (Insomnia, restlessness, coughing, drooling, etc.)	Apparently lowering of metabolism changes availability of ionized calcium for tissue use.
8. Excessive secretions (Drooling, thin, watery saliva, watering of eyes and nose)	Probably neurological reaction, loss of autonomic control.
9. Circulatory disturbances (Leg cramps, tight feeling in chest, dull heart pain)	Blood viscosity.
10. Cranial symptoms (Headaches, irritability, throbbing sensations)	Viscosity of cerebro-spinal fluids.
11. Gastric hyperacidity (Acid rebound, symptoms immediately after eating)	Combats excessive hydrochloric acid secretions, mechanism probably neurological.

Symptom Characteristics: Usually involve muscular spasticity, joint stiffness or neurological response in one category; circulatory disturbances via blood or cerebro-spinal fluid viscosity in another category.

Laboratory Tests — **Note:** A decrease in inorganic phosphorus occurs in active rickets; increased in hypoparathyroidism and in chronic nephritis. Intestinal absorption may be faulty when serum phosphorus is low.

Clinical Tests

Test:	Need Shown By:
a. Endocardiograph	Bradycardia
b. Reflex tests	Diminished
c. Blood Coagulation Test	Clotting time less than 2 minutes.
d. Sulkowitch Reagent Test	Increased turbidity shows calcium loss (phosphorus excess, possibility); absence of turbidity shows high lkaline diet, faulty absorption

PHOSFOOD LIQUID

Administration	
	Dosage: 10 to 20 drops one to three times per day. Phosfood makes a pleasant beverage when sweetened. May be added to either fruit juice or water. Best results are obtained when taken between meals or upon arising or retiring.
	Effect: Neurological involvement's respond almost immediately, stomach spasms and nausea for example. Some types of bursitis, muscle stiffness and joint pains may show favorable response in two or three days, circulatory disturbances should evidence response in 10 days to two weeks.
	Side Effect: Hyperthyroid cases cannot tolerate phosphoric acid as this may increase the metabolic rate and sensitivity to Phosfood would lead one to suspect this etiology. Hypersensitivity may develop from the use of either acid or alkaline minerals in excess, and as cold sores and fever blisters may result from a deficiency of alkaline minerals, so an excess of acid minerals may bring them on. Remedy in such cases is Organic Minerals and Calcium Lactate. In the case of hyperthyroidism, Prolamine Iodine would be added.

Synergists:	Activity Contributed:
Prolamine Iodine	(See "Side-Effects" above)
Organic Minerals	(See "Side-Effects" above)
Calcium Lactate	(See "Side-Effects" above)
Soybean Lecithin	Fat metabolism cholesterol antagonist
Bio-Dent	Bone determinants, arthritic factors
Biost	Phosphatase metabolizing enzyme, particularly on raw food deficient diets

GENERAL CONSIDERATIONS

Phosphorus acts as an accelerator control of the autonomic nervous system and the glands. Its nutritional effects may be listed as follows:

a. Aids in preventing excessive hydrostatic pressure of the blood (and possibly cerebro-spinal fluid) by lowering its viscosity, thus improving circulation.
b. Combats calcium bicarbonate deposits in soft tissues.
c. Essential in calcium metabolism
d. Combats alkalosis
e. Remedy for excess flow of hydrochloric acid

CLINICALLY ASSOCIATED CONDITIONS

GASTRO-INTESTINAL
URINARY
   <u>Liver and Gallbladder</u>
      Gallbladder Disorders
   <u>Kidney and Bladder</u>
      Kidney Stones
      Urinary Incompetence
NERVOUS AND
PSYCHOGENIC
   <u>Functional</u>
      Autonomic Unbalance
      Colitis, Ulcerative
      Dysphagia
      Headaches
      Salivary Disorders
      Ulcers, Gastric
   <u>Vaso-Motor</u>
      Blood Pressure
      Changes
METABOLIC DISORDERS
   <u>Intermediate Processes</u>
      Cramps

METABOLIC DISORDERS
   <u>Collagen Diseases</u>
      Arcus senilis
      Arteriosclerosis
      Arthritis
      Bursitis
      Cataracts
   <u>Acid-Base Balance</u>
      Acids, Craving for
      Alkalosis tory
      Urine, pH of
   <u>Water Balance</u>
      Edema
   <u>Respiratory</u>
      Bronchitis
      Emphysema
   <u>Body Weight</u>
      Appetite Decreased
EXOGENIC DISORDERS
   <u>Toxic</u>
      Nightmares

EXOGENIC DISORDERS
   <u>Traumatic</u>
      Strictures
VASCULAR DISORDERS
   <u>Circulatory Diseases</u>
      Intermittent
   Claudication
      Cold Hands and Feet
      Buerger's Disease
      Hemorrhoids
      Phlebitis
      Varicose Veins
   <u>Heart Disorders</u>
      Angina Pectoris
      Myocarditis
GENETIC
   <u>Female Disorders</u>
      Amenorrhea

PITUITROPHIN PMG

(PITUITARY CYTOTROPHIN)

Label: Cytotrophic Extract of Beef Pituitary—A tissue extract intended to supply the specific determinant factor of the above mentioned organ, and to aid in improving the local nutritional environment for that organ. Manufactured under U.S. Patent No. 2,374,219. One to three tablets per day, as directed. (One tablet per day should be maximum for first week)

Tissue or Function Supported   Pituitary gland

CLINICAL CONSIDERATIONS
Prominent Clinical Signs And Symptoms

Symptoms:	Possible Etiological Background:
1. Fatigue ("Nervousness", exhaustion from excessive mental stress and overactivity)	General state of glandular insufficiency.
2. Stress intolerance (Instability, inability to work under "pressure"; and other symptoms related to thyroid function)	The pituitary is in the etiological background of most thyroid cases, either hypo- or hyperactive.
3. Digestive complaints (Gastrointestinal involvements such as ulcers, colitis, diarrhea, gastritis)	Possibly related to sex hormone, liver and pancreas influence as well as general glandular insufficiency over which pituitary has governing influence.
4. Metabolic disorders (Fluid balance, blood sugar levels, weight distribution, growth, etc. Typical examples: headaches [migraine], edema, obesity, vasomotor disturbances, etc.)	Trophic control of pituitary, probably under influence of adrenal.
5. Delayed healing response (Inflammatory, ulcerative or festering lesions which fail or are slow to heal)	Adrenal-gonad diathesis may be primarily concerned via trophic pituitary influence.
6. Nervous manifestations (Autonomic storms, tachycardia, dysphagia, photophobia, pyloric spasms and other symptom of autonomic unbalance.	Influence of pituitary through the adreno-sympathetic nervous system.

Symptom Characteristics: Usually involve mental processes and metabolic changes (including healing, blood sugar and fluid balance problems, fat distribution, etc.) Most common characteristic is fatigue associated with nervousness)

	Tests:	Need Shown By:
Laboratory Tests	a. Basil Metabolic Rate	Either increased or decreased
	b. Blood Sugar	Increased, but may be decreased also
	c. 17-Ketosteroid Test	Above or below normal (14 to 16 mg)
Clinical Tests	Signs and Symptoms of Glandular Dysfunction	See Clinical Appraisal Manual
Administration	**Dosage:** 1 to 6 per day, use step-ladder dosage until level of relief is obtained.	
	Effect: Usually immediate and beneficial, producing a definite increase in feeling of well-being..	
	Side Effect: Where extreme deviations of blood sugar exist, a side effect may be produced, apparently caused by lowering of the blood sugar levels, in which case the pancreas should be supported (Pancreatrophin or Zypan) before resuming full dosage of Pituitrophin.	

Synergists:	Activity Contributed:
Chlorophyll Complex (perles)	Sex hormone precursors
Pancreatrophin	Local environment of cells
Trace Minerals B_{12} or Manganese B_{12}	Manganese is mineral factor necessary for pituitary Activity, (as iodine is for thyroid)

PITUITROPHIN PMG

GENERAL CONSIDERATIONS

We may consider Pituitrophin as having a role in all endocrinopathies and may be considered as the universal protomorphogen, acting as a synergist to most of the cytotrophic extracts. It is useful in all cases where fullest response is desired or where other measures may prove lacking.

The effects have been particularly noted:
- Beneficial for digestive processes
- Influence in blood sugar problems
- Promotion of healing processes

The most prominent indication for its need is "nervous" fatigue associated with the stomach ulcer syndrome. Another strong indication is in thyroid cases, the pituitary almost invariably being an intervening factor whether hypo- or hyperthyroidism is concerned. The trophic effects upon the gonads are also to be considered.

CLINICALLY ASSOCIATED CONDITIONS

GASTROINTESTINAL-URINARY
  Stomach and Intestines
    Colitis, Mucous
  Liver and Gallbladder
    Digestion Faulty
NERVOUS AND PSYCHOGENIC
  Functional
    Asthenia
    Autonomic Unbalance
    Colitis, Ulcerative
    Dysphagia
    Migraine Headaches
    Nervous Strain
    Ulcers, Gastric
  Metabolic
    Alcoholism
    Tranquilizing effects
  Mentality
    Backwardness in Children
METABOLIC DISORDERS
  Intermediate Processes
    Carbohydrate Metabolism
    Diabetes Mellitus
    Drowsiness
  Collagen
    Arteriosclerosis
  Acid-Base Balance
    Ketosis
  Water-Balance
    Ascites
    Dropsy
    Edema
    Edema of Ankles

METABOLIC DISORDERS
  Blood
    Leukopenia
  Body Weight
    Obesity
EXOGENIC DISORDERS
  Virus
    Herpes Zoster
  Inflammation
    Diarrhea
VASCULAR DISORDERS
  Circulatory
    Bed Sores
    Leg Ulcers
SKIN DISORDERS
    Alopecia
GENETIC
  Female Disorders
    Amenorrhea
    Menopausal Symptoms
SPECIFIC DEFICIENCY
  Glandular
    Goiter
    Sterility
    Gynecomastia

PNEUMOTROPHIN PMG

Label: Pneumotrophin-Cytotrophic Extract of Beef Lung—A tissue extract intended to supply the specific determinant factors of the above mentioned organ and to aid in improving the local nutritional environment for that organ. For experimental use in cooperation with conventional Therapeutic methods. One to three tablets per day, or as directed. (One per day should be maximum dosage for first week.)

Tissue or Function Supported   Lung tissue.

CLINICAL CONSIDERATIONS
Prominent Clinical Signs And Symptoms

Symptoms:

1. Respiratory Disorders (Such as bronchitis, asthma, chronic coughs, "chest colds", cigarette coughs)
2. Convalescent Stages (Of pneumonia, colds, flu, grippe, etc.)
3. Pulmonary Involvements (Of congestive heart failure, adrenal insufficiency, anoxia, etc.)
4. Pulmonary Accidents (Such as industrial hazards, fire, fumes, dust inhalation, etc.)
5. Acid-Base Unbalance (Respiratory acidosis and alkalosis)

Possible Etiological Background:

Like all Cytotrophic Extracts, **Pneumotrophin** involves the protomorphogen reaction. See "Introduction to Protomorphology" by Royal Lee for details. The physiology of the lungs includes the exchange of gases influential in regulation of acid-base balance and as such is involved in a wide variety of disorders where the alkaline-acid balance is concerned. Also, the superimposed burden upon the lungs brought about by adrenal insufficiency (pulmonary hypertension) is to be considered, and, in a similar vein, we must consider the pulmonary edema of congestive heart failure as indicative of specific lung support, even though the etiological background and basic cause is the heart.

Symptom Characteristics: The obvious pulmonary symptoms are, of course, the primary consideration, but this should be extended to include the lungs as a regulatory organ in acid-base disorders and as an eliminative organ. Superimposed burdens such as heart failure (edema) should not preclude lung tissue support.

Laboratory and Clinical Tests: None known. (Reliance upon case history and biochemical factors concerned constitutes the scope of diagnostic possibilities).

Administration		
	Dosage:	See label (above).
	Effect:	Often spectacular in cases of chronic bronchitis, cigarette cough, and some types of asthma. Two to three weeks should be allowed before concluding effectiveness. See "Emphysema" in Manual of Clinical Trophology for supportive considerations.
	Side Effect:	Histamine reactions may occur in early stages of therapy, the patient often feeling like he is coming down with a cold. This is not serious and shows a specific need for the therapy.

Synergists:

	Activity Contributed:
a. Adrenamin	Adrenal relation to respiratory disorders
b. Calcium Lactate	Ionizable calcium
c. Phosfood	By lowering blood viscosity, improves pulmonary circulation where indicated.

GENERAL CONSIDERATIONS

Two important functions of the lungs are: Maintenance of acid-base disorders, and, maintenance of water balance (insensible perspiration), showing that the lungs are important eliminative organs for water and waste acids (carbonic acid). The lungs eliminate about 350 cc. daily as compared with 600 cc. via the urine. As such the lungs need to be considered in many phases of body activity other than those which may arise from the consideration of pulmonary considerations alone, edema, for example.

To illustrate, let us consider a congestive heart failure case with pulmonary edema. The rationale, of course, would be to direct the therapy towards improvement in the heart itself and this is the correct procedure, since heart failure

PNEUMOTROPHIN PMG

GENERAL CONSIDERATIONS

is the cause of the pulmonary situation. However, neglect of treatment of the secondarily stressed organ is not justified on the same basis since now a malicious cycle is in effect and the pulmonary embarrassment puts further stress on the heart and <u>both</u> must be treated. We have observed dramatic improvement in congestive heart failure cases (with pulmonary edema) where this two-fold therapeutic approach has been applied. For complete schedule in pulmonary involvements see "Emphysema" in the Manual of Clinical Trophology.

CLINICALLY ASSOCIATED CONDITIONS

METABOLIC DISORDERS
- <u>Intermediate Processes</u>
  - Acid-base Disorders
  - Oxygen Metabolism
  - Drowsiness
- <u>Respiratory</u>
  - Bronchitis
  - Emphysema
  - Coughs, Chronic
- <u>Allergies</u>
  - Asthma

PROLAMINE IODINE

(ORGANIC IODINE TABLETS)

Label: Organic Iodine for nutritional use only. Each tablet contains 3 mgs., Iodine as Prolamine Iodine (Organically combined in vegetable source protein). (I tablet contains the normal nutritional requirements for one month.) Dose to replace Iodine reserves: 1 to 3 tablets per day or for such time as directed.

Tissue or Function Supported   Trace mineral component concerned with general metabolism.

CLINICAL CONSIDERATIONS
Prominent Clinical Signs and Symptoms

<u>Symptoms:</u>

1. Diminished Secretions (Saliva, nasal secretions, sweat gland activity)
2. Hyperirritability (Tachycardia, tremors)
3. Increased Metabolism (Excessive appetite, weight loss)
4. Personality Aberrations (Irritability of aged, instability)
5. Activity Intensification (Excessive intensity, "frightened face" appearance)
6. Virus Infection, History (Polio, encephalitis, brucellosis, etc.)
7. Fibrotic Lesions (Prostate disease, ligamentous involvements, etc.)

<u>Possible Etiological Background:</u>

will be noted, symptoms listed concern hyperthyroidism primarily. This is in conformity with the widely reported benefits to iodine administration in hyperthyroidism (Lugol's solution is usually used). While this is true, we must not forget the important qualification usually given in the discussion of iodine therapy which is: "Try it and see!" In other words, iodine administration often shows a clinical response in situations where clinical evidence may be lacking, again a situation where a Therapeutic Test may prove invaluable. With these thoughts in mind, we would lend credence to indications in the hypermetabolic state, but not use it as a differential factor in excluding the wide scope of its beneficial possibilities.

Symptom Characteristics: Diminished secretions, hypermetabolic state and hyperirritability associated with tachycardia are outstanding points of clinical evaluation for need.

	Test	Test Shown By:
Laboratory Tests	a. Basal Metabolism b. Protein Bound Iodine c. Cholesterol Test	Increased Values Increased Values Low or normal
Clinical Tests	Test a. Pulse Rate b. Reflex Test c. Observation	Test Shown By: Tachycardia Hyperactivity Tremors (protruding tongue test)
Administration	**Dosage:** 3 per day in initial stages, gradually reduced upon symptomatic response…observe pulse rate: tachycardia may result in iodism; decrease in pulse rate shows favorable response.	
	Effect: Two effects are noted: (1) relaxing, tranquilizing effect; (2) tonic effect. Both of these effects are quite marked in susceptible cases.	
	Side Effect: Iodism is marked by tachycardia, skin irritation, thinning of secretions (watery eyes, nose, and saliva), nervousness and headache. When these, or other adverse symptoms, are brought about by iodine administration, it indicates a sensitivity to iodine (or excessive ingestion) and it should be discontinued. Most patients are aware of iodine sensitivity and should be questioned in this regard. Probable need in iodism is for Calcium Lactate.	

<u>Synergists:</u>   <u>Activity Contributed:</u>

1. Thyroid Cytotrophin   Local Nutritional Environment of Cells
2. Calcium Lactate   Source Ionizable Calcium
3. Parotid Cytotrophin   We have reasons to believe chromosome factors provided by salivary secretions offer determinants necessary for assimilation of heretofore unsuspected non-vitamin biochemical factors which appear to be influential in thyroid activity, as clinical observations in the use of **Parotid Cytotrophin** would lead us to believe, for example, the beneficial effects in the treatment of underdeveloped children

PROLAMINE IODINE

GENERAL CONSIDERATIONS

The total effects of iodine deficiency may be such as to effect every tissue in the body due to its widespread distribution in the intracellular chemistry. It is thus present in most cells, but, of course, highest in thyroid tissue, lesser amounts in adrenals and pituitary.

Because of the diffuse distribution of iodine in the human economy its deficiency may take many clinical forms, specific thyroid dysfunction being but one of them. However, the time-honored position iodine holds as one of the experienced clinicians favorite remedies, especially for the aged, places it high on the list of nutritional substances which have been proven to be empirically effective.

The rationale for clinical application is as follows:

1. In general, we may expect the administration of iodine to increase secretions, thus it is an important factor where impaired circulation is concerned. Since it probably does this by "thinning" the secretions, its importance in lymphatic drainage is realized.

2. Benefits of iodine administration are widely reported in hyperthyroidism, favorable response in suspected cases being considered as a pathognomonic sign. This effect, we believe, should be extended to include hyperactivity of the adrenals and pituitary. This is especially true during menopause, as well as a possible factor in menstruation disorders, and, with the increase of thyroid activity in pregnancy (particularly the third trimester), it becomes an important consideration in this category as well.

3. The geriatric patient is usually a favorable prospect for iodine administration, apparently the aging processes increasing the metabolic rate as evidenced by weight loss, nervous irritability, mental aberrations and restlessness so characteristic of these patients.

CLINICALLY ASSOCIATED CONDITIONS

NERVOUS AND PSYCHOGENIC
- Functional
  - Nervous Strain
- Mentality
  - Backwardness in Children
- Metabolic
  - Appetite Decreased
  - Obesity

EXOGENIC DISORDERS
- Infections
  - Lymph Node Infections
- Inflammation
- Mastitis
- Sinusitis
- Strictures

VASCULAR DISORDERS
- Circulatory Diseases
- Phlebitis

GENETIC DISORDERS
- Female
  - Menopausal Symptoms
  - Uterine Congestion

GLANDULAR DISEASES
- Goiter

ASSOCIATED PRODUCT:
Trace Minerals B$_{12}$: (See Page 177, Trace Minerals B$_{12}$)

Note: *Sometimes there is confusion when a product will have a different name depending on which one of Dr. Lee's company's it originated from. Please check the list of name changes in the front of the book*

PROSTATE PMG

(PROSTATE CYTOTROPHIN)

Label: Cytotrophic Extract of Beef Prostate—A tissue extract intended to supply the specific determinant factors of the above mentioned organ and to aid in improving the local nutritional environment for that organ. For experimental use in cooperation with conventional Therapeutic methods. One to three tablets per day, or as directed. (One per day should be maximum dosage for first week.)

Tissue or Function Supported — Prostate gland

CLINICAL CONSIDERATIONS
Prominent Clinical Signs And Symptoms

Symptoms referable to prostate disease such as:
1. Nocturia
2. Dribbling
3. Low back pain
4. Leg pains
5. Fatigue
6. Loss of libido
7. Constipation

Possible Etiological Background:
Our impression is that the etiological background involves the thyroid gland, probably associated with a hyperactivity normally occurring with the aging processes, but attended with loss of integrity of the thyroid hormones produced. Hyperthyroidism is associated with hypertrophy and fibrosis and **Vitamin F Complex** is known to aid in normalizing thyroid function.

Symptom Characteristics: Associated with the hypermetabolic clinical picture, irritability, instability and hypersensitivity being characteristic.

	Test:	Need Shown By:
Laboratory Tests	a. Urinary 17-Ketosteroids	Slightly diminished
	b. Serum Acid Phosphatase	(May be elevated in carcinoma of prostate with metastasis to bone)
Clinical Tests	Physical Examination	Palpation
Administration	**Dosage:** 1 to 3 per day.	
	Effect: Depends upon synergists employed and chronicity and acuteness of the case, less favorable with venereal history.	
	Side Effect: None known.	

Synergists:	Activity Contributed:
a. Vitamin F Complex	Iodine Synergists
b. Adrenamin	(C and G Complexes with Adrenal Cytotrophin)
c. Prost-X	Enzymatic Factors (Phosphatase source)
d. Pituitary Cytotrophin	Trophic Influence on Endocrines
e. Thyroid Cytotrophin	Local Nutritional Environment of Cells

GENERAL CONSIDERATIONS

Prostate Cytotrophin has proved beneficial in the treatment of disorders of the prostate gland, particularly when used in cooperation with **Vitamin F Complex**. The common occurrence of this disorder in older men shows enough possibilities to recommend its use prophylactically. For further information see pages 586 to 591, *Practical Endocrinology*, by Harrower.

CLINICALLY ASSOCIATED CONDITIONS

<u>Male Disorders</u>
  Prostate disease
  Sterility

ASSOCIATED PRODUCTS:
  Prost-X: (See Page 153, **Prost-X**)

PROST-X

Label: Enzymatic Extract of the Bovine Prostate Gland. Each capsule contains Prostate Phosphatase with tillandsia extract. For experimental use in determining its value in correcting states of metabolic unbalance due to malnutrition.

Tissue or Function Supported Supplies phosphatase, a prostatic enzyme which is a factor in calcium metabolism.

CLINICAL CONSIDERATIONS
Prominent Clinical Signs And Symptoms

Symptoms	Possible Etiological Background:
1. Symptoms referable to deviations in calcium metabolism, such as: 2. Pain of arthritis, stiff joints and sore muscles. 3. Prostate disease (Nocturia, dribbling, leg and back pains, painful coitus, etc. 4. Gonads (male hormone) (Male climacteric, loss of libido, aging processes)	Loss of sex hormone activity at the climacteric and inability of the thyroid (and adrenals) to compensate in respect to calcium metabolism is a frequent cause of disturbance in calcium metabolism and may be a source of considerable discomfort of both sexes. The prostate gland is a rich source of phosphatase, an enzyme which metabolizes calcium. Phosphatase, otherwise, is found in highest amounts in growing bone tissue. All of which points to the likelihood of deficiency of this factor in the aged.

Symptom Characteristics: Pain, particularly the transient variety, is, we find, frequently related to disturbances in calcium metabolism for which **Prost-X** has proved clinically effective in some cases.

Note: We frequently find cases where calcium administration not only fails to relieve obvious calcium deficiency symptoms, but actually seems to aggravate them. This most often occurs in the patient with a sex hormone problem, particularly prominent in the climacteric, and calls for the calcium metabolizers of which **Prost-X** may be important in either sex, judging results by clinical response.

Laboratory and Clinical Tests REMARKS: While the serum phosphatase rises when metastasis to bone occurs laboratory tests which may be applied to the deficiency state

Administration	**Dosage:** 1 to 3 per day, as determined by symptomatic response.
	Effect: Prompt when indicated, pain from this cause being usually relieved within a few hours; libido often quickly restored; prostate disease (hypertrophy) benefited.
	Side Effect: Prostate phosphatase has, in some cases, been known to aggravate muscular cramps; therefore, tillandsia has been added to supply hormone precursors of the Vitamin E complex to offset this effect.

Synergists:	Activity Contributed:
Vitamin F Complex	Calcium diffusing influence
Prostate Cytotrophin	Local nutritional environment of cells
Pituitary Cytotrophin	Trophic influence on endocrines

GENERAL CONSIDERATIONS

Considerations are as follows:

1. While considered as a valuable adjunct in prostate disorders, it may also be used as an adjunct in either sex where symptomatic response is evident as phosphatase, its contained enzyme, is a calcium metabolizer.
2. Indicated, along with synergists, in male sex hormone deficiency syndrome, particularly when accompanied with symptoms of hypothyroidism.

CLINICALLY ASSOCIATED CONDITIONS

METABOLIC DISORDERS	EXOGENIC DISORDERS	MALE DISORDERS
Arthritis, Rheumatoid Bones, Pain in Bursitis	<u>Traumatic</u> Pain, Nutritional Aspects	Prostate Diseases

ASSOCIATED PRODUCTS:

Prostate Cytotrophin: The effects of **Prost-X** are independent of activity of the prostate, containing as it does, the enzymatic principles involved. **Prostate Cytotrophin**, on the other hand, contains the protomorphogen principles which influence the local nutritional environment of the cell and depends upon the response of the organ to these factors. (See Page, 151, **Prostate PMG**)

PROTEFOOD

Label: Contains food protein concentrates high in heat labile amino acids known to be essential to life, plus 60 mg. per capsule of Ribo-Nucleic acid. One capsule per day is considered maximum by the maker as necessary to improve the amino acid pattern of the average diet.

Tissue or Function Supported Protein metabolism.

CLINICAL CONSIDERATIONS
Prominent Clinical Signs and Symptoms

Symptoms:	Possible Etiological Background
1. Debilitation (Emaciation, weight loss, recuperation, decreased appetite and others)	Where dietary deficiency of protein is not the problem, may be due to inability to metabolize protein because of incomplete amino acid pattern.
2. Flabbiness of Flesh (hanging flesh, looseness, wasting, particularly under arms and abdomen)	May be dietary deficiency, usually complicated by diminished gastric secretion (proteolytic enzymes of pancreas) as well as protein metabolism deviations.
3. Chronic Fatigue (Usually accompanied by decreased appetite, loss of taste for meat)	Incomplete amino acid pattern preventing utilization of proteins of the blood by tissues.
4. Edema (Ascites, swollen ankles, water-logged tissues, etc.)	Hydrostatic pressure of blood secondary to protein metabolism.
5. Muscular Weakness (Also atrophy)	Protein metabolism insufficiency.

Symptom Characteristics: Syndrome progresses through following stages: first, fatigue, next loss of appetite and finally wasting of tissues (with or without edema). Muscle cells are particularly concerned. Deficiency frequently accompanies anemia and may be considered pathognomonic of achlorhydria, where dietary deficiency is not the problem.

Laboratory Tests	Test: Creatine (Urine)	Need Shown By: Normal value about 3 to 7 (except during menstruation, pregnancy, postnatal and in children). Increased excretion is found in muscular wasting.
Clinical Tests	Test: Physical Examination	Need Shown By: Evidence of muscular dystrophy, weakness, flabbiness, etc.
Administration	**Dosage:** One per day seems maximum required to produce optimum benefits.	
	Effect: Appetite improvement and relief of fatigue may be immediate. Long-term usage may be required in profound deviations in protein metabolism as in wasting diseases.	
	Side Effects: None known	

Synergists:	Activity Contributed:
a. Zypan	Digestive catalyst
b. Nutrimere	Dietary protein source
c. Calcium Lactate	Low serum calcium is usually found in hypoproteinemia.

GENERAL CONSIDERATIONS

The following points are to be considered in application to clinical problems:

1. Where the diet is high in low quality proteins and does not furnish a complete amino acid pattern, these incomplete amino acids may be absorbed and carried by the bloodstream but are not utilized by the tissues because of their incomplete structural pattern. This may result in a high blood viscosity with such symptoms as decreased appetite, loss of muscular tone, and circulatory disturbances.

PROTEFOOD

GENERAL CONSIDERATIONS

2. Protefood in such circumstances has the effect of completing the amino acid pattern which promotes utilization of the protein by the tissues. (This may result in a temporary drop of the plasma protein level, a physiological effect).

3. By the same line of reasoning, Protefood is especially helpful where a high protein intake places extra demands upon the utilization of protein.

4. The function of Protefood is, therefore not to supply quantitative amounts of protein to the dietary economy (which should be obtained from the diet), but rather to promote utilization of ingested proteins as described above.

5. A marked tonic effect is often produced by the use of this product-patients noticing less requirement for sleep, increased stamina, and appetite improvement.

CLINICALLY ASSOCIATED CONDITIONS

NERVOUS AND PSYCHOGENIC
   Functional
      Asthenia
   Metabolic
      Alcoholism
   Mentality
      Backwardness in children

METABOLIC DISORDERS
   Growth and Repair
      Aging Processes
      Deafness
      Healing, Promotion of
      Nails, Integrity of
   Intermediate Processes
      Protein Metabolism
   Collagen Diseases
      Bones, Pain in

METABOLIC DISORDERS
   Water-Balance
      Edema
   Blood
      Anemia
      Epistaxis
      Leukopenia
   Body Weight
      Appetite Decreased

EXOGENIC DISORDERS
   Traumatic
      Stroke, Recovery from

VASCULAR DISORDERS
   Circulatory Disorders
      Bed Sores
      Cold Hands and Feet
      Leg Ulcers

GLANDULAR
   Sterility

RENATROPHIN PMG

(KIDNEY CYTOTROPHIN)

Label: Cytotrophic Extract of Beef Kidney—A tissue extract intended to supply the specific determinants of the above mentioned organ and to aid in improving the local nutritional environment for the organ. For experimental use in cooperation with conventional Therapeutic methods. One to three tablets per day, or as directed. (One per day should be maximum dosage for first week).

Tissue or Function Supported — Kidney tissue.

CLINICAL CONSIDERATIONS
Prominent Clinical Signs And Symptoms

Symptoms:

1. Urinary Symptoms (Burning sensations, variation in urine volume, urinary incompetence, etc.)
2. Fluid Balance (Edema, ascites, localized edema, ankles, eyes, etc., pitting edema)
3. Blood Pressure Changes (Hypertension and severe hypotension, below 75 mm. Systolic)
4. Toxemia (Uremia, kidney overload)
5. Anemia (Found in chronic nephritis)
6. Reflex Pains (Back and leg pains)

Possible Etiological Background:

Widely rated as most important organ in homeostasis and, in this respect, two functions are outstanding, 1) maintenance of acid-base balance and, 2) elimination of toxic wastes. At lower levels of dysfunction, the systemic evidence is usually vague due to the vast reserve capacity of this organ. However, this obscurity of symptoms should not be allowed to minimize the important keystone position that the kidney holds in the armament of the bodies defenses. Support of liver function (protein metabolism) and Vitamin A (epithelial factor) should be considered in all cases of kidney dysfunction.

Symptom Characteristics: **Symptom Characteristics:** History usually shows recurrent attacks as well as liver dysfunction, in addition to obvious urinary symptoms. Demineralization, fluid balance, acid-base disorders, toxemia and hyperirritability are also indicative.

	Test:	Need Shown By:
Laboratory Tests	Urinalysis	Albuminuria, cells, casts, etc.
Clinical Tests	a. Hydrion Papers b. Uristix	Persistent alkaline or acid urine Albuminuria
Administration	**Dosage:** 1 to 3 per day.	
	Effect: Laboratory tests important to check progress. Diuresis may be produced in some cases. Synergistic support is important.	
	Side Effect: None known	

Synergists:	Activity Contributed:
Vitamin A-C-P Complex	Epithelial and connective tissue integrity
Chlorophyll Complex (perles)	Detoxification and healing
Betacol	Liver metabolism
Arginex	Kidney overload (enzyme factors)
Vitamin G Complex	Cell proliferation
Vitamin F Complex	Calcium diffusing factors

Note: While the above synergists are listed in the order of their usual importance, any or all of these synergists may be of primary importance in any one case. Where immediate results are lacking, therefore, we suggest the eventual results are lacking, therefore, we suggest the eventual schedule to be extended to include as wide variety of these synergists as practicable.

GENERAL CONSIDERATIONS

The physiological functions of the kidney include the following:

1. Homeostasis (retention and excretion of metabolites)

RENATROPHIN PMG

GENERAL CONSIDERATIONS

2. Maintaining acid-base balance (most important organ)
3. Regulation of fluid balance
4. Excretion of waste products of metabolism

The nutritional effects of **Kidney Cytotrophin** may be listed as follows:

1. Indicated in almost all hypertensive patients because of closely associated kidney problems. The hypotensive patient also ahs increased need for kidney support because of possible lack of blood supply to this part.
2. Useful as a prophylaxis in recurrent nephritis.
3. Allergic reactions, trauma, shock, and burns place extra stress on kidney function, indicating need for support to this organ.
4. In *Practical Endocrinology* by Harrower (page, 592) an interesting review of the edema of myxedema (hypothyroidism) as related to thyroid function is discussed. The reviewer of kidney pathology (nephritis, specifically) should find these observations as meritorious avenues of investigation.

CLINICALLY ASSOCIATED CONDITIONS

GASTROINTESTINAL-URINARY
    Kidney and Bladder
        Albuminuria
        Kidney Stones
        Nephritis
        Urinary Incompetence
        Uremia
NERVOUS AND PSYCHOGENIC
    Functional
        Sweat Gland Activity
    Vasomotor
        Blood Pressure Changes

METABOLIC DISORDERS
    Intermediate Processes
        Salt Metabolism
    Collagen
        Gout
    Acid-Base Balance
        Acidosis
        Alkalosis
        Urine, pH of
    Water Balance
        Ascites
        Dropsy
        Edema

RIBO-NUCLEIC ACID (RNA)

Label: Ribo-Nucleic Acid from Yeast; prepared for nutritional use. Probable maximum dosage 1 to 2 tablets per day.

Tissue or Function Supported   Protein metabolism.

CLINICAL CONSIDERATIONS
Prominent Clinical Signs And Symptoms

<u>Symptoms:</u>
1. Hypothyroid symptoms (Coldness of extremities, coarse hair, thick skin, inability to tolerate stress)
2. Emaciation (Prominence of bones or rib cage, weight loss)
3. Lowered resistance (Frequent colds, fevers of long standing nature)

<u>Possible Etiological Background:</u>
The mechanism of protein synthesis for tissue use is believed to be dependent upon ribonucleic acid metabolism and the integrity of the protein complex where this factor is deficient may account for the observed clinical results.

Symptom Characteristics: The nature is such that tissue integrity, particularly muscle tissue, and the metabolic processes are usually the only clinical manifestation of need.

	Test:	Need Shown By:
Laboratory Tests	Creatine	Excretion, pathologically
Clinical Tests	Weight Check	Progressive loss indicates possible need; gain shows response to therapy.

Administration	**Dosage:**	Dosage should be doubled every day until 12 tablets per day are used if necessary to obtain control of symptom of cold hands and feet.
	Effect:	Often very important in promoting normal thyroid function; cold hands and feet may quickly clear on adequate dosage, emaciation symptoms require longer periods.
	Side Effect:	None known.

<u>Synergists:</u>
a. Protefood
b. Thytrophin
c. Pituitrophin

<u>Activity Contributed:</u>
Protein Metabolism Factors
Local Nutritional Environment of Cells
Trophic Effects of Pituitary

GENERAL CONSIDERATIONS

General considerations are as follows:
1. Nucleic acid is normally found in all cell cytoplasm. It is part of the protomorphogen complex of every living cell, assuming its role in the enzymatic structure in relation to protein synthesis.
2. Leukocytosis is inhibited by nucleic acid deficiency. Therefore, Nucleic Acid may be important when infections are present, especially chronic infections or fevers of long standing.
3. We have found that people susceptible to colds usually build up resistance to colds by the use of this product.
4. Most important use, however, is to improve thyroid activity in patients with lowered metabolism who complain of cold extremities and have difficulty keeping warm.

CLINICALLY ASSOCIATED CONDITIONS

NERVOUS AND PSYCHOGENIC
   <u>Functional</u>
      Asthenia
METABOLIC DISORDERS
   <u>Blood</u>
      Leukopenia

EXOGENIC DISORDERS
   <u>Infections</u>
      Febrile Diseases
VASCULAR DISORDERS
   <u>Circulatory</u>
      Cold Hands and Feet

RIBO-NUCLEIC ACID (RNA)

SOYBEAN LECITHIN PERLES

Label: 385 mgs. perles containing 200 mgs. of Lecithin per perle.

Tissue or Function Supported Nerve, blood and fat metabolism (cholesterol antagonist)

CLINICAL CONSIDERATIONS
Prominent Clinical Signs And Symptoms

Symptoms:	Possible Etiological Background:
1. Joint-muscle symptoms (Stiffness of joints, particularly mornings; bursitis, cramps, soreness, myositis, etc.)	Possible phosphorus deficiency states related to calcium carbonate deposits and viscosity of synovial fluids.
2. Vasomotor disturbances (Hypertension and hypotension)	Related to transportation of fat and its deposition, also, neurological integrity in which lecithin may participate as nerve factor.
3. Digestive symptoms (Gallbladder syndrome, nausea, intolerance to fats, etc.)	Lecithin compliments the action of bile by its emulsifying properties, as well as promoting nerve integrity for establishment of neurological control.
4. Mental symptoms (Arteriosclerotic syndrome, irritability, repetitiousness, depression, forgetfulness and others)	Associated with the circulatory mechanisms, probably impaired by cholesterol deposition in areas governing blood supply to brain.
5. Lowered metabolism (Fatigue, emaciation, "nervousness", etc.)	Lecithin contains phosphorus and choline, lipotrophic factors related to thyroid function, both of which may be deficient in the hypothyroid case, usually attended with secondary liver dysfunction and anemia--low blood protein as well.

Symptom Characteristics: Distinct clinical manifestations of lecithin deficiency states are not clearly defined. It should be considered as a reliable factor in all arteriosclerotic cases and as a valuable adjunct in gallbladder and liver disorders involving the neurological mechanisms, valued clinically in these respects for its ability to produce a tonic effect.

	Test:	Need Shown By:
Laboratory Tests	Total Cholesterol	Normal range. 120 to 260 mg/100 cc. Elevated values show need for lecithin, found in xanthomatosis, certain liver diseases and hypothyroidism.

	Test:	Need Shown By:
Clinical Tests	a. Reflex tests	Particularly diminished gagging reflex
	b. Range of motion	"Stretch" tests (leg, shoulder, back, etc.)
	c. Skin examination	Abnormal fat-like growths
	d. X-Ray	"Spurs"
	e. Sulkowitch Reagent	Clear solution

Administration	**Dosage:** 6 per day or as directed. This dosage may be used routinely and has been found adequate to produce satisfactory results.
	Effect: The tonic effect and improvement in joint stiffness are usually evident within two weeks; however, no "dramatic" effects are to be expected from the use of this product, long-term use being required for best results.
	Side Effect: Ordinarily Lecithin produces no side-effects. However, because of its high phosphorus content its use must be considered in conditions where this factor may aggravate decalcification or an already elevated phosphorus level such as in osteoporosis, hyperthyroidism, latter stages of pregnancy (when phosphorus levels are believed to be increased), elevated metabolism and others.

SOYBEAN LECITHIN PERLES

Synergists:	Activity Contributed:
1. Ferrofood	Antianemia factor
2. Cyruta Cholesterol metabolism	
3. A&F with Betafood	Bile-thinning factor

GENERAL CONSIDERATIONS

The principle constituents of Lecithin are choline and phosphorus. See **Choline** and **Phosfood** Bulletins for further information applying to these constituents.

The nutritional effects of Lecithin may be considered as follows:

1. Lecithin acts as an emulsifier of fats. Thus, in the local environment of the intestinal tract it supplements the emulsifying action of bile, promoting the absorption of fat-soluble vitamins and aiding in fat digestion. Systemically it acts as a transporter of fats and is a cholesterol antagonist.
2. Lecithin is a constituent of cell membrane where its counterpart is cholesterol to which it is antagonistic.
3. Choline, one of its constituents, acts as a lipotrophic agent and through its physiological detergent effect promotes capillary circulation.
4. Due to common excess use of saturated fats, Lecithin is widely indicated, especially in hypercholesterolemia with its associated hypertension and arteriosclerotic involvements.
5. Lecithin has been reported as a remedy for anemia.
6. Lecithin has a known tonic effect which is particularly enhanced in the geriatric patient.

CLINICALLY ASSOCIATED CONDITIONS

NERVOUS AND PSYCHOGENIC
   Functional
      Asthenia
      Hyperirritability
      Nervous Strain
   Metabolic
      Torticollis
   Vasomotor
      Blood Pressure Changes
      Dizziness
      Hypotension
METABOLIC DISORDERS
   Growth and Repair
      Aging Processes
   Intermediate Processes
      Carbohydrate Metabolism
      Diabetes Mellitus
      Cholesterol Metabolism
METABOLIC DISORDERS
   Collagen Diseases
      Arcus Senilis
      Arteriosclerosis
      Arthritis, Hypertrophic
      Bursitis

Collagen Diseases
   Cataracts
   Collagen Diseases
   Disc Lesions
Acid-Base Balance
   Alkalosis
Blood
   Anemia
Body Weight
   Obesity
VASCULAR DISORDERS
   Circulatory Diseases
      Buerger's Disease
      Intermittent Claudication   Phlebitis
   Heart Disorders
      Myocarditis
SKIN DISORDERS
   Psoriasis

ASSOCIATED PRODUCT:
Phosfood Liquid: (See notes Under Associated Products, Product Bulletin on **Phosfood**, page, 143).

SPLEEN PMG

Label: Cytotrophic Extract of Beef Spleen—A tissue extract intended to supply the specific determinant factors of the above mentioned organ, and to aid in improving the local nutritional environment for that organ. For experimental use in cooperation with conventional therapeutic methods. Mfg. under Patent No. 2,374,219. One to three tablets per day, as directed. (One per day should be maximum dosage for first week.)

Tissue or Function Supported	Spleen

CLINICAL CONSIDERATIONS
Prominent Clinical Signs And Symptoms

Symptoms:	Possible Etiological Background:
1. Allergic Reactions (Hives, canker sores, cold blisters, etc.)	Control of mineral metabolism disturbances in allergic reactions is considered possible.
2. Lymph Node Swelling (Neck, breasts, groin, etc.)	Relation to lymphatic system is noted.
3. Edema (Transient variety, compensatory type involving blood volume)	Regulatory effect on blood volume.
4. Blood Dyscrasias (Anemia, polycythermia, lymphocytosis, leukopenia, etc.)	Believed to be a factor in control of hemoglobin and R.B.C.'s.
5. Demineralization (Hyperirritability most common finding)	Possible relation to colloidal state in mineral metabolism.
6. Lowered Resistance (Susceptibility to infections, boils, etc.)	Possible relation to activity of leukocytes.

Symptom Characteristics: Involvements of R.E. system are most common findings (lymphatic system, blood integrity). Fluid balance (edema) and allergic reactions are also indicative.

	Test:	Need Shown By:
Laboratory Tests	Blood Count (Differential)	Deviations from normal findings
Clinical Tests	a. Palpation b. Examination	Lymph node swelling, spleen enlargement Hydration or dehydration

Administration	**Dosage:** 1 to 3 per day.
	Effect: Difficult to evaluate by symptoms of patient.
	Side Effect: None known.

Synergists:	Activity Contributed:
a. Thymex	Aids in phagocytosis
b. Cataplex A-C-P	Epithelial-Connective Tissue Factors

GENERAL CONSIDERATIONS

The following are extracts from *Practical Endocrinology*, Henry R. Harrower, M.D., pages 181 to 183:Harrower reports functions as follows:

1) Disposal of red blood cells
2) Generator of leukocytes
3) Development of immunity
4) Resistance to infection
5) Action on intestinal peristalsis
6) Metabolism of iron

"The nutritional influence of spleen therapy, mentioned many times in the literature, is not explained by specific effect that it possesses. The explanation of Charles Bayle, now of Paris, is original, his conclusions being based on years of patient experimentation on animals while carrying on an extensive consulting practice at Cannes on the Riviera. Bayle's theory is this:

SPLEEN PMG

GENERAL CONSIDERATIONS

The blood contains the mineral elements in two forms:

1) Those in colloid state suitable for cellular appropriation and thus not suited for elimination by the kidneys, and

2) The mineral cellular wastes, which are dissolved in the plasma and destined for elimination.

If these elements lose their colloidal form, they are promptly eliminated, and a condition of demineralization obtains. The capacity to maintain the mineral salts in a colloidal state is evidently of considerable importance, and, according to Bayle, its regulation seems to belong to the spleen.

On page 182: (Studies cited to show influence of spleen action simulating activity of parathyroid hormone). Removal of the spleen from dogs was followed by hypocalcemia. When a desiccated spleen extract was fed to these splenectomized dogs, the low calcium index was promptly raised to normal, although identical treatment to parathyroidectomized dogs had no such effect on the calcium figure.

Quoting from the journal of the American Medical Association (Sept. 27, 1930, xcv, P. 182 & 937):

From the studies here discussed it appears that the spleen is likewise concerned in calcium metabolism. Furthermore, it appears that the results might even be interpreted to mean that, in the absence of the parathyroid glands, the spleen can take over their function in preventing tetany. These intricate relationships between organ systems illustrate the ends to which the organism as a whole will go in order to preserve the vital equilibrium; furthermore they indicate, in some measure, the inherent difficulties in outlining effective therapy."

Our observations on the above data: In "An Introduction to Protomorptiology", by Royal Lee, it is stated that it is the mineral component of the protein which produces the reaction in allergic states…and that a protein which has lost its mineral component (as Bayles outlines above) is denatured. Further that these mineral components as combined proteins (enzymes known as protomorphogens and Natural Tissue Antibodies) are active principles regulating the processes of growth and repair and the important principle of the allergic reaction as it pertains to these processes. (A discussion in greater detail is given in the above mentioned booklet.) The influence of spleen on calcium metabolism may be but one manifestation of these principles, which could theoretically be extended to include all of the colloidal trace minerals active as combined minerals in the various enzyme systems. Investigation along these lines may reveal a much wider application of spleen therapy than has been suggested here.

CLINICALLY ASSOCIATED CONDITIONS

GASTROINTESTINAL-URINARY
   Liver and Gallbladder
      Hepatitis
      Jaundice
      Liver Disease
NERVOUS AND PSYCHOGENIC
   Functional
      Colitis, Ulcerative
      Epilepsy
      Migraine Headaches
METABOLIC DISORDERS
   Blood
      Anemia, Pernicious
      Leukopenia

Allergies
   Histamine Reactions
   Hives
EXOGENIC DISORDERS
   Infections
      Febrile Diseases
      Lymph Node Infections
   Toxic
      Boils
SKIN CONDITIONS
   Pruritis
   Psoriasis

ASSOCIATED PRODUCTS:

Ferrofood: (See Product Bulletin on **Ferrofood**, page, 97).

SUPER-EFF

Label: Vitamin F2 Complex, as unsaturated fatty acids in natural forms from beef and flax lipids. A product not accepted at this time by official opinion as having nutritional importance. Suggested dosage: 1 to 3 capsules per day.

Tissue or Function Supported Promotes the availability of hydrolysable inorganic phosphorus to form phosphogen and adenosine triphosphate.

CLINICAL CONSIDERATIONS
Prominent Clinical Signs And Symptoms

<u>Symptoms:</u>

1. Energy Mechanisms (Neurological response as related to such reactions as:
    a. Tachycardia
    b. Pruritis
    c. Appetite loss
    d. Nausea
2. Chromosome Insulation (Toxic reactions as related to intercellular mechanisms as:
    a. Myositis
    b. Allergic
    c. Inflammatory
    d. Nephritis
    e. Lymphatic
    f. Anemia
3. Healing Mechanisms Determinant integrity as related to:
    a. Atrophy
    b. Emaciation

<u>Possible Etiological Background</u>

Because of the cyclic nature of the reactions concerned with the metabolism of adenosine triphosphate (ATP), the tracing of these reactions assumes gigantic biochemical proportions as given in the Kreb's cycle. These pathways, though of little more than academic interest to the clinician, provide the means whereby energy is produced within the muscle cell, and probably of significance in nerve reactions as well. While little is known about these extremely complicated reactions, it is obvious that nutritional support must play an important role. In this respect, F2 or Super-EFF. has provided much clinical evidence to show that its role, in part, is in providing enzyme precursors which assist in establishing its integrity.

Symptom Characteristics: Muscular tissue-the inter-cellular metabolism—is concerned, clinically manifest by rate, degree of activity or nutrition to the muscle fiber cells.

	Test:	Need Shown By:
Laboratory Tests	Creatine Test (Urine)	Presence pathologically
Clinical Tests	Therapeutic Test	Administration of 1 or 2 Super-EFF capsules in tachycardia shows appreciable decrease in rate in 20 minutes.
Administration	**Dosage:** 1 to 3 per day depending upon clinical evidence of response.	
	Effect: Usually immediate in tachycardia and loss of appetite when due to this cause. In other conditions, response takes longer and is more dependent upon synergists as listed below.	
	Side Effect: None known.	

<u>Synergists:</u>   <u>Activity Contributed:</u>
 a. Myotrophin}
 b. Organic Minerals}   See "Neuromuscular Disorders" in the Therapeutic Foods Manual
 c. Cataplex G}
 d. Inositol}

GENERAL CONSIDERATIONS

The nutritional effects may be listed as follows:
1. Acts as an insulating layer or wrapper for the determinant factors that guide the reactions of healing and construction, an important factor in anemia's for example.
2. The above effect has been found clinically useful in promotion of healing and inflammatory conditions, particularly those involving the lymphatic system.

SUPER-EFF

GENERAL CONSIDERATIONS

3. Apparently synergistic with Inositol which has a potentiating effect in the energy mechanisms (ATP) of the muscle tissue as evidenced by beneficial effect in tachycardia.
4. Benefits as an alterative as evidenced by improvement of poor appetite, one of the first signs of impaired health.

CLINICALLY ASSOCIATED CONDITIONS

NERVOUS AND PSYCHOGENIC
    Functional
        Tachycardia
    Metabolic
        Neuro-Muscular Disorders
METABOLIC
    Growth and Repair
        Healing, Promotion of
    Blood
        Anemias
    Body Weight
        Appetite Decreased

EXOGENIC
    Inflammation
        Mastitis
VASCULAR
    Circulatory
        Tinnitus Aurium
SKIN CONDITIONS
    Pruritis
    Purpura
GLANDULAR
    Sterility

THYMEX

Label: Enzymatic Extract of the Bovine Thymus Gland. Each tablet represents approximately 3 grams of fresh glandular material in enzymatic activity. For experimental use in determining its value in correcting states of metabolic unbalance due to malnutrition. Mfg. Under U. S. Patent No. 2,374,219. 1 to 3 tablets per day or as directed.

Tissue or Function Supported Intended to promote phagocytic and lymphatic activity-and thus stimulate healing and defense against bacterial invasion.

CLINICAL CONSIDERATIONS
Prominent Clinical Signs And Symptoms

Symptoms:	Possible Etiological Background:
1. Skin Conditions (Infectious psoriasis, boils, acne, ulcers)	Lymphatic activity and healing process.
2. Infectious Conditions (Particularly bone, mastoiditis, osteomyelitis, etc.)	Phagocytosis and resistance factors.
3. Healing (Exuberant granulation tissue, festers, chronic lesions)	Healing reactions.
4. Allergic Reactions (Intolerance to milk, particularly children)	Antibody integrity.
5. Inflammatory Conditions (Mastitis, tonsillitis, rheumatoid arthritis, etc.)	Lymphatic activity.
6. Hyperglandular Activity (Hyperthyroidism, hyperadrenal, etc.)	Regulatory influence in these situations, according to clinical reports.

Symptom Characteristics: Follow same pattern taken by the mechanisms of healing, resistance, and glandular hyperactivity.

	Test:	Need Shown By:
Laboratory Tests	Blood	Leukopenia
Clinical Tests	Blood pressure	Increase
	Temperature Pulse	Increase
	Palpation	Lymph node congestion
	Observation	Skin lesions

Administration	**Dosage:** 1 to 3 per day, long-term use should be recommended, continuing administration after initial benefits as a prophylactic measure.
	Effect: Usually shows benefits within one week, although up to three weeks should be given before evaluation this effectiveness.
	Side Effect: These are of very low incidence. Mild fever may occur in some types of low grade infections; fatigue may be aggravated in hypoglandular conditions, indicating need for Drenatrophin or Drenamin.

Synergists:	Activity Contributed:
1. Chlorophyll Complex	Support of detoxification systems
2. Cataplex A-C-P	Epithelial and connective tissue integrity
3. Calcium Lactate	Ionized calcium source
4. Pituitrophin	Trophic influence on endocrines
5. Super-EFF	Cell protective phospholipids aid in healing processes

GENERAL CONSIDERATIONS

Despite the fact that the thymus plays a decided part in the endocrine balance, as yet virtually no leading endocrinologist will admit that the thymus is an endocrine organ. One consideration is that the physiology of the thymus has had to be studied largely in connection with abnormalities. For example, it has been suggested that since studies made by autopsy have been largely on diseased bodies, that the normal thymus may be quite active and evident. We can state that it is becoming increasingly evident to us that the postulated effects by investigators over 30 years ago seem to be born out by clinical observations made after the introduction of more potent extracts.

THYMEX

GENERAL CONSIDERATIONS

Thus, we may divide our general considerations into two phases: first, those effects we have observed from actual clinical application of these extracts, and, second, those which have been postulated, as follows:

Clinical results which have been observed and have been favorable in the following:

1. Skin conditions, particularly those involving infection, such as infectious psoriasis.
2. Bone conditions, particularly osteomyelitis.
3. Infectious states, particularly lymphatic stasis.

Postulated effects reported in *Practical Endocrinology*—by Harrower—

Page 190: "By six or seven years" (of age) "the thymus is a negligible 'rest', essentially epithelial in character, this may be 'resurrected', however, in certain cases of hyperthyroidism.

Page 191: "In experimental animals with the thymus removed the muscles are flabby, the animals are pasty and bloated…and become sedentary in their habits. The gait is awkward and the bones bend under the weight of the body, so that the dogs have clumsy squat appearance. The appetite is increased, and the animals eat voraciously without discrimination.

Page 193: "With the idea that the internal secretion of the true thymus is locked up in the giant epithelial cells, and on the supposition that this thymic internal secretion preserves normal epithelial health throughout the body, i.e., that it controls and helps to keep up normal epithelial growth and cell repair, I set myself the task of isolating the true thymic hormone.

We may make some interesting observations in regard to the above abstracts. First, we have noted clinical improvement in hyperthyroid states from the use of this product, and, of equal importance in this respect, a production of fatigue in some patients indicating either thyroid or adrenal relationship. Many references in the literature refer to bony changes and the relation of the thymus to calcium metabolism; also the increased appetite and loss of tissue integrity may be significant insofar as some types of obesity are concerned. We have made the clinical observation that obese persons rate very high as calcium deficient subjects, so the hypothesis presents itself: increased appetite, calcium deficit (hyperirritability), and obesity. Investigation of this aspect may prove thymic extracts to be of merit, although we have no clinical evidence to date. We do have clinical evidence, however, of benefits in skin disorders, tending to substantiate the epithelial premise outlined above.

The above information is provided as a profile of the areas of possible physiological effects which may provide the observer with a new perspective of its potentialities.

CLINICALLY ASSOCIATED CONDITIONS

NERVOUS AND PSYCHOGENIC
  Functional
    Colitis, Ulcerative
    Ulcers, Gastric
  Mentality
    Backwardness, in Children
METABOLIC DISORDERS
  Growth and Repair
    Osteoporosis
  Collagen Disease
    Arthritis, rheumatoid
  Blood
    Leukopenia
  Allergies
    Hives
EXOGENIC DISORDERS
  Infections
    Febrile Diseases
    Lymph Node Infections
    Pneumonia
    Rheumatic Fever

Virus Infections
  Colds, Flu, Grippe
Virus Infections
  Earache
  Herpes Simplex
  Herpes Zoster
  Lumbago
Toxic Disorders
  Boils
  Poison Ivy and Oak
  Inflammation
  Sinusitis
  Tonsillitis
Toxic Disorders
  Diarrhea
  Gingivitis
  Periodontoclasia
Traumatic
  Sedimentation Rate

THYMEX

CLINICALLY ASSOCIATED CONDITIONS

VASCULAR DISORDERS
   <u>Circulatory</u>
      Bed Sores
      Buerger's Disease
      Leg Ulcers
SKIN DISORDERS
   Acne
   Dermatitis
   Eczema
   Psoriasis

GENETIC DISORDERS
   <u>Female</u>
      Endocervicitis
      Leukorrhea
      Vaginitis

ASSOCIATED PRODUCTS:
Thymus PMG: Preferred primarily for children, particularly where intolerance to milk products is noted. Otherwise, Thymex is usual product of choice. (See Page, 171)

THYMEX

THYMUS PMG

(THYMUS CYTOTROPHIN)

Label: Cytotrophic Extract of Beef Thymus—A tissue extract intended to supply the specific determinant factors of the above mentioned organ and to aid in improving the local nutritional environment for that organ. For experimental use in cooperation with conventional Therapeutic Methods. One to three tablets per day, or as directed. (One per day should be maximum dosage for first week.)

Tissue or Function Supported   Thymus

CLINICAL CONSIDERATIONS
Prominent Clinical Signs And Symptoms

Symptoms:
1. Debilitating Diseases (Myasthenia gravis, muscular weakness, etc.)
2. Hyperthyroidism (Grave's Disease)
3. Leukopenia

Possible Etiological Background:
It is known that changes occur in thymus tissue during periods of stress, atrophy being observable. Autopsies on the healthy body—soldiers during World War II—revealed a much larger thymus gland than was considered normal by prior methods taken largely on diseased bodies. Thymocytes—the thymus cell—resembled lymphocytes. These may break down in great numbers during illness and provide mechanism for the immune reaction…closely related to the allergic reaction.

Symptom Characteristics: Follow pattern of resistance to stress, thus may arise following severe mental or physical stress.

Laboratory Tests and Clinical: None known.

Administration
- **Dosage:** See label.
- **Effect:** At least three weeks should be given before evaluating its effectiveness.
- **Side Effect:** Rare but occurrence may be related to adrenal glands, indicating need for Adrenamin.

Synergists:	Activity Contributed:
a. Vitamin A-C-P Complex	Epithelial and Connective Tissue Integrity
b. Calcium Lactate	Ionizable calcium
c. Pituitary Cytotrophin	Trophic Influence on Endocrines

GENERAL CONSIDERATIONS

Note: The enzymatic extract of Thymus, **Thymex**, is often effective where the glands fail to respond to Thymus Cytotrophin. (See Product Bulletin on **Thymex** for details.) Generally, the **Thymus Cytotrophin** is indicated in the younger patient, **Thymex** in the older.

CLINICALLY ASSOCIATED CONDITIONS

NERVOUS AND PSYCHOGENIC
   Mentality
      Underdeveloped children
METABOLIC DISORDERS
   Growth and Repair
      Osteoporosis
   Blood
      Leukopenia

EXOGENIC DISORDERS
   Infections
      Febrile diseases
   Virus Infections
      Colds, flu, grippe, etc.
   Toxic Conditions
      Boils
   Inflammation
      Sinusitis
      Tonsillitis
      Gingivitis, etc.

VASCULAR DISORDERS
   Circulatory
      Bed sores
      Leg ulcers
SKIN DISORDERS
      Acne
      Hermatitis, etc.

THYMUS PMG

THYTROPHIN PMG

Label: Cytotrophic Extract of Thyroid—A tissue extract intended to supply the specific determinant factor of the above mentioned organ, and to aid in improving the local nutritional environment for that organ. For experimental use in cooperation with conventional Therapeutic Methods. Manufactured under U.S. Patent No. 2,374,219. One to three tablets per day, as directed. (One per day should be maximum dosage for first week.)

Tissue or Function Supported   Thyroid Gland

CLINICAL CONSIDERATIONS
Prominent Clinical Signs And Symptoms

Reference is made to Therapeutic Foods Manual under "Signs and Symptoms" where complete discussion of clinical picture of thyroid aberrations is given. The following data pertains to classical symptoms of hypo-and hyperthyroidism:

Symptoms:

A. HYPERTHYROIDISM

1. Tachycardia (Found in 100% of cases, pathognomonic sign)
2. Tremors (Particularly tremors of protruding tongue)
3. Sweating (Tendency to moist skin, particularly palms of hands and soles of feet)
4. Weight Loss (General distribution, increased appetite and linear build)
5. Vertigo (Balance mechanism, ability to balance on one leg standing on chair)
6. Personality Stability (Frightened appearance, intensity outstanding, venture conscious)

Possible Etiological Background:

As would be expected in an elevated metabolic state, phosphorus (the acid mineral) is predominant over calcium (alkaline). As a general rule, cholesterol may be expected to be decreased or normal; fat, however, high in localized deposits, behind eyeballs, for example. Calcium loss is characteristics (Sulkowitch Reagent test). Iodine (or thyroxin according to the Protein Bound Iodine Test) i.e., blood iodine or circulating thyroid hormone is usually high. These biochemical circumstances are discussed hypothetically under "Clinical Considerations" which follow. The point to be made here is that through the above mechanisms, the pathological manifestations of hyperthyroidism are expressed, i.e., as fibrosis or fatty deposits, oxygenation increased (increased B.M.R.), hyperirritability (calcium loss), etc.

Symptom Characteristics: Tachycardia is most outstanding finding. The characteristic intensity shown by personality presentation is usually easily recognized; exopthalmia may or may not be present.

Symptoms:

B. HYPOTHYROIDISM

1) Weight Gain (Particularly upper body, breasts and arms)
2) Mental Dullness (Inability to work under mental stress and strain)
3) Hair and Skin Symptoms (Coarse hair, thick skin, thick lips and tongue)
4) Lowered Temperature (Cold hands and feet, need for more warmth than average person, etc.)
5) Parasthesias (Numbness, tingling sensations)
6) Fingernails (Ridged, thick, brittle)

Possible Etiological Background:

Pathognomonic of hypothyroidism is an elevated cholesterol the remainder of the findings listed above are in the main, the opposite of hyperthyroidism i.e., elevated calcium in relation to phosphorus, decreased blood iodine, etc. These, also, are discussed under "Clinical Considerations". The mental picture of the hypothyroid case is often the most important factor in differential diagnosis, here the outstanding quality being the inability to tolerate pressure situations and to make immediate decisions. As hypothyroidism, as usually presented clinically, is indistinct from a symptomatic viewpoint, the mental consideration may be of considerable importance.

Symptom Characteristics: The hypothyroid case may be difficult to recognize clinically, however with other significant findings, an inability to withstand mental pressure as outlined above may be the only differentiating factor.

THYTROPHIN PMG

LABORATORY AND CLINICAL TESTS: The following notes are supplied as being pertinent in the differential diagnosis and clinical management of the non-thyroid metabolic dysfunction patient and the thyroid cases.

NON-THYROID DISEASES ACCOMPANIED BY HYPERMETABOLISM SIMULATING HYPERTHYROIDISM:
1. Leukemia
2. Anxiety States
3. Cardiac Failure   INCREASED BMR - PBI NORMAL
4. Hypertension

NON-THYROID DISEASES ACCOMPANIED BY HYPOMETABOLISM SIMULATING HYPOTHYROIDISM:
1. Obesity
2. Anorexia Nervosa
3. Nephrosis   DECREASED BMR - PBI NORMAL

THYROID DYSFUNCTION ACCOMPANIED BY HYPERMETABOLISM OF VARIOUS ORIGINS:
1. Graves Disease
2. Toxic Adenoma
3. Acromegaly   INCREASED BMR - PBI INCREASED
4. Pregnancy
5. Therapy
6. Iodine or thyroxine
7. Irradiation
8. Thyrotoxicosis factitia
9. Acute Thyroiditis

THYROID DYSFUNCTION ACCOMPANIED BY HYPOTHYROIDISM OF VARIOUS ORIGINS
1. Myxedema
2. Pituitary Myxedema
3. Thyroiditis, chronic   DECREASED BMR – PBI DECREASED
4. Anti-thyroid drugs
5. Iodine deficiency states

CONDITIONS IN WHICH THE B.M.R. IS INCREASED: (Other than the above)
1. Severe pain
2. Fevers (about 7% for each degree F.)
3. Paralysis agitans
4. Chorea
5. Chills and convulsions
6. Pernicious anemia

CONDITIONS IN WHICH B.M.R. IS DECREASED: (Other than above)
1. Allergies
2. Undernutrition (fasting)
3. Chronic arthritis

A valuable screen-test to differentiate hyperthyroidism from similarly manifest diseases is to take the pulse rate during sleep. In hyperthyroidism, the rate is constant throughout the 24 hour period. In most other conditions, there is a decrease during sleep, especially true if neurosis.

Administration	**Dosage:** 1 to 3 per day, increasing dosage does not seem to produce added benefits.
	Effect: This may be obscure for the reasons outlined below under "General Considerations" and may depend upon supportive therapy as appropriate.
	Side Effect: None specifically known, however variations in pulse rate would be the specific indication, tachycardia indicating increased thyroid activity, bradycardia decreased activity

<u>Synergists:</u>   <u>Activity Contributed:</u>
a. Pituitrophin   Trophic Effects
b. Drenamin   Adrenal Support

THYTROPHIN PMG

GENERAL CONSIDERATIONS

The nutritional effects of the thyroid gland may be listed as follows:
1. Calcium-Phosphorus ratio regulator.
2. Oxygenation factor.
3. Factor in elimination of toxins.
4. Regulation factor in cellular metabolism.
5. Factor in cholesterol metabolism.

A suitable hypothesis for rationalization of thyroid therapy is presented as follows:

The relation of the activity of the thyroid with calcium-phosphorus and cholesterol metabolism is the most obvious effect to be observed.

1. In general we may say that the activity of the thyroid follows the blood levels of these as follows:

    a. Increased thyroid activity: Balance in favor of phosphorus (Increased need for calcium) Cholesterol decreased

    b. Decreased thyroid activity. Balance in favor of calcium (Increased need for phosphorus) Cholesterol increased

2. According to clinical experience the following biochemical factors act to influence thyroid function as follows:

    a. <u>Iodine:</u> Acts as a depressant for thyroid activity as evidenced by use of Lugolls (potassium iodide).Solution in hyperthyroidism.

    b. <u>Unsaturated Fatty Acids:</u> Acts to increase thyroid activity as evidenced by ability to lower blood cholesterol levels (probably through thyroid stimulation).

3. By this rationalization, iodine (Cataplex F) and calcium (Calcium Lactate) would be recommended in hyperthyroidism. And, unsaturated fatty acids without iodine added (Cataplex F Perles) and Soybean Lecithin (as source of phosphorus) would be indicated in hypothyroidism.

4. Thytrophin is indicated in both hypo- and hyperthyroidism on a clinical basis depending upon symptomatic response of patient.

While the above hypothesis is far from complete, it does form a basic range of activity which clinical experience has shown to be sound. In all cases where the thyroid is being considered, the important axis of the thyroid-adrenal-pituitary should be kept in mind. Considerable evidence exists to show that clinical disturbances manifest as thyroid problems are often superimposed burdens brought about by adrenal or pituitary dysfunction.

CLINICALLY ASSOCIATED CONDITIONS

NERVOUS AND PSYCHOGENIC
<u>Functional</u>
    Asthenia
METABOLIC DISORDERS
<u>Growth and Repair</u>
    Nails, Integrity of
<u>Collagen Diseases</u>
    Arteriosclerosis
    Arthritis, Hypertrophic
    Dupuytrens's Contracture
METABOLIC DISORDERS
<u>Blood</u>
    Leukopenia
VASCULAR DISORDERS
<u>Circulatory Diseases</u>
    Cold Hands and Feet
    Tinnitus Aurium

GENETIC DISORDERS
<u>Female Disorders</u>
    Amenorrhea
<u>Male Disorders</u>
    Prostate Disease
EXOGENIC DISORDERS
<u>Traumatic</u>
    Strictures
SPECIFIC DEFICIENCY DISEASES
<u>Glandular</u>
    Goiter
    Sterility

THYTROPHIN PMG

TRACE MINERALS B_{12}

Label: Each tablet contains: 250 mgms. Manganese B_{12}, 20 mgms. Zinc Phytate, 0.8 mgm. Copper Phytate, 5 mgms. Iodine organically combined with vegetable protein, 5.0 mcgm. Vitamin B_{12} for Organic Cobalt with organic trace mineral complex from molasses. For the correction of a nutritional deficiency of these minerals as established by diagnostic procedure. Dose: 2 to 3 daily, or as directed.

Tissue or Function Support	Enzyme system activators as related to trace mineral deficiencies.

CLINICAL CONSIDERATIONS
Prominent Clinical Signs And Symptoms

Symptoms:	Possible Etiological Background:
1. Hyperthyroid Syndrome (Tachycardia, inability to gain weight, elevated B.M.R. and pulse rate, tremors, emotional instability, etc.).	Disturbance in iodine metabolism, hyperthyroidism (usually benefited by administration of iodine).
2. Connective Tissue Integrity (Joint pains, bursitis, disc lesions, fallen arches, low back pain, etc.).	Loss of integrity of ligamentous structures in which manganese deficiency may play important role.
3. Resistance of Infections (Low grade fevers, viral infections, brucellosis, Poliomyelitis, etc.).	The reported benefits probably due to activation of enzyme systems.
4. Anemias (Blood dyscrasias, anemia)	Cobalt as B_{12}, as well as other trace minerals enter into integrity of hematopoietic system.

Symptom Characteristics: Hyperactivity of thyroid and pituitary with increased metabolic rate may be most easily observed clinical characteristics. Secondarily, anemias, infectious states and connective tissue disorders are observed as trace mineral entities.

	Test:	Need Shown By:
Laboratory Tests	Protein Bound Iodine	Over 8
	B.M.R.	Above 15+
Clinical Tests	Physical Findings Tachycardia, tremors, weight loss, emotional instability, poor balancing ability, etc.	
Administration	**Dosage:** 1 to 6 per day, higher dosage being indicated in elevated metabolic states, pulse rate criterion.	
	Effect: Varies with acuteness and chronicity of condition; generally in elevated B.M.R. effect is augmented by low-fat diet, particularly where exophthalmos is present.	
	Side Effects: Some patients are sensitive to iodine in which case **Manganese B_{12}** may be used where the consideration is ligamentous problems. Iodism is marked by eczema, coryza, excess salivation, tachycardia and weakness (thin secretions). Reactions to **Trace Minerals B_{12}** generally indicate a need for **Calcium Lactate**.	

Synergists:	Activity Contributed:
1. Vitamin E Complex, Ostogen Wafers, Soybean Lecithin, Calcifood	In connective tissue disorders.
2. Calcium Lactate	In hypermetabolic states.
3. Chlorophyll Complex (perles), and Vitamin C Complex	In infectious conditions

GENERAL CONSIDERATIONS

Trace mineral deficiency is a common occurrence. We recommend reading, "The Trace Elements" by Warren L. Anderson, LF 71, for a comprehensive review of this subject. (The author reviewed over 500 research papers and consulted more than 50 leading specialists in this field in the preparation of this article).

The clinical picture presented by commonly occurring trace mineral deficiencies is rather indistinct, however, this is beginning to clear as research continues. For example, recent reports show benefits in brucellosis, poliomyelitis and encephalitis, at least from the prophylactic viewpoint. Of course, iodine, a trace mineral has long been known to be a factor in thyroid physiology being known to be of specific value in the prevention of goiter and useful in

TRACE MINERALS B_{12}

hypermetabolic states due to thyroid dysfunction. Manganese, another trace mineral, reported to be concerned with pituitary physiology, has in our experience been shown to be beneficial in various aspects related to the treatment of collagen-type diseases, loss of integrity of fascia, ligaments and tendons, for example. It would, therefore, seem reasonable to rationalize that these trace elements are beneficial where fibrosis or sclerosis, or other changes in the connective and supportive tissues are involved.

Trace minerals are described as "enzyme system activators" and the widespread practice of administering iodine to the aged on an empirical basis with reported benefits tends to show the activating influence of at least this one trace mineral in this respect. (Note: Potassium iodide is usually given to these patients. We recommend the organic trace mineral complex as found in Trace Minerals $B_{12,}$ including iodine.).

CLINICALLY ASSOCIATED CONDITIONS

NERVOUS AND PSYCHOGENIC
   <u>Metabolic</u>
      Neuromuscular Disorders
METABOLIC DISORDERS
   <u>Collagen Diseases</u>
      Arcus Senilis
      Arteriosclerosis
      Arthritis, Hypertrophic
      Bursitis
      Cataracts
      Disc Lesions
      Ligaments, Deformity of
      Dupuytren's Contracture

EXOGENIC DISORDERS
   <u>Infections</u>
      Brucellosis
   <u>Inflammation</u>
      Sciatica
   <u>Traumatic</u>
      Strictures
GLANDULAR
      Goiter

ASSOCIATED PRODUCTS:

Prolamine Iodine: (See Product Bulletin on **Prolamine Iodine Tablets**, page, 143)

Manganese, B_{12}:   Available where these factors are desired without the contained iodine in Trace Minerals B_{12}, where the patient may be sensitized to iodine (which, incidentally, is usually the case in hypothyroidism).

USF OINTMENT

Label:	Each ounce contains 3 grams unsaturated fatty acids from flax and beef lipoids with soy lecithin, lanolin, and special lard in vehicle of soy oil and beeswax. For local application in skin disorder due to a deficiency of this vitamin. Medical authorities have not yet accepted USF Ointment (Vitamin F) as essential to human nutrition.
Tissue or Function Supported	Supplies skin lipids for its integrity.

CLINICAL CONSIDERATIONS
Prominent Clinical Signs And Symptoms

<u>Symptoms:</u>

1. Skin and Scalp Integrity (Dry skin, dandruff, brittle hair, etc.)
2. Dermatitis (Allergic eczema, irritated skin)
3. Burns (X-Ray, industrial, sunburn)
4. Infantile dermatitis (Diaper rash, etc.)
5. Chapped lips

<u>Possible Etiological Background:</u>

The normal epidermis contain cholesterol, lecithin and unsaturated fatty acids, amount them, USF Ointment. (This complex of skin factors is supplied for local application in USF Ointment). A deficiency or faulty metabolism of these factors may result in various skin disorders

Symptom Characteristics: Applied topically. Non-toxic and has no contraindication as an unguent.

GENERAL CONSIDERATIONS

Shepherd* emphasized the importance of the ratio of the skin lipids which, for the normal epidermis, are in the proportion of one part of cholesterol to one part of lecithin to three parts of total unsaturated fatty acids, among them USF Ointment. He next emphasized the value of restoring fats to the skin in the proportion intended by nature. Our formula was compounded with this ratio as a basis.

* *Reprint No. 11, "Vitamin F Ointments," Lee Foundation for Nutritional Research, gives a complete discussion of the developmental phases of this product.*

USF OINTMENT

UTROPHIN

(UTERUS CYTOTROPHIN)

Label: Cytotrophic Extract of Beef Uterus—A tissue extract intended to supply the specific determinant factors of the above mentioned organ and to aid in improving the local nutritional environment for that organ. For experimental use in cooperation with conventional Therapeutic methods. Mfg. under U.S. Patent No. 2,374,219. One to three tablets per day, or as directed. (One per day should be maximum dosage for first week).

Tissue or Function Supported	Uterus

CLINICAL CONSIDERATIONS
Prominent Clinical Signs And Symptoms

<u>Symptoms:</u>

1. History of Abortion (also threatened abortion)
2. Endocervicitis (Leukorrhea, vaginitis from this cause)
3. Uterine cysts (Chocolate cysts, fibroids, etc.)
4. Uterine displacement (Bearing down sensation, back pain when from this cause)
5. Menstruation symptoms (Excessive or scanty mense)
6. Sterility (Some types)
7. Uterine congestion (menstruation cramps, when from this cause)

<u>Possible Etiological Background:</u>

The effect of **Uterus Cytotrophin** must be considered largely from its effects on the local environment of the uterus itself. Dysfunction of uterine tissue usually involves the trophic effects of estrogens, which are governed by pituitary and liver influences, though produced by the ovaries. Thus the etiological background of uterine problems may be quite complex and all predisposing possibilities need to be considered, not the least of these may be the thyroid. However, regardless of the inciting factor or factors, **Uterus Cytotrophin** serves to relieve the stress of faulty nutritional environment at the site of the difficulty and should therefore be employed in all situations involving this organ.

Symptom Characteristics: Unfortunately, uterine dysfunction may remain guised in an asymptomatic cloak, many cases of long standing endocervicitis remaining undiagnosed until after serious consequences have occurred.

	Test:	Need Shown By:
Laboratory Tests	Cervix Uteri Smear	Pus cells, Papanicolaou findings, etc.
Clinical Tests	Pelvic Examination	Evidence of inflammation, erosions, leukorrhea, etc.

Administration	**Dosage:** See "General Considerations" for rationalization of why low initial dosage should be given. Where reactions occur, **Calcium Lactate** is beneficial, and, in these cases, dosage should be reduced to ¼ tablet every six hours, gradually increased as tolerance is noted by the patient.
	Effect: In threatened abortions has been very satisfactory. In other conditions, effect may depend upon supportive therapy as described under "Synergists" below.
	Side Effects: See "General Considerations" for explanation, **Calcium Lactate** mitigates these reactions in the majority of cases.

<u>Synergists:</u>	<u>Activity Contributed</u>
a. Pituitary Cytotrophin	Trophic Effects of Pituitary Gland
b. Ovex	Ovarian Extract (aqueous)
c. Ovary Cytotrophin	Local Tissue Nutritional Environment
d. Betacol (or Liver Cytotrophin)	Liver Detoxification Effect (estrogens)
e. Thyroid Cytotrophin	Metabolic Activity Factor (oxygenation)
f. Vitamin A-C-P Complex	Epithelial and Connective Tissue Integrity

GENERAL CONSIDERATIONS

The hyperplastic activity of menstruation, as well as the traumatic possibilities of childbirth, even under normal conditions, show the uterus to be particularly vulnerable to stress situations and the female lacking the ability to

UTROPHIN

GENERAL CONSIDERATIONS

meet these requirements—and lacking symptomatic evidence to be concerned—accounts for the long-standing causes of subacute endocervicitis which stand as a cancer producing hazard. Therefore, for this—if for no other reason—**Utrophin** may be indicated in most women for prophylaxis alone.

By the same line of reasoning, we may find an organ which is highly sensitized (by standards of the protomorphogen reaction), and the administration of **Utrophin** under these circumstances may produce a preponderance of antibody formation with marked reactions, increased nervousness, for example. This is a histamine reaction—**Anti-Pyrexin** and **Calcium Lactate** are indicated—and shows the definite need of the patient for the product. These reactions are not serious and subsequent progress of the patient is accelerated after this initial phase.

CLINICALLY ASSOCIATED CONDITIONS

FEMALE DISORDERS

Abortion	Dysmenorrhea	Leukorrhea	Uterine Congestion
Amenorrhea	Endocervicitis	Menstruation Symptoms	Sterility

VASCULIN

Label: A tissue extract intended to supply the specific determinant factors of heart muscle with nutritional factors concentrated from Alfalfa, Mushroom, Green Buckwheat Leaf, Green Peas (whole plant), Fresh Bone Flour and Liver. This product is intended to improve vascular tone. Dosage: 3 to 12 tablets per day, or as directed.

Tissue or Function Supported   Heart tissue and vascular system.

CLINICAL CONSIDERATIONS
Prominent, Clinical, Signs And Symptoms

Symptoms:	Possible Etiological Background:
1. Congestive Heart Failure (Anoxia, orthopnea, reduced exercise tolerance, etc.) 2. Blood Pressure Changes (Both hypo- and hypertension) 3. Chronic Fatigue 4. Muscular Weakness 5. Capillary Fragility	Heart overload due to deficiency of Vitamin C factors which influence the oxygen-carrying capacity of the blood, as well as participate in protein metabolism, together with specific tissue determinant factors of heart muscle, cooperate in relieving nutritional states of deficiency

Symptom Characteristics: Indicated in a wide variety of conditions involving the muscular and vascular systems.

Laboratory Tests	None known.	
Clinical Tests	Test a. Blood Pressure Test b. Endocardiograph c. Pulse Rate d. Observation	Need Shown By: Hypo- or hypertension Indications of heart failure Tachycardia or bradycardia Evidence of vascular lesions
Administration	**Dosage:** 3 to 12 per day	
	Effect: A general increase in the feeling of well-being, acting as a tonic, is usually noted by the patient..	
	Side Effect: These are rare, the only possibility to our knowledge would be where the heart muscle extract may lower the blood sugar by its beneficial effects on muscle metabolism..	

Synergists:	Activity Contributed:
a. Vitamin G Complex	Enzyme Precursors (cholinesterase).
b. Vitamin B Complex	Lactic Acid Oxygenation Influence
c. Vitamin E Complex	Connective Tissue Integrity

GENERAL CONSIDERATIONS

The nutritional effects may be listed as follows:

a. Supplies Vitamin C Complex factors for promoting tissue repair and increasing the oxygen carrying capacity of the blood.

b. Supplies specific heart tissue extract beneficial t muscles.

Rationalization for clinical use is as follows:

1. Where heart muscle is unable to meet its demands, being fatigued in its performance, **Vasculin** is indicated.
2. General fatigue and muscular weakness, particularly if associated with cardiovascular breakdown, are indications for its need.

VASCULIN

CLINICALLY ASSOCIATED CONDITIONS

METABOLIC
  Legs, Weakness of
  Neuromuscular Disorders
TRAUMATIC
  Stroke, Recovery from
CIRCULATORY
  Bed Sores
  Intermittent Claudication
HEART DISORDERS
  Heart Abnormalities
SKIN
  Purpura

WHEAT GERM OIL PERLES

Label: Cold processed wheat germ oil. A good source of the fat soluble vitamins of the wheat berry, principally Vitamin E. The daily requirement of Vitamin E and its necessity for human nutrition has not been established by the consensus of medical opinion – 1 to 2 Perles per day or as directed.

Tissue or Function Supported   Acts as anti-abortive factor and is concerned with oxygen metabolism.

CLINICAL CONSIDERATIONS
Prominent Clinical Signs And Symptoms

Symptoms:	Possible Etiological Background
1. Capillary Engorgement (Bruising easily, "black and blue spots", purpura)	Apparently two factors are concerned: first, the well-known effects of Vitamin E as an anti-oxidant, and, second, the interrelationship between unsaturated fatty acids and iodine metabolism applying here to the hypothyroid state. The combined effects may account for many of the beneficial effects reported from the use of wheat germ oil.
2. Lowered Metabolism (Chronic fatigue, loss of vigor)	
3. Anoxia-type Symptoms (Frequent sighing and yawning, tachycardia, hyperirritability)	
4. Tissue Integrity (Bleeding gums, tendency to pyhorrhea, other gum symptoms)	
5. Cramps (Types brought on by exertion, "charley-horse" varieties)	

Symptom Characteristics: The pattern follows the characteristic clinical picture of lowered metabolism, where, for example, in obesity insufficient oxygen or thyroid hormone would be available to metabolize fats. This situation is almost invariably accompanied by loss of integrity of the vascular network showing lack of capillary tone, as evidenced by the most common clinical sign-of capillary engorgement, "black and blue spots" or bruising easily.

	Test:	Need Shown By:
Laboratory Tests	CO_2 Combining Power	A screen-test for acidosis, common in anoxia.
Clinical Tests	Breath Holding Test	Lowered oxygen reserves may be roughly indicated by breath-holding test, an ability to hold the breath for at least 20 seconds.

Administration	**Dosage:**	6 per day for a week or two produces adequate results in most cases.
	Effect:	Fatigue and skin lesions, as described above, usually clear up within a week or two and there is usually a marked increase in stamina.
	Side Effect:	None known. Where oils or fats are not tolerated however, bile salts or some other liver stimulating factors (**DiSodium-Phosphate**) may be necessary to promote absorption.

Synergists:	Activity Contributed:
1. Sodium Citrate	Anti-acidosis factor
2. Betacol	Promotes liver function
3. Ferrofood	Anti-anemia factors
4. Sesame Seed Perles	Supplies Vitamin T (platelet factor)

GENERAL CONSIDERATIONS

A general rationale for use of wheat germ oil may be obtained by applying the following information to clinical situations:

1. Oxygen acts to constrict the capillaries (carbon-dioxide and lactic acid to dilate them). If sufficient oxygen is not available, congestion brought about by even slight trauma cannot be expelled and the commonly found "black and blue" spots result and the patient complains of bruising easily.

WHEAT GERM OIL PERLES

GENERAL CONSIDERATIONS

2. **Wheat Germ Oil** is about 75% unsaturated fatty acids and as such is believed to have an effect on iodine metabolism, acting to increase thyroid activity in this respect. This may account for the relief of fatigue often expressed by patients using wheat germ oil in the diet.

3. The above mechanisms may act together to produce a special type of muscle cramp. This can be differentiated by other cramps by its characteristic of being brought on by exertion (exercise) or stimulation (massage), producing the typical "charley-horse" type of cramp of the athlete.

Differential Diagnosis:

There are several conditions which simulate the above descriptions symptomatically and must be differentiated. These conditions, described below, may exist concomitantly or as separate entities and require treatment as indicated:

	Characterized By:
Acidosis	Tachycardia, breathlessness, hyperirritability.
Anemia	Pallor, as well as the above symptoms.
Hypothyroidism	Obesity, thick skin, coarse hair, inability to work under pressure, etc.

Note: Use in the case of miscarriages **Wheat Germ Oil** should be considered, for best results a program should be started at least 3 months before conception. Read Nutrition and Physical Degeneration by Dr. Weston Price (See Page, 310).

CLINICALLY ASSOCIATED CONDITIONS

NERVOUS AND PSYCHOGENIC
  Metabolic
    Neuro-Muscular Disorders
    Tremors, muscular
  Mentality
    Backwardness in children
METABOLIC DISORDERS
  Growth and Repair
    Eye conditions
    Gums, receding of
  Intermediate Processes
    Cramps
    Oxygen metabolism
  Collagen Diseases
    Arcus Senilis
  Acid-Base Balance
    Acidosis
  Respiratory
    Bronchitis
  Allergies
    Asthma
EXOGENIC DISORDERS
  Toxic
    *Worms, intestinal

EXOGENIC DISORDERS
  Inflammation
    Denture irritation
    Gingivitis
    Periodontoclasia
  Vascular Disorders
    Angina Pectoris
    Heart Abnormalities
SKIN DISORDERS
  Purpura
  Telangiectasis
FEMALE DISORDERS
  Amenorrhea
  Leucorrhea
  Menopausal Symptoms
  Menstruation Symptoms
  Pregnancy Schedule
GLANDULAR
  Adrenal insufficiency
  Goiter
  Sterility

*Vermifuge effect of wheat germ oil has been reported.

ZYMEX

Label: An enzyme complex from special cultures of lactic acid forming microorganisms. Grown on wheat and extracted beet leaf. Malted barley used as an excipient. For experimental use as an aid to digestion and to alter the intestinal flora.

Tissue or Function Supported   Rehabilitation of the intestinal flora.

CLINICAL CONSIDERATIONS
Prominent Clinical Signs And Symptoms

<u>Symptoms:</u>

1. Gastro-Intestinal Symptoms (Diarrhea, constipation, malassimilation [weight loss], biliousness, heartburn, etc.)
2. Diseases Associated with Toxemia (Such as drug addiction, cancer, epilepsy, uremia, diabetes, celiac disease, liver and kidney disease, etc.)
3. Symptoms related to Toxemia (Such as tachycardia, fever, halitosis, body odor, skin, pallor, diarrhea, etc.)
4. Specific Type of Diarrhea (Where symbiotic relations of intestinal flora have been disrupted by antibiotics)

<u>Possible Etiological Background:</u>

Judging from its usefulness in a wide variety of clinical situations associated with the toxic state, both local intestinal and systemic effects of detoxification must be considered. This effect is, no doubt, related to enzymatic factors similar to the action f Arginex. The effect of Zymex in promoting favorable intestinal flora contributes materially in liver and kidney conditions by tending to eliminate this source of toxic overload. The widespread incidence of toxemia in the etiological background of many diseases indicates that this product has a broad scope of application.

Symptom Characteristics: Although specific gastrointestinal symptoms are usually accepted as indication for need of Zymex, application should not necessarily be restricted to this category of disorders. History of exposure to toxic situations or presence of toxic manifestations is also to be considered as possible indication for its need.

	Test:	Need Shown By:
Laboratory Tests	Urinalysis	Indicanuria
Clinical Tests	Bromthymol blue Indicator Test	Stool on alkaline side of pH, normal 6.8 to 7

Administration	**Dosage:** Normally, 2 to 4 per day is sufficient to influence intestinal environment in uncomplicated cases. Diarrhea may require doubling this amount for a few days to bring symptoms under control. Increased dosage in initial stages of therapy is usually desirable.
	Effect: Depends upon chronicity. Usually rapid in gastrointestinal disorders, dependent upon dosage; longer treatment is required where systemic involvements are the problem.
	Side Effect: None known.

<u>Synergists:</u>	<u>Activity Contributed</u>
Zypan	Digestive catalyst
Arginex	Kidney-liver overload
Okra Pepsin E_3	Anti-gastritis factors
Chlorophyll Complex (perles)	Detoxification-healing aid

Note: Specific liver support is often indicated in these cases, as follows: Betacol, Choline and Betafood.

GENERAL CONSIDERATIONS

The following nutritional effects are to be considered:
1. Zymex is an essential part of every detoxification program.
2. As an intestinal detoxicant, it is especially indicated in cases of diarrhea following antibiotic therapy.
3. Undesirable intestinal environment is usually a secondary condition to be dealt with in cases of liver and kidney disease, and these cases can be aided by the use of Zymex to relieve the stress on the liver-kidney detoxification system.

ZYMEX

GENERAL CONSIDERATIONS

Note: that many diseases are directly associated with toxic conditions, particularly those related to metabolic diseases. Zymex has proved very beneficial in the detoxification necessary in these cases. Some typical examples are: **Drug Addiction, Diabetes, Uremia, Epilepsy, Cancer, Celiac Disease**

While Zymex is not concerned directly with the treatment of the above diseases, its use in promoting detoxification is recommended in these and similar toxic situations.

CLINICALLY ASSOCIATED CONDITIONS

GASTROINTESTINAL-URINARY
- Stomach and Intestine
  - Colitis, Mucous
  - Flatulence

NERVOUS AND PSYCHOGENIC
- Functional
  - Chorea
  - Epilepsy
- Metabolic
  - Alcoholism
- Lesions
  - Cerebral Palsy
  - Multiple Sclerosis

METABOLIC DISORDERS
- Allergies
  - Sneezing Attacks

EXOGENIC DISORDERS
- Toxic
  - Boils
  - Halitosis
  - Nightmares
- Inflammation
  - Diarrhea
  - Sciatica
- Traumatic
  - Cancer, Relief of Pain in

DERMAL DISORDERS
- Acne Vulgaris
- Eczema
- Psoriasis

ZYMEX II

Label: Contains enzymatic factors from figs and almonds that act as a vermifuge digesting the parasite. Non-toxic in the dosage recommended. Adult dosage: 4 to 6 capsules per day for one week, or as directed.

Tissue or Function Supported   Acts to digest intestinal parasites by proteolytic enzyme activity.

CLINICAL CONSIDERATIONS
Prominent, Clinical Signs And Symptoms

Symptoms:

The list of possible situations where intestinal parasites may be a factor includes the following:

1. Flatulence
2. Abdominal pain and tenderness
3. Epigastric gnawing and distress ("Stomach ache" as expressed by children)
4. Nervousness
5. Loss of weight
6. Constipation or diarrhea (usually the latter)
7. Irregular fever
8. Urticaria
9. Dizziness
10. Pruritis ani
11. Mucous in stools
12. Blood in stools
13. Nausea
14. Vomiting
15. Gnawing of teeth
16. Restlessness in sleep
17. Sore mouth and gums

Possible Etiological Background:

Many children developing worms are deficient in ordinary salt, sodium chloride being a time-honored remedy for worms. Also, intestinal parasites are a common cause of appendicitis, especially in children.

The variously reported extremely high percentages of the incidence of worms or intestinal parasites would lead one to suspect this etiological background in many conditions heretofore receiving little consideration in this respect.

Symptom Characteristics: Aside from those symptoms directly traceable to gastrointestinal origin, reflex response from the neurological aspects of the irritation they may cause should be the outstanding consideration.

Laboratory Tests   There has been far too little laboratory work in routine examination of patients to check up on this infestation problem.

Clinical Tests   In children, parents should be instructed to examine anal area at night when child is asleep for evidence of pinworms.

Administration	
Dosage:	See label above.
Effect:	Digestion of proteins is improved as well as relief of symptoms caused by parasites when indicated.
Side Effect:	None known.

Synergists: **Activity Contributed:**

a. Sodium Chloride Tablets   Time-proved remedy
b. Wheat Germ Oil Perles   Reported vermifuge activity
c. Zymex   Intestinal Detoxicant
d. Zypan   Digestive
e. Cholacol II   Adsorbent (filtering effect)

GENERAL CONSIDERATIONS

For a complete discussion of **Vermidase Capsules (Zymex II)** and the problem of intestinal parasites and their control, see Applied Trophology, Vol. 2 – No. 10, October –1958. A few pertinent extracts from this article are given below:

ZYMEX II

GENERAL CONSIDERATIONS

"In trying to eliminate these parasites the use of poisons has been the usual practice. These poisons are far less satisfactory than the enzyme method".

"It so happens that there are also some plant enzymes that digest insect protein. (Enzymes are highly selective in their action; here we have one that digests the insect protein (chitin) without correspondingly affecting the human tissue.) The plants apparently use these enzymes in their self-defense against insects. Ripe figs when fresh contain an enzyme to digest worms. This accounts for the fact that a fig on a tree never has a worm in it."

"We have been informed by a prominent dentist that he found, over a number of years of careful checking, that many of his patients complaining of poorly fitting dentures were in fact, having mouth lesions due to giardia lamblia infestation instead of improperly fitted plates."

CLINICALLY ASSOCIATED CONDITIONS

GASTROINTESTINAL-URINARY
   <u>Liver and Gallbladder</u>
      Hepatitis
METABOLIC DISORDERS
   <u>Growth and Repair</u>
      Mouth-Tongue Disorders
   <u>Intermediate Processes</u>
      Protein Metabolism
   <u>Body Weight</u>
      Appetite Decreased

EXOGENIC DISORDERS
   <u>Infections</u>
      Vincents Infection
   <u>Toxic</u>
      Worms
   <u>Inflammation</u>
      Denture Irritation
      Gingivitis
      Periodontoclasia

ZYPAN

Label: Each tablet contains: Pancreatin 1.5 grs., Pepsin (1:3000) 1.5 grs., Betaine Hydrochloride 2.75 grs., and Ammonium Chloride .15 grs. This product is intended to improve protein digestion. Dose: 1 – 2 tablets with each meal or as directed.

Tissue or Function Supported Source of hydrochloric acid and associated factors beneficial in digestive enzyme systems, promoting activity in hypofunction of the pancreas.

CLINICAL CONSIDERATIONS
Prominent Clinical Signs And Symptoms

Symptoms:

1. Chronic Indigestion (Symptoms usually occur several hours after eating, but may be continuous)
2. Anemia (Seldom occurs in normal diets without hypochlorhydria)
3. Calcium Deficiency (Insomnia, cramps, nervousness, etc.)
4. Protein Deficiency (Emaciation)

Possible Etiological Backgrounds:

Predisposing factors:

a. "Salt-Free diets, either prescribed or self-imposed.
b. Excessive use of alkalizers, antacids, "soda-mints", etc.
c. Protracted hydrochloric acid loss from longstanding hyperacidity, vomiting or diarrhea or hypermotility of the intestines.
d. Increased metabolic requirements such as pregnancy, aging processes, glandular hyperactivity or abnormal nervous tension.
e. Congenital weakness.

Symptom Characteristics: Gastro-intestinal symptoms are usually –though not invariably—present, typical clinical picture as follows: Several hours after eating, patient experiences lower bowel gas, full feeling, sour stomach or heartburn. Constipation alternating with diarrhea is common. Halitosis and foul-smelling stools, appetite changes, particularly loss of taste for meat, are common complaints.

Note: Many of the above symptoms may be entirely lacking. In these cases, pallor, fatigue, emaciation and other non-specific indications may be due to protein, calcium and iron since these are best utilized in an acid medium and their assimilation and absorption may be faulty due to hypochlorhydria. This can be a common occurrence.

Laboratory Tests Note: While laboratory tests showing diminished gastric secretion may be used, the inconvenience to the patient encountered by these tests is considerable, as well as entailing an expense.

Clinical Tests Note: In a much more practical vein than the above, is the therapeutic or clinical test which may be performed with little discomfort and expense to the patient and still provide diagnostic information not available from a laboratory gastric analysis. This applies, of course, only to uncomplicated clinical situations and does not discount the value of laboratory test in selected cases. For complete information as to procedure in making this functional test, see "Achlorhydria" in the Therapeutic Foods Manual.

Administration	**Dosage:** There are a few products in which regulation of dosage assumes such an important role. Symptomatic response is the criterion of levels required, see "Achlorhydria", Therapeutic Foods Manual. He number of tablets per meal is the important factor. Thus, 3 to 6 tablets at any one meal may give symptomatic evidence of response, whereas, the same number of tablets dispersed over three meals may fail in this respect to show observable evidence. IT is best to use the following step ladder dosage first day, 3 with evening meal; second day, 3 with evening and noon meals; third day, 3 evening, noon and breakfast. By the same measure, reduction in dosage should follow the same reversed course. Usually within 6 weeks, 2 or 3 tablets with evening (or protein meal) course will be sufficient, later reduced to symptomatic levels.
	Effect: Relief of gastrointestinal symptoms when from this cause is usually immediate; in absence of gastrointestinal symptoms-anemia's and emaciation, for example—long term dosage is recommended..
	Side Effect: Various reactions which may occur have a specific diagnostic value. For complete information on this subject, see "Achlorhydria," Therapeutic Foods Manual.

ZYPAN

Synergists:	Activity Contributed:
a. Pancreatrophin	Application of the protomorphogen principles (Discussion under General Considerations, below)
b. AF Betafood	Improves bile flow (lowers viscosity)
c. Cholacol	Stimulates bile flow
d. Cal-Amo	Combats alkalosis
e. Choline	Anti-cholic effect, detergent action

GENERAL CONSIDERATIONS

IMPORTANT COMMENT: Notice that to potentiate the effects described below on an experimental basis, it would be necessary to use both **PANCREATROPHIN** and the product being discussed here, **ZYPAN** (Zypan supplements the external secretions of the pancreas, Pancreatrophin gives nutritional support to the entire organ by improvement of local nutritional environment of cells.)

Insufficiency of the pancreas and deficiency of hydrochloric acid may be considered one of the most commonly omitted diagnoses, in the patient suffering from chronic fatigue, emaciation, lowered resistance and a variety of general symptoms not directly associated with sufficiency of the gastric secretions.

Substance in fact to the above statement is provided by Harrower on page 482 of his book, "*Practical Endocrinology*", which reads, in part, as follows:

> "The frequency with which diabetics suffer from concomitant infections is well known…small pimples often become serious boils…and may spread with amazing rapidity. Infections that may ordinarily be considered trivial frequently becoming quite serous in the diabetic.
>
> In experimental work on animals it has been found that the removal of the pancreas in one step is almost invariably fatal. The significant fact is that these animals do not die of shock or loss of the digestive services of the pancreas, but from severe sepsis-the wound will not heal. This may be obviated by the implantation, in the abdominal wall, of a small piece of pancreatic tissue, preferably from the tail of the pancreas…even a small graft is enough to preserve the immunizing response to infection. This seems to afford the best kind of evidence of a relation between the internal secretion of the pancreas and the power to overcome bacterial infection.

CLINICALLY ASSOCIATED CONDITIONS

GASTROINTESTINAL-URINARY
   <u>Stomach and Intestine</u>
      Achlorhydria
      Alimentary Canal Flora
      Colitis, Mucous
      Flatulence
   <u>Liver and Gallbladder</u>
      Biliary Stasis
      Constipation
      Digestion Faulty
      Gallbladder Disease
      Indigestion, Acute
      Liver Disease
NERVOUS AND PSYCHOGENIC
   <u>Vaso-Motor</u>
      Dizziness
METABOLIC DISORDERS
   <u>Intermediate Processes</u>
      Carbohydrate Metabolism
      Diabetes Mellitus
      Reactions to Foods
   <u>Acid-Base Balance</u>
      Acids, Craving for
      Ketosis
   <u>Blood</u>
      Anemia, Pernicious
      Anemia, Secondary
   <u>Allergies</u>
      Asthma
   <u>Body Weight</u>
      Obesity
EXOGENIC DISORDERS
   <u>Toxic</u>
      Halitosis
   <u>Inflammation</u>
      Diarrhea
   <u>Traumatic</u>
      Cancer, Relief of Pain in
      Stroke, Recovery from
SKIN DISORDERS
   Psoriasis
FEMALE DISORDERS
   Pregnancy Schedules
SPECIFIC DEFICIENCY DISEASES
   Cheilosis
   Glossitis
   Conjunctivitis
   Pellagra

PORTFOLIO

OF

PRODUCT BULLETINS

DISCONTINUED ITEMS

CHLOROPHYLL, AQUEOUS CAPSULES

(DISCONTINUED)

Label: Water Soluble Chlorophyll, with physiological buffer salts. Capsules may be emptied into a measured amount of distilled water for an Aqueous solution, or may be swallowed intact with a glass of water for internal dosage. Each capsule is equal to one teaspoonful of 2% Aqueous Chlorophyll Solution. Three capsules to four ounces of distilled water gives a 25% Chlorophyll Solution (proper concentration for irrigation purposes).

Tissue or Function Supported   Detoxification.

CLINICAL CONSIDERATIONS
Prominent Clinical Signs And Symptoms

Symptoms:

1. Toxic Manifestations (Body odor, halitosis, strong odor to urine or stool, sallow appearance of skin, etc.)
2. Metabolic Wastes (Excess smoking, drinking and eating; metabolic diseases as gout, diabetes, arthritis, hypertension, etc.)
3. Kidney and Bladder Disorders (Urine volume deviations, pain in lower abdomen (bladder), burning on urination, etc.)
4. Blood Dyscrasias (Anemia, uremia and toxemia of various types)
5. Intestinal Toxemia (Resulting in inflammation, irrigation (gastritis), toxic end products)
6. Local Application (Irrigations and compresses as in sinusitis, vaginitis, ulcers, gingivitis, burns, bleeding gums, etc.)
7. Alterative (Tonic effect)

Possible Etiological Backgrounds:

The etiological background of the action of chlrophyll is rather indistinct, although its effectiveness on an empirical basis as a reliable remedy in the treatment of many disorders is well established. We may state that its effects seem to be through its ability to detoxify and as a cell proliferating factor. The absence of evidence as to untoward effects points to the finding of a safe remedy worthy of trial in a wide variety of ailments as an adjunct if not as a specific in their treatment. The usual absence of chlorophyll rich foods—mostly green leafy vegetables—in the average diet, also leads to the conclusion of a wide-spread deficiency of this apparently important nutrient. Thus, Chlorophyll with an absence of toxicity and a high potential for benefits is to be considered as a broad-spectrum nutritional factor of unusual merit.

IMPORTANT: See Product Bulletin on **Chlorophyll Perles** (Fat-Soluble) page 89 for further information.

Symptom Characteristics: The indications are more general than specific, toxic overload being the primary consideration. This is generally due to liver or kidney insufficiency or to intestinal toxemia.

	Test:	Need Shown By:
Laboratory Tests	Urinalysis	Indicanuria; albuminuria
Clinical Tests toxemia	Pulse Rate	Tachycardia, as related to

Administration	**Dosage:** One capsule per day seems to produce appreciable results in most cases, 2 per day apparently shows maximum benefits in the initial stages of administration. It has been reported that best results are obtained when capsules are dissolved in water when used internally. Much higher dosage than the above has been used by some clinicians with reported success, particularly in such conditions as gastric ulcers and colitis. (We believe that **Chlorophyll Perles** added to the schedule is advisable in these cases and that in this event the increased dosage would be unnecessary).
	Effect: In toxic conditions, a marked tonic effect is usually experienced for the first few days of use, decreasing as toxemia is relieved and other factors attain prominence, at which time **Chlorophyll Perles** should be administered as the basic chlorophyll supplement.
	Side Effect: None known.

CHLOROPHYLL, AQUEOUS CAPSULES

Synergists:	Activity Contributed:
Thymex	Aids phagocytosis
Arginex	Liver-Kidney overload
Zymex	Detoxification factor

GENERAL CONSIDERATIONS

Note: Chlorophyll Capsules (Aqueous) differ from **Chlorophyll Perles (Fat-Soluble)**. **Chlorophyll Capsules** do not contain vitamins or other fat-soluble factors as do **Chlorophyll Perles**. Their principle advantage is in their solubility and thus are, perhaps, quicker acting on the detoxification mechanisms. However, the more physiological of the two products is **Chlorophyll Perles**, which should be the product of choice for internal use.

1. **Chlorophyll Capsules** act as detoxification factors.

2. 2The organs of stress seem to be overloaded kidneys which receive the brunt of toxemia and, in this respect, **Chlorophyll Capsules** with **Arginex** have performed very satisfactorily.

3. The effects of local application in aqueous solutions are excellent. Irrigations, wet compresses or douches may be used, but note that at least 5 minutes of contact must be maintained for each area treated. Some typical conditions amenable to such treatment are as follows:

Sinusitis	Skin Irritations	Wound Healing
Vaginitis	Gingivitis	Burns
Ulcers	Bleeding Gums	Infections

Chlorophyll Ointment may be used where applicable, its staining effect being greater and thus may be limited for cosmetic reasons.

Atomizer-type bottles are available for use with Chlorophyll Capsules in sinusitis and other conditions where atomizing might be advantageous.

CLINICALLY ASSOCIATED CONDITIONS

GASTROINTESTINAL-URINARY
   <u>Liver and Gallbladder</u>
      Hepatitis
      Jaundice
   <u>Kidney and Bladder</u>
      Cystitis
      Urinary Incompetence
      Uremia
EXOGENIC DISORDERS
   <u>Infections</u>
      Febrile Diseases
      Lymph Node Infections
   <u>Toxic</u>
      Halitosis

VASCULAR DISORDERS
   <u>Circulatory</u>
      Bed Sores
      Varicose Veins
SKIN DISORDERS
   Pruritis
FEMALE DISORDERS
   Vaginitis

ASSOCIATED PRODUCTS:

Chlorophyll Complex: (See Product Bulletin on **Chlorophyll Complex**, page, 69).

CYROFOOD D

(DISCONTINUED)

Label: Contains soybean flour, peanut and rice bran, concentrates from beet, carrot, alfalfa, mushrooms, peas (whole plant), yeast, beef kidney, veal bone, and cereal germ. Each heaping teaspoon full contains 166 i.u. vitamin D from fish liver lipoid (one-third adult minimum daily requirements). For adults: 2 to 8 level teaspoons per day.

Tissue or Function Supported	A special formula of essential foods intended to support the general nutritional requirements of the diabetic, i.e., low calorie, highly concentrated essential nutrients of selected low heat treated foods.

CLINICAL CONSIDERATIONS
Prominent Clinical Signs And Symptoms

Symptoms:

1. Remarks: The diagnosis of diabetes, of course, depends upon blood sugar evaluations, and it will be assumed that such diagnosis will have been made prior to the consideration of the use of Cyrofood D in the diet.
2. Concomitant Features:
    a. Hypertension
    b. Arteriosclerosis
    c. Coronary disease
    d. Fatty degeneration of:
        1.) Liver
        2.) Kidney
        3.) Heart
    e. Obesity

Possible Etiological Background

The diabetic is confronted not only with the problem of regulation of the blood sugar, but also with related disturbances in fat metabolism- usually ostensibly reflected as obesity, but systemically manifest as fatty degeneration involving such vital organs as the liver, kidney, and heart , as well as arteriosclerosis. As such, hypertension, liver and gallbladder disease, coronary disease, and nephritis or nephrosis result with a high incidence in these patients. Since fat metabolism has been shown to be under the influence of nutritional factors, it is important that essential foods, such as found in Cyrofood D, be included in the dietary regime of the diabetic patient.

Symptom Characteristics: Symptoms pertaining to diabetes do not necessarily apply since Cyrofood D is provided as a generally beneficial essential food in support of the metabolism, independent of whatever choice of therapy the physician may be using for the treatment of the disease per se.

Laboratory and Clinical Tests	Test: Blood Sugar Urinalysis	Need Shown By: Routine Findings
Administration	**Dosage:** See label above.	
	Effect: The affect is not to be traced through observation of blood sugar levels as these are presumed to be influenced by more specific remedies, but rather through long-term observation of the general nutrition of the patient, where material benefit is usually noted.	
	Side Effect: None Know.	
Synergists:	**Activity Contributed:** (See Pancreatrophin Bulletin, page, 139)	

GENERAL CONSIDERATIONS

As discussed above, the general nutrition of the diabetic is an indispensable consideration in the management of each case. We believe that Cyrofood D provides the physician with an essential food complex of selected ingredients which goes far in satisfying this requirement, emphasis being made of the fact that its ingredients are low-heat processed and that these, with their preserved enzymes, vitamins, minerals, and proteins, are particularly important in fortifying this aspect of the diabetic diet.

CLINICALLY ASSOCIATED CONDITIONS

(See comments under "Characteristic Symptoms" above)

NUNUCLEO-PROTEIN

(DISCONTINUED)

Label: 75 mg. per capsule. Dosage: As a nutritional protein supplement, 1 to 3 capsules per day, or as directed.

Tissue or Function Supported   A nonspecific nutritional factor useful in normalization of cell metabolism.

CLINICAL CONSIDERATIONS
Prominent Clinical Signs And Symptoms

Symptoms:
Various metabolic and degenerative
Diseases of a chronic nature, particularly emaciation
(wasting diseases).

Possible Etiological Background:
Indicated primarily as an adjunct to basic therapies where ordinary measures have failed to produce satisfactory results.

Symptom Characteristics: These are difficult to evaluate except that a morbid mental state seems characteristic of the pattern, otherwise as indicated above.

Laboratory and Clinical Tests   None known.

Administration

Dosage: Higher dosage in early stages, later reduced to clinical indications necessary to maintain level of response.

Side Effect: Symptoms which are possibly referable to the pituitary have occurred. These include vertigo, headache, nausea and other vague symptoms. In these cases it is suspected that trace minerals, particularly iodine and manganese, should be used in the form of **Trace Minerals B12**.

Synergists:
a. Vitamin G Complex
b. Organic Minerals
c. Super-EFF
d. Spleen Cytotrophin

Activity Contributed:
Enzyme activator (cholinesterase)
Organic Potassium Source
Chromosome Protective Phospholipids
Natural Tissue Antibody Factor

GENERAL CONSIDERATIONS

Very complex acids containing phosphorus-nucleic acids-combined with proteins are designated nucleo-proteins; they occur in particularly large amounts in the thymus and pancreas and are believed to be important constituents of the nuclei of both animal and plant cells although their physiological function is not understood. Clinically, we have had reports that one of the general effects of **Nucleo-Protein** is to improve the thinking processes, promoting a feeling of well-being and stability which may be lacking in states of debility.

CLINICALLY ASSOCIATED CONDITIONS

NERVOUS AND PSYCHOGENIC
  Mentality
    Brain, Dysfunction of
METABOLIC DISORDERS
  Growth and Repair
    Healing, Promotion of
  Collagen
    Arthritis, Rheumatoid
  Blood
    Anemias

Body Weight
  Appetite Decreased
EXOGENIC DISORDERS
  Toxic
    Delirium
    Nightmares
  Traumatic
    Stroke, Recovery from
VASCULAR DISORDERS
  Circulatory Diseases
    Bed Sores
    Leg Ulcers

POTASSIUM BICARBONATE

(DISCONTINUED)

Label: Potassium Bicarbonate U.S.P. Contents: 10 ounces

Tissue or Function Supported   Systemic alkalizer

CLINICAL CONSIDERATIONS
Prominent Clinical Signs And Symptoms

Symptoms:

1. Infectious diseases (Flu, grippe, pneumonia, bronchitis and other diseases imposing upon adrenal function)
2. Dehydration (Fluid loss from diarrhea, pernicious vomiting, emaciation, etc.)
3. Gastric hyperacidity (Excessive secretion of HCl, relief of symptoms only)
4. Acidosis (Anoxia, hyperirritability, tachycardia from this cause)
5. Diminished urination (Acts as physiological diuretic in indicated cases)
6. Arthritic diathesis (Gouty type of arthritis, excess uric acid, faulty excretion)

Possible Etiological Background:

Action is via adrenal stimulation, probably by means of the following: when potassium rises in the blood beyond a minimum level, the adrenals are called upon to promote its excretion. When **Potassium Bicarbonate** is introduced, the adrenals are called upon thus and their activity is increased. This is a physiological effect as normally potassium is lost from the tissue guardianship into the circulation during periods of stress and tissue breakdown as would be expected in these conditions. However, where potassium is initially deficient in the cell, this may not occur in sufficient quantities, hence the rationale of potentiating this effect with **Potassium Bicarbonate**. This rationalization should only be applied where the adrenals are functionally stable, otherwise see "Side-Effects" below.

Symptom Characteristics: Involve primarily temporary loss of integrity of adrenals and as such useful in initiating immediate response in acute situations. Otherwise, **Organic Minerals** as a source of organic potassium should be used.

Laboratory and Clinical Tests   Use with caution in hypotension, see "Side-Effects" below

Administration

Dosage: ½ teaspoonful in water once or twice daily seems to be maximum dosage required, once daily being adequate in most cases. Higher dosage is seldom recommended.

Effect: In gastric hyperacidity it is very effective in relieving the burning sensation; in systemic disorders it is often very effective in bringing about a reversal of the course of flu, severe colds, etc.; in gout and arthritis its activity is indicated by strong odor to urine which it produces in applicable cases.

Side Effect: It should never be used in cases where a high blood potassium is suspected. This would be possible in such states as hypoadrenia (low blood pressure). Addison's Disease, congestive heart failure, bradycardia (heart block), or where the patient is in danger of shock or in an extremely debilitated state. T he side-effect would be evidenced by a feeling of "heebie-jeebies"—as expressed by the patient—or hyperirritability.

Synergists: **Activity Contributed:**

Note: Organic Minerals, the organic form of potassium from alfalfa and sea lettuce, differs from the inorganic forms (Potassium Bicarbonate) in that it does not possess the adrenal stimulating effect in as high a degree, but is utilized more readily by the cells, a more basic physiological effect. **Organic Minerals** should, therefore, always be used in long-term therapy, **Potassium Bicarbonate** only for short periods of time, less than a week (except in gout, where longer use may be advisable).

GENERAL CONSIDERATIONS

Nutritional effects may be listed as follows:

a. Simulates the effects of adrenalin
b. Systemic alkalizer
c. Physiological diuretic
d. Combats effects of gastric hyperacidity

POTASSIUM BICARBONATE

GENERAL CONSIDERATIONS

Rationalization for clinical application is as follows:
1. Potassium bicarbonate is apparently dependent upon adrenal response for its effects and as such should be administered in accordance with side-effects outlined above.
2. It has proved useful in gout and, as such, may be considered a factor in uric acid metabolism.
3. Judging from benefits shown in fibrosis clinically, a synergistic effect is obtained when **Potassium Bicarbonate** and **Phosfood** are used together—note separate dosage, each taken at different times of the day, preferably on an empty stomach.

CLINICALLY ASSOCIATED CONDITIONS

<u>Liver and Gallbladder</u>
    Indigestion, Acute

<u>Collagen Diseases</u>
    Gout

<u>Virus Infections</u>
    Colds, Flu, Grippe

<u>Inflammation</u>
    Diarrhea

SODIUM CITRATE

(DISCONTINUED)

Label: Sodium Citrate (for food use); Contents: 9 Ounces.

Tissue or Function Supported Sodium deficiency states

CLINICAL CONSIDERATIONS
Prominent Clinical Signs And Symptoms

<u>Symptoms:</u>

1. Symptoms of acidosis, such as:
   a. Irregular respiration
   b. Frequent sighing, gasping
   c. Dehydration
   d. Excessive perspiration (NaCl loss)
2. Symptoms of potassium excess, such as:
   a. Hypotension
   b. Bradycardia
   c. Neurasthenia
   d. Intolerance to potassium-rich foods
3. Low salt diets (Low sodium diets)
4. Addisons Disease (Weight loss, bronzing of skin, hypotension, etc.)

<u>Possible Etiological Background:</u>

Hypoadrenia most common cause, potassium retained and sodium excreted in adrenal insufficiency.

For complete discussion, see "Acidosis" in the Manual of Clinical Trophology, also discussion under "Salt Metabolism".

Lee Foundation Reprint No. 96, "A New Theory of Diet in the Treatment of Coronary Thrombosis"- Klein, provides interesting information in respect to blood volume, applicable where sodium deficiency states are encountered.

Symptom Characteristics: Strongest consideration should be given to sodium deficiency states in hypotension or normal blood pressure, seldom occurs in hypertension on persons with hypertensive tendencies, fluctuations.

	<u>Test:</u>	<u>Need Shown By:</u>
Laboratory Tests	CO_2 Combining Power	Decrease
Clinical Tests	Breath Holding Test (Screen Test)	Inability to hold breath for at least 20 seconds (acidosis test)
Administration	**Dosage:** 1 or 2 tsp. daily for a few days. Subsequent dosage should be limited to ½ tsp. once or twice daily.	
	Effect: Quickly relieves symptoms of acidosis.	
	Side Effect: May aggravate alkalosis symptoms (see **Cal-Amo** Bulletin) or aggravate fluid retention in hyperadrenia or other situations where sodium retention is present. In either even, **Adrenamin** would act to support adrenal dysfunction then shown to be present.	

<u>Synergists:</u>	<u>Activity Contributed:</u>
a. Adrenamin	Adrenal Determinants and Related Factors
b. Kidney Cytotrophin	Local Environment of Cells

GENERAL CONSIDERATIONS

Sodium Citrate breaks down in the blood stream into the bicarbonate form and as such acts as the principle blood buffer salt, sodium bicarbonate, and thus combats acidosis. While the supplying of this salt does not correct the basic cause of the deficiency-which is usually renal or adrenal in origin- it is extremely useful in handling temporary or transient phases in the treatment of acidosis.

CLINICALLY ASSOCIATED CONDITIONS

NERVOUS AND PSYCHOGENIC
<u>Functional</u>
    Sweat Gland Activity
    Hypotension
    Shock

Intermediate
    Salt Metabolism
<u>Acid-Base Disorders</u>
    Acidosis
<u>Glandular</u>
    Adrenal Insufficiency

SODIUM CITRATE

SPECIAL SECTION

ON

CLINICAL NUTRITION

THERAPEUTIC FOOD COMPANY
OF
MILWAUKEE WISCONSIN USA

SPECIAL FORMULA PRODUCTS

These Special Formula products were developed in the late 1950's at the request of physicians who were using a number of products in certain combinations on a regular basis. These formulas consist of combinations of Standard Process products and make a nutritional regimen easier for both the doctor and the patient. Approximate percentages in the formulas, with space for doctor's notes follow.

Formula:	Product:	Approximate Composition:
Albaplex (0900)	Betacol	40%
	Renatrophin PMG	20%
	Arginex	20%
	Cataplex A-C	10%
	Thymex	10%
Notes:		
Allerplex (0975)	Pneumotrophin PMG	20%
	Drenatrophin PMG	20%
	Cataplex A-C	20%
	Betacol	20%
	Antronex	20%
Notes:		
Cardio-Plus (2065)	Cataplex C	32%
	Cataplex G	32%
	Cardiotrophin	23%
	Cataplex E2	14%
Notes:		
Cholaplex (2525)	Orchex	40%
	Cataplex G	21%
	Cataplex F	16%
	Cyruta	9%
	Cholacol	7%
Notes:		
Circuplex (2650)	Phosfood	33%
	Niacinamide B6	33%
	Ribonucleic Acid	33%
Notes:		

SPECIAL FORMULA PRODUCTS

Formula:	Product:	Approximate Composition:
Congaplex (2900)	Cataplex A-C	29%
	Thymex	25%
	Calcium Lactate Fortified	37%
	Ribonucleic Acid	9%
Notes:		
Cardio-Plus (2065)	Cataplex C	32%
	Cataplex G	32%
	Cardiotrophin PMG	23%
	Cataplex E2	14%
Notes:		
Diaplex (3550)	Zypan	30%
	Arginex	30%
	A-F Betafood	12%
	Betacol	8%
	Pituitrophin PMG	10%
	Pancreatrophin PMG	10%
Notes:		
Drenamin (3650)	Cataplex C	48%
	Cataplex G	27%
	Drenatrophin PMG	25%
Notes:		
Emphaplex (3950)	Catalyn	16.65%
	Drenamin	45.90%
	Pneumotrophin PMG	12.50%
	Phosfood	16.65%
	Protefood	8.30%
Notes:		
e-Poise (4030)	Catalyn	85%
	Ferrofood	10%
	Tillandsia	5%
Notes:		

SPECIAL FORMULA PRODUCTS

Formula:	Product:	Approximate Composition:
Iplex (5100)	Cataplex A-C	30%
	Cataplex G	20%
	Cyruta	20%
	Ostrophin PMG	10%
	Phosfood	10%
	Oculotrophin PMG	10%
Notes:		
Ligaplex I (5200)	Manganese B12	40%
	Cataplex E	25%
	Ostrophin PMG	25%
	Cataplex A-C-P	10%
Notes:		
Ligaplex II (5275)	Cyro-Yeast	16%
	Cardiotrophin PMG	16%
	Ostrophin PMG	16%
	Manganese B12	16%
	Super-EFF	16%
	Cataplex E	20%
Notes:		
Livaplex (5375)	A-F Betafood	30%
	Hepatrophin PMG	21%
	Betacol	15%
	Spanish Black Radish	13%
	Chezyn	12%
	Antronex	9%
Notes:		
Min-Chex (5525)	Min-Tran	65%
	Orchex	35%
Notes:		
Ostarplex (6350)	Betacol	30%
	Phosfood	30%
	Ostrophin PMG	20%
	Cataplex G	10%
	Cal-Amo	10%
Notes:		

SPECIAL FORMULA PRODUCTS

Formula:	Product:	Approximate Composition:
Rumaplex (7275)	Catalyn	20%
	Arginex	20%
	Betacol	10%
	Brewer's Yeast	10%
	Prost-X	10%
	Calcifood	10%
	Ostrophin PMG	10%
	Calcium Lactate Fortified	10%
Notes:		
Senaplex (7350)	Betacol	40%
	Cyro-Yeast	40%
	For-Til B12	10%
	Protefood	10%
Notes:		
Vasculin (8165)	Cardiotrophin PMG	35%
	Cataplex E	33%
	Cataplex B	17%
	Cataplex C	15%
Notes:		

ORGAN AND GLANDULAR PRODUCTS

WHOLE DESICCATED PRODUCTS

PRODUCT NAME	SOURCE BOVINE	DESICCATED EXTRACT PER TABLET
Adrenal, Dessicated	adrenal	130 mg
E-Manganese	anterior pituitary	165 mg
Neuroplex (per two capsules)	hypothalamus	35 mg
	anterior pituitary	30 mg
	spleen	100 mg
Spleen, Desiccated	spleen	350 mg

CYTOSOL EXTRACTS

PRODUCT NAME	SOURCE BOVINE	CYTOSOL EXTRACT PER TABLET
Hypothalmex	hypothalamus	140 mg
Orchex	testis	88 mg
Ovex	ovary	120 mg
Prost-X	prostate	20 mg
Thymex	thymus	130 mg

SPECIAL FORMULA PRODUCTS

PMG EXTRACTS

PRODUCT NAME	SOURCE BOVINE	PMG EXTRACT PER TABLE
Cardiotrophin PMG	heart	120 mg
Dermatrophin PMG	epithelia	60 mg
Drenatrophin PMG	adrenal	60 mg
Hepatrophin PMG	liver	430 mg
Hypothalamus PMG	hypothalamus	145 mg
Mammary PMG	mammary	120 mg
Myotrophin PMG	heart muscle	120 mg
Neurotrophin PMG	brain	145 mg
Oculotrophin PMG	eye	125 mg
Orchic PMG	testis	195 mg
Biost	bone, marrow, spinal cord	225 mg
Ostrophin PMG	bone, marrow, spinal cord	225 mg
Ovatrophin PMG	ovary	125 mg
Pancreatrophin PMG	pancreas	95 mg
Parotid PMG	parotid	190 mg
Pituitrophin PMG	pituitary	45 mg
Pneumotrophin PMG	lung	20 mg
Prostate PMG	prostate	190 mg
Renatrophin PMG	kidney	190 mg
Spleen PMG	spleen	115 mg
Thymus PMG	thymus	185 mg
Thytrophin PMG	thyroid	45 mg
Utrophin PMG	uterus	125 mg
Paraplex	Pituitary	10 mg
	thyroid	10 mg
	adrenal	15 mg
	pancreas	25 mg
Symplex F	pituitary	10 mg
	thyroid	10 mg
	adrenal	15 mg
	ovary	30 mg
Symplex M	pituitary	10 mg
	thyroid	10 mg
	adrenal	15 mg
	testis	45 mg

©1996 – 2010 International Foundation for Nutrition and Health, All Rights Reserved

ASSOCIATED PRODUCTS

Product Name	Contains	Also Contains	Related Products
A C Carbamide			Vitamin F, Arginex
AF Betafood		Cataplex A, Cataplex F, Betafood	Zypan, Choline, Soy Bean Lecithin
Antronex		Yalcriton	Orchex, Calcium Lactate, Cataplex F, Betacol
Arginex			A-C Carbamide, Clorophyll (perles), Phosfood Liquid, Zymex
Betacol		Hepatrophin PMG	Choline, Zypan, A-F Betafood, Disodium Phosphate, Hepatrophin PMG
Betafood		Betaine	Choline, Zypan or Betaine Hydrochloride
Betaine Hydrochloride	Zypan		Zypan, Pancreatrophin PMG, Cal-Amo, Cholacol, Cholacol II, Okra Pepsin E₃
Bio-Dent	Biost		Ostogen, Catalyn, Biost, Ostrophin PMG
Biost	Cyrofood		Calcifood Wafers, Bio-Dent, Cyrofood, Ostrophin PMG
Cal-Amo			Renatrophin PMG, Drenamin, Thytrophin PMG
Calcifood Wafers	Ostrophin PMG		Calcium Lactate, Bio-Dent, Biost
Calcium Lactate	Cataplex D, Organic Minerals		Cataplex F, Cataplex D Nutrimere, Min-Tran
Casol			Cataplex D, Cataplex F, Zypan, Lactic Acid Yeast
Cardio-Plus		Cataplex È₂, Cataplex G, Cardiotrophin PMG	Organic Minerals, Calcium Lactate, Betafood
Cadiotrophin PMG Myotrophin PMG			Organic Minerals, Calcium Lactate, Betafood
Catalyn	Cyrofood Powder, Cyrofood	Natural vitamin complex and trace minerals	Organic Minerals, Calcium Lactate, Chlorophyll Complex (perles)
Cataplex A	Cataplex A-C, Cataplex A-C-P, Catalyn		Cataplex È, Chlorophyll Complex (perles), Cataplex G, Calcium Lactate
Cataplex A-C	Catalyn, Cataplex A-C-P		Cataplex G, Chlorophyll Complex (perles), Calcium Lactate, Arginex, Betacol
Cataplex A C P	Cataplex A-C taken with Cyruta-Plus	Cataplex A, Cataplex C, Cyruta Plus	Cataplex G, Chlorophyll (perles), Calcium Lactate, Arginex, Betacol
Cataplex B₁₂	Ferrofood, Manganese B₁₂, Trace Minerals B₁₂		Ferrofood, Super Eff, Chlorophyll Complex (perles), Wheat Germ Oil, Manganese B₁₂
Cataplex B	Catalyn		Organic Minerals, Calcium Lactate, Cataplex G
Cataplex C	Cataplex A-C, Cataplex A C P, Catalyn		Calcium Lactate, CataplexG

ASSOCIATED PRODUCTS

Product Name	Contains In	Also Contains	Related Products
Cataplex D	Cyrofood D, Biost, Catalyn		Cataplex F, Chlorophyll Complex (perles), Calcium Lactate
Cataplex E2	Cardio-Plus		Cataplex G, Organic Minerals, Orchex
Cataplex E	Chlorophyll Complex (perles), Cataplex E2, Catalyn		Trace Minerals-B12, Thymex, Cataplex F, Pituitrophin PMG
Cataplex F	Catalyn, A-F Betaood, Cataplex F (perles) (without iodine)		Calcium Lactate, Cataplex F (perles), Thytrophin PMG
Cataplex F Perles			Thytrophin PMG, Super-Eff, Soy Bean Lecithin, Pituitrophin PMG
Cataplex G	Drenamin, Cardio-Plus, Betacol, Niacinamide B6		Organic Minerals, Choline, Betacol, Drenamin, Cardio-Plus
Chlorophyll Complex (perles)			) Chlorophyll Ointment, Cataplex G, Cataplex A-C-P, Ferrofood
Chlorophyll Ointment			A-C Carbamide, Cataplex F Ointment, Chlorophyll Complex (perles
Cholacol II		Bile Salts (Cholacol) Collinsonia and Bentonite	Zypan, Zymex, Okra Pepsin E3, Organic Minerals
Cholacol		Collinsonia, Bile Salts	Betafood, Zypan, Di-Sodium Phosphate
Choline			Betacol, Betafood, Di-Sodium Phosphate, Zypan
Collinsonia (Root)	Cholacol		Cyruta-Plus, Phosfood Liquid, Cataplex B, Cataplex G, Chlorophyll Complex (perles)
Congaplex			Organic Minerals, Min-Tran, A-C Carbamide, Cataplex C
Cyrofood			Organic Minerals, Calcium Lactate, Chlorophyll Complex (perles)
Cyruta		Inositol	Soy Bean Lecithin, Phosfood Liquid
Cyruta Plus	Cataplex A C P	Vitamin P factors of the C Complex	Chlorophill Complex (perles), Phosfood Liquid
Dermatrophin PMG			Cataplex A-C-P, Cataplex G, Chlorophyll (perles), Cyruta, Pituitrophin PMG
Di-Sodium Phosphate			Betacol, Organic Minerals, Zypan, Betafood
Drenamin		Cataplex C, Cataplex G, Drenatrophin PMG	Organic Minerals, Drenatrophin PMG
Ferrofood		Spleen, Vitamin B12, Iron, etc.	Zypan, Chlorophyll Complex (perles), Soy Bean Lecithin, Spleen PMG
For-Til B12	Chlorophyll Complex (perles)		Chlorophyll Complex (perles), Pituitrophin PMG

ASSOCIATED PRODUCTS

Product Name	Contains In	Also Contains	Related Products
Gastrex			Pituitrophin PMG, Chlorophyll Complex (perles)
Hepatrophin			Betacol, Choline, Betafood
Inositol (tablets)	Cyruta		Myotrophin PMG, Organic Minerals, Cataplex G, Super Eff, Cataplex È, Arginex
Iplex			Cataplex G, Organic Minerals, Cataplex A-C-P, Wheat Germ Oil (perles), Calcium Lactate (see General Considerations, page 107
Lactid Acid Yeast	Cyro-Yeast		Cataplex A-C-P, Inositol, Chlorophyll Complex (perles), Pituitrophin PMG
Mammary PMG			
Manganese Phytate-B_{12}	Trace Minerals-B_{12}		Trace Minerals-B_{12}
Min-Tran			Organic Minerals, Orchex
Myotrophin PMG Cardiotrophin PMG			Organic Minerals, Calcium Lactate, Betafood
Neurotrophin PMG			Cataplex G, Organic Minerals, Orchex, Cataplex B, Zymex, Inositol (tablets), Protefood
Niacinamide-B_6	Orchex		Organic Minerals, Cataplexx B, Calcium Lactate
Okra, Pepsin &E_3			Zypan, Di-Sodium Phosphate, A-F Betafood, Gastrex
Orchex		Niacinamide B_6	Cataplex G, Calcium Lactate, Organic Minerals, Niacinamide B_6, Orchic PMG
Orchic PMG			Cataplex È, Chlorophyll Complex (perles), Pituitrophin PMG
Organic Bound Minerals			Drenamin, Min-Tran
Ostrophin PMG			Biost, Bio-Dent, Calcifood Wafers, Calcium Lactate
Ovatrophin PMG			Ovex (see General Considerations, pages 135-136
Ovex			Cataplex F (perles), Pituitrophin PMG, Thytrophin PMG, Calcium Lactate, Prolamine Iodine, Soy Bean Lecithin, Drenamin
Pancreatrophin PMG			Zypan, Sea Salt
Parotid PMG			Pituitrophin PMG, Thytrophin PMG, Pancreatrophin PMG Cataplex F, Cataplex G, Cataplex A-C-P
Phosfood Liquid			Prolamine Iodine, Organic Minerals, Calcium Lactate, Soy Bean Lecithin, Biost (Bio-Dent), Calcifood Wafers
Pituitrophin PMG			Chlorophyll Complex (perles), Pancreatrophin PMG, Trace Minerals-B_{12}, or Manganese B_{12}
Pneumotrophin PMG			Drenamin, Calcium Lactate, Phosfood

ASSOCIATED PRODUCTS

Product Name	Contains In	Also Contains	Related Products
Prolamine Iodine			
Prostate PMG			Prost X, Cataplex F, Drenamin, Pituitrophin PMG, Thytrophin PMG
Prost X			Cataplex F, Prostate PMG, Pituitrophin PMG
Protefood		Ribonucleic Acid	Zypan, Nutrimere, Calcium Lactate
Renatrophin PMG			Cataplex A-C-P, Chlorophyll Complex (perles), Betacol, Arginex, Cataplex F, Cataplex G
Ribonucleic Acid (RNA)	Protofood		Protofood, Thytrophin PMG, Pituitrophin PMG
Soy Bean Lecithin		Choline, Phosphorus	Ferrofood, Cyruta, A-F Betafood, Phosfood Liquid
Spleen PMG	Ferrofood		Thymex, Cataplex A-C-P, Ferrofood
Super-Eff			Mytrophin, Organic Minerals, Cataplex G, Inositol
Thymex			Thymus PMG, Chlorophyll Complex (perles), Cataplex A-C-P, Calcium Lactate, Pituitrophin PMG, Super-Eff
Thymus PMG			Cataplex A-C-P, Calcium Lactate, Pituitrophin PMG
Thytrophin PMG			Pituitrophin PMG, Drenamin, (see General Diretions, page173)
Trace Minerals B_{12}		Manganese B_{12} Organic Iodine	Cataplex E, Calcifood Wafers, SoyBean Lecithin, Biost, Calcium Lactate, Chlorophyll Complex (perles), Cataplex C
USF Ointment			
Utrophin PMG			Pituitrophin PMG, Ovex, Ovatrophin PMG, Betacol(or Hepatrophin PMG), Thytrophin PMG Cataplex A-C-P
Vasculin		Cataplex B, Cataplex C, Cardiotrophin	Cataplex G, Cataplex B, Cataplex E
Wheat Germ Oil Perles		Wheat Germ Oil	Betacol, Ferrofood, Sesame Products
Zymex			Zypan, Arginex, Okra Pepsin E_3, Chlorophyll Complex(perles), Betacol, Choline, Betafood
Zymex II			Wheat Germ Oil Perles, Manganese B_{12}
Zypan			Betaine Hydrochloride, Pancreatrophin PMG, A-F Betafood, Cholacol, Cal-Amo, Choline

Note: *Catalyn contains the Vitamin Complex and Trace Minerals, but depending on the severity of the situation, the straight complexes are needed, either in conjunction with Catalyn or with synergistic or related products. Refer to the Product Bulletins for more information on the Related Products.

Where the term Vitamin appears, it is understood that we are referring to our natural complexes.

DRUGS AND WHOLE FOOD SUPPORT

The following information is supplied for the purpose of practical clinical application where these entities are required. There are no contra indications for food therapy and in most cases it supports the effects of drugs and lessons possible toxicity which may be produced where drugs are being used.

DRUG THERAPY

ASPIRIN
Antipyretic and relieves many of the minor aches and pains, develops full effect in about 30 minutes, eliminated in urine, effects persist about 3 hours from single dose.

ADRENAL CORTEX EXTRACT
Used in Addison's disease; overdosage produces symptoms similar to edema of heart failure.

ADRENALIN
Adrenergic effect; antiallergic effect and used in serious hypersensitivity reaction and in asthmatic attacks.

ALCOHOL
Often prescribed for its sedative effect on some, as an appetite stimulant, although this effect varies in individuals. It tends to be fattening due to its high caloric content. It is an important fact that alcoholics do not eat much other foods.

ALOE
A constituent of many commonly used laxatives, acting as a mild cathartic, but in large doses may produce renal irritation.

ALUMINUM HYDROXIDE MIXTURES
A form of aluminum gel used as an antacid. Prolonged use may interfere with calcium absorption and impaction of the gel in the intestine may cause obstruction.

AMINOPHYLLINE
Diuretic, antispasmodic and respiratory stimulant, used to dilate coronary arteries, although many doubt its usefulness here. Gastrointestinal distress is common from its use.

AMPHETAMINE
"Benzedrine", often used to counteract sleepiness, narcolepsy, mental fatigue, orthostatic hypotension; tends to elevate blood pressure and may produce insomnia.

PHYSIOLOGICAL COUNTERPART

Etiology must be sought; spasticity usually a complicating factor, usually a deficiency of ionizable calcium for which Calcium Lactate is recommended; Prostex has been found useful in pain; also Cal-Amo for pain brought on by alkalosis situations; the use of Anti-Pyrexin in allergic reactions.

ADRENAMIN – ADRENAPLEX
Adrenamin or Adrenaplex supplies the non hormone fractions of the adrenal glands and is an important adjunct in all adrenal therapy, whether specific hormones are used or not. Attention should be given to sufficient salt intake in these cases.

POTASSIUM BICARBONATE
Useful in simulating the effects of adrenalin. Supportive in this respect, is Adrenamin, Adrenaplex and Antipyrexin. Note: Adrenalin opposes histamine in its effects.

HONEY
Honey duplicates many of the beneficial effects of alcohol without its detrimental effects. Honey is a well-known alterative in heart conditions and is a well tolerated carbohydrate which is also rich in nutrients many of which have not been isolated. The uncooked varieties of honey should be recommended, Tupelo Honey has particular merit in many respects.

LACTIC ACID YEAST – ACIDOPHILUS YEAST
Constipation is best treated by physiological means, one of the best being to supply Lactic Acid Yeast preparations which normalize the pH of the colon and supply bulk forming elements.

CHOLACOL II
Containing montmorillonite is completely natural adsorbent which controls acidity by absorption and is not alkalizing in its effects, retains moisture and thus promotes motility to stool.

VITAMIN G COMPLEX – CATAPLEX G
Simulates these effects through physiological mechanisms, a safe and effective means of promoting coronary integrity with no contra-indications which may be used indefinitely.

PROTEFOOD OR PROTEDYN – ADRENAMIN OR ADRENAPLEX
Simulate these effects by providing protein metabolizers and adrenal hormone precursors, there are no known contraindications for their use.

DRUGS AND WHOLE FOOD SUPPORT

DRUG THERAPY

AMYL NITRATE
When inhaled, dilates smooth muscle, especially coronary arteries, used in angina pectoris, effects persist for short time only, causes intense and rapid lowering of the blood pressure which may lead to headaches and shock-like reactions. <u>Patient should be sitting when inhaling vapors.</u>

ANTIBIOTICS
It is essential that they be used with discrimination; side-effects are suppress bacterial activity essential to health; pave way for superinfections (antibiotic resistant infections) and systemic reactions, skin lesions, etc.

ANTIHISTAMINES
They are not curative. They provide only systematic relief and their action never extends over the few hours following their administration, patient must be warned of drowsiness; there is no way of determining their effectiveness beforehand.

ARSENIC COMPOUNDS
In syphilis it has been virtually displaced by penicillin, all have serious toxic potentialities.

ASCORBIC ACID
Large doses may lead to GI upsets, although generally considered to be non-toxic, does not correct the lesions of scurvy – although its lack is said to cause scurvy.

ATROPINE
The active principle of belladonna, an anticholinergic and mydriatic, a vagal antagonist, paralyzing or depressing nerves of the parasympathetic nervous system; diminishes secretions of saliva and gastric juices, suppresses respiration and accelerates heart, used in peptic ulcer.

BARBITUATES
Produce sedation, hypnosis, somnolence depending upon dose given; continued use may lead to dependence with withdrawal symptoms; a favorite drug for suicide.

DICUMAROL (BISHYDROXYCOUMARIN)
Lengthens prothrombin time by decreasing prothrombin content of blood, used to prevent clots, particularly in coronary patients; overdosage may lead to internal hemorrhage, must be used in conjunction with daily blood checks.

PHYSIOLOGICAL COUNTERPART

VITAMIN G COMPLEX OR CATAPLEX G
Acts as physiological relaxant. May be safely taken in standing position, if we may be permitted to say so. Synergistic in this effect is Vitamin E2, the combination of which is effective in the relief of the pains of angina in the majority of cases, no contraindications to their use.

THYMEX, VITAMIN C COMPLEX OR CATAPLEX C AND CALCIUM LACTATE
The natural resistance of the body in its highest state seldom encounters an overwhelming infection, which is the only reason antibiotics are indicated. Natural resistance encompasses many factors, but the Vitamin C is of particular note. Thymex, Vitamin C and Calcium Lactate often succeed in handling these situations.

ANTI-PYREXIN
It is a completely physiological antihistamine because it is an extract of liver tissue. Its effects are extended over a long period of time and in addition it is beneficial in other metabolic processes such as detoxification through liver function.

Arsenic containing wallpapers and paints (green color) have been used with serious results simply by being in the environment, care of depressed feelings in certain likely areas should be noted.

VITAMIN C COMPLEX OR CATAPLEX C
Does correct the symptoms of scurvy and is completely non-toxic, being considered as a food source item and not a synthesized compound in its chemically pure form, therefore nutritional, not pharmaceutical in its classification and effects.

PHOSFOOD OR PHOSPHADE
The beneficial action of Phosfood or Phosphade simulates these effects by physiological means. This action is augmented by Calcium Lactate. These may be safely used to control symptoms ordinarily shown to be belladonna indications by drug methods.

ORCHEX
Orchex and other nutritional adjuncts produce a feeling of well-being seldom requiring drug sedation in ordinary living; a well-fed body does not require sedation in normal circumstances.

BETAFOOD OR BETARIS AND PHOSFOOD OR PHOSPHADE
Betacol acts to normalize liver function, the basic cause; Betafood and Phosfood act to lower the viscosity of the blood, a circumstance, we believe, is necessary before blood clotting is likely to occur. High protein diets are not recommend as this also tends to thicken blood.

DRUGS AND WHOLE FOOD SUPPORT

DRUG THERAPY	PHYSIOLOGICAL COUNTERPART
BROMIDES Used for sedation and hypnosis; slowly eliminated and may cumulate; skin eruptions are common; psychological manifestations may be quite serious; value as sedative is questionable.	See "Barbiturates"
CALCIUM CARBONATE Used as gastric antacid; liberates gas on contact with acid; tends to produce constipation.	See "Aluminum Hydroxide Mixtures"
CARBON TETRACHLORIDE Widely used against hookworm and other intestinal parasites; highly toxic, may cause liver, kidney or nerve injury.	**VERMIDASE** Is a completely non-toxic vermifuge which is dependent upon the enzyme action of natural substances for its action; may be safely used for as long as desired with additional benefits because of its protein digesting enzymes.
CASCARA SAGRADA Like all laxatives, tends to induce dependence when used regularly.	See "Aloe"
CHARCOAL, ACTIVATED Tends to adsorb gases, but of doubtful value.	See "Aluminum Hydroxide Mixtures"
CHLORAL HYDRATE Hypnotic and sedative	See "Barbiturates"
COCAINE (NOVOCAIN OR PROTEIN) A potent local anesthetic widely used in dentistry, dangers from rapid absorption are great, under control of Federal Narcotic Laws.	**CHLOROPHYLL OINTMENT** Applied locally does much to promote healing and relieve pain after extraction.
CORTOTROPHIN May induce diabetes, interfere with control of congestive heart failure, cause psychic disturbances, skin eruptions, etc.	See "Adrenal Cortex Extract"
CORTISONE Gastric ulcers have been reported from long continued use. Does not cure.	See "Adrenal Cortex Extract"
DEHYDROCHOLIC ACID Stimulates flow of bile and hastens filling of gallbladder, not its emptying; contraindicated in biliary obstruction. May induce asthmatic attacks in patients with asthma, use carefully in hepatitis.	**BETAFOOD OR BETARIS** By reason of its non-stimulatory effect and bile thinning action is beneficial and may be safely used in all gallbladder disorders; Zypan aids in its effects, Betaine Hydrochloride being beneficial in initiating sphincter release by reason of its acid nature.
DESOXYCORTICOSTERONE Overdosage may lead to edema, pulmonary congestion and signs of cardiac failure.	See "Adrenal Cortex Extract"
DIETHYL STILBESTROL Stilbestrol – potent estrogenic drug, in common with other estrogens, may produce excessive uterine bleeding.	**OVARY CYTOTROPHIN OR OVEX** Are basic nutritional products which may be used on a physiological basis, for the purpose of improving local environment which will in many cases restore function of this organ.

DRUGS AND WHOLE FOOD SUPPORT

DRUG THERAPY	PHYSIOLOGICAL COUNTERPART
DIGITALIS Nausea and vomiting are the early signs of intoxication. Potassium may be used for treatment of digitalis poisoning.	**ORGANIC MINERALS OR MINAPLEX** Potassium is the natural regulator of the heartbeat, for which Organic Minerals is recommended. Calcium Lactate augments the effects of digitalis.
ERGOT Causes potent constriction of uterus, overdosage may cause gangrene.	Physiological care both before and after delivery is usually effective in producing normal childbirth, obviating the need for oxytocics.
ESTROGENS Uterine hypertrophy and bleeding in improper dosage.	See "Diethyl Stilbestrol", similar drug
EXCHANGE RESINS Precipitate various ions (alkaline or acid) and used to control diets.	**CHOLACOL II** With montmorillonite, acts to precitate potassium and is useful in elevated potassium levels, as in Addison's disease.
FERROUS SULFATE May cause G.I. distress, stools turn dark green or black.	**FERROFOOD OR FERROPLUS** Is a complex of ingredients with less irritating iron in small amounts, more useful in the treatment of nutritional anemias.
FOLIC ACID Should not be substituted for liver extracts in pernicious anemia. Of no value in aplastic anemia or iron deficiency anemias.	See "Ferrous Sulfate"
GLUTAMIC ACID HYDROCHLORIDE Releases hydrochloric acid on contact with water, providing this acid on hypacidity.	**BETAINE HYDROCHLORIDE** This is, we believe, the more basic physiological form and should be combined with pepsin and other gastric enzymes for fullest effect.
GOLD SALTS Used in arthritis; many toxic effects including, baldness, anemia, bronchitis, conjunctivitis, nephritis, hepatitis and others.	**BETACOL AND BETALCO AND OSTOGEN OR BIOST TABLETS** Arthritis is believed to be a nutritional disease by many prominent European doctors. We believe it to be a cooked food disease. Betacol and Ostogen offer best clinical results, although each case is different.
GONADOTROPHIN, CHORIONIC Its value in all but cryptorchism remains to be seen. Excessive dosage may induce pseudo-puberty and precocious sexuality.	**PITUITARY CYTOTROPHIN** The use of Pituitary Cytotrophin has simulated many of the effects by completely physiological mechanisms, related Cytotrophins may be necessary, of course.
HEPARIN Anticoagulant, clotting time must be carefully followed.	See "Dicumerol", similar drug.
HEXESTROL Synthetic estrogen.	See "Estrogen".
HYDROCORTISONE Should not be used in infectious arthritis.	See "Adrenal Cortical Extracts".
MAGNESIUM HYDROXIDE Milk of Magnesia. Salts of magnesium are relatively nonirritating and poorly absorbed. They act both as intestinal antacids and laxatives given in relatively large doses. When magnesium is absorbed in large amounts, it acts as a strong depressant, the antidote for which is calcium given slowly intravenously.	That milk of magnesia, used as a laxative, does become adsorbed in large amounts in many cases is evidenced by the many reports of epistaxis from habitual users. We, no doubt, __ere have a disturbance in the blood clotting mechanism of which calcium plays such an important role. Therapy is discontinuation of the drug and use of Calcium Lactate to supply the drug induced deficiency.

DRUGS AND WHOLE FOOD SUPPORT

DRUG THERAPY	PHYSIOLOGICAL COUNTERPART
MAGNESIUM TRISILICATE Widely used in stomach ulcers and as antacid.	See "Magnesium Hydroxide".
MANNITOL HEXANITRATE Slower action than nitroglycerin, longer lasting, may depress bone marrow.	See "Aminophylline", similar drug.
MECHLORETHAMINE (Nitrogen Mustard) Restrains growth of several tumors but does not cure them, may be used in areas where X-Ray and radium are not available.	Nutritional support important in all such cases.
MENTHOL Systemic action is that of central nervous system depressant, producing convulsions and death when used in very large areas of skin in topical applications.	Mustard poultices much safer, only effect being local irritation and rubefaction.
MEPROBAMATE Equanil, Miltown, etc. One of a number of new drugs said to be valuable in anxiety states, they should be used with considerable circumspection as their value remains to be established and their toxicity and potential for addiction has not been determined.	**ORCHEX** Any number of nutritional remedies, the most common of which is calcium, may be used to control certain anxiety states, which if not caused by nutritional deficiencies, are certainly aggravated by them. Outstanding in this respect is Orchex, with its contained B_6, an established antispasmodic in deficiency states, with Calcium Lactate its results have been outstanding.
MERCURIAL DIURETICS Mercuhydrin, contraindicated in acute nephritis, frequent use presents danger of low-salt syndrome.	**ARGINEX AND BETACOL OR BETALCO** Outstanding kidney remedy in overload, is Arginex, augmented by Betacol or Betalco and Vitamin G Complex or Cataplex G (liver) satisfactory supportive therapy here reduces the likelihood of need for such mercurial diuretics except in the most advanced an emergency cases.
MERCURIC CHLORIDE Rapidly produces irreversible kidney damage, extremely rapidly absorbed from all mucous membranes, use as a vaginal douche is dangerous for that reason, has little place in modern pharacopeas.	N/A
METHANTHELINE Banthine – There is real danger of glaucoma in sensitive patients, widely used drug in stomach disorders.	See "Atrophine", similar drug.
METHYLCELLULOSE Used to stimulate bowel activity by increasing intestinal bulk, should not be used where there is intestinal obstruction.	**LACTIC ACID YEAST OR ACIDOPHILUS YEAST** Is the completely physiological method of correcting constipation, bile salts (Cholacol) stimulate liver function and bile flow, Di-Sodium Phosphate for obstinate cases.
METHYLROSANILINE Gentian Violet, contraindicated internally in patients with serious heart or kidney or liver disease, nausea and even vomiting may occur after internal use.	**VERMIDASE** Natural remedy, see "Carbon Tetrachloride" for legend.
MORPHINE One of the most useful, yet dangerous drugs; overdosage may cause serious depression of respiration. Frequent use leads easily to addiction, especially in alcoholics or depressed patients, narcotic laws abide.	**CARBAMIDE AND ZYMEX** Toxic effects may be mitigated by concomitant use of Carbamide (urea) which narcotics tend to depress, particularly true in withdrawal states in drug addiction. Zymex very useful as detoxicant.

DRUGS AND WHOLE FOOD SUPPORT

DRUG THERAPY	PHYSIOLOGICAL COUNTERPART

NAPHAZPLINE
Privine, use reduction of swelling in nasal mucosa, excessive use may lead to local irritation and "rebound" congestion.

CHLOROPHYLL
A non-toxic remedy which may be safely used, small amounts of tannic acid potentiate the healing and constricting effect.

NEOSTIGMINE
Prostigmin – Causes stimulation of parasympathetic by preventing destruction of acetylcholine; may induce asthmatic attacks, nausea, vomiting and depressed blood pressure.

VITAMIN G COMPLEX OR CATAPLEX G
Supplies the natural precursors of cholinesterase, the enzyme which is necessary for normal synapse of the cholinergic system, may be safely used indefinitely, augmented in its effects by potassium, Organic Minerals or Minaplex.

NIKETHAMIDE
Coramine – A convulsant drug for respiratory and cardiac stimulation, for which action, however, there is little substantial proof, and in many circles the drug has been largely discontinued.

CALCIUM LACTATE
The natural cardiac stimulant is Calcium Lactate or other similar calcium preparations such as calcium gluconate.

PANTOPON
Mixture of narcotic alkaloids. All its important effects are derived from its morphine content and it has no real value over morphine other than its name which is generally not associated with morphine in the mind of the layman. This makes it often possible to prescribe a potent narcotic with the patient and relatives remaining in ignorance of its real nature.

Apparently placebos, deceptive labeling and other forms of deception and substifuge are acceptable medical practice. This approach is not only not necessary with natural therapy, but is looked upon with considerable askance.

PAPAVERINE
Relaxes smooth muscles in coronary states, vascular conditions, etc. In the conditions for which it is used, the situation is often irreversible and therefore little may be expected from one drug in such instances. Narcotic, inject slowly, overdosage may cause faintness.

The proper treatment consists of nutritional therapy instituted as a preventative measure when first signs are shown, revealed by Endocardiograph readings showing dysfunction before pathological changes occur.

PARALDEHYDE
A potent sedative and hypnotic commonly used for noisy and obstreperous alcoholics; use with caution in liver disease; rapid injection may cause pulmonary edema or cardiac failure.

Many reports show interrelationship between alcoholism and nutrition. Supportive therapy for liver should be given, not therapy which should be "sued with Caution" in liver conditions.

PETROLATUM (Mineral Oil)
Base or vehicle in ointments, sprays, etc., laxative in constipation; may prevent absorption of fat soluble vitamins; inhalation may cause lipoid pneumonia.

See "Aloe", laxative discussion.

PHENOBARBITOL
Luminal – As for all other barbiturates, may lead to habituation.

N/A

PHENOL
Carbolic acid – Although freely used for years, now recognized as relatively dangerous material for use in or on the patient, highly toxic and caustic.

N/A

PHENOLPHTHALINE
Cathartic, may be habit forming, small doses have been highly toxic, commonly used in candy chewing gum and other forms of hidden laxatives.

N/A

DRUGS AND WHOLE FOOD SUPPORT

DRUG THERAPY	PHYSIOLOGICAL COUNTERPART
PHEYLEPRHINE Neo-Synephrine	See "Atropine", similar drug.
PHYSOSTIGMINE Parasympathetic stimulant.	N/A
PIPERAZINE Vermifuge	N/A
PLACEBO Any preparation administered to satisfy the patient's desire or symbolic need for medication rather than for a pharmacologic action.	Many nutritional preparations labeled by force of court action "as having no value in human nutrition" are done so because of macabe interests who at the same time use placebos at their discretion.
PLANTAGO SEED Psyllium Seed	N/A
PODOPHYLLUM RESIN COMPOUNDS Potent skin irritant, used for treatment of granuloma inquinale and "venereal" warts, avoid contact with open flame.	N/A
QUINIDINE Cardiac depressant, may cause nausea, ringing of ears, dizziness, etc., (cinchonism), substitute for quinine.	N/A
RELAXIN (RELEASIN) A new hormone, utility remains to be established.	N/A
SQUILL Cardiac stimulant, has all the dangers of digitalis treatment.	N/A
STRYCHNINE Highly toxic causing tetanic convulsions, there are some medications which contain small amounts, not toxic to adults (such as laxatives which contain strychnine) which may be fatal if taken in sufficient numbers by children.	N/A
SUCROSE Occasionally used as diuretic which action it exerts by preventing reabsorption of water in the kidneys, there is evidence that repeated intravenous sue of this material may cause permanent kidney damage.	N/A
SULFONAMIDES Now a large list, perhaps 6000 have been screened, the danger of bone marrow depression is a real one and must be watched for by regular red and white cell counts. Kidney damage must also be considered.	N/A
SYNTHETIC OLEOVITAMIN D There is danger from large overdosage. Manufacturer must indicate whether preparation contains calciferol or other forms of Vitamin D.	N/A
TANNIC ACID Astringent on skin – use has been discontinued because of liver damage from extensive use.	N/A

DRUGS AND WHOLE FOOD SUPPORT

DRUG THERAPY	PHYSIOLOGICAL COUNTERPART
TRANQUILIZERS Their value in the treatment of the run-of-the-mill anxiety symptoms is highly questionable and may even be hazardous in the long run.	N/A

OPTIMAL TIME TO TAKE NUTRITIONAL SUPPLEMENTS

After Meals

Lactic Acid Yeast	Ferrofood	Cardio-Plus	For-Til B_{12}
Cyro-Yeast	Protefood	Chlorophyll	Zypan
Vitamin A	Betafood	Cholacol	All Tissue Extracts
Vitamin A & C	Betacol	Choline	
Vitamin A-C-P	Super-EFF	Comfrey, Pepsin & E_3	
Vitamin D	Vitamin E_2	Inositol	
Vitamin E	Ostogen	Nucleo-Protein	
Vitamin F	Adrenamin	Organic Iodine	
A & F Betafood	Allorganic Trace Minerals	R.N.A.	
Wheat Germ Oil	Betaine Hydrochloride	Zymex	
Vitamin F Perles	Cal-Amo	Vasculin	

Before or After Meals

Cyroplex	Cyruta	Lecithin	Vitamin B_{12}
Vitamin B	Cyruta A	Manganese – B_{12}	
Vitamin C	Calcifood A	Niacinamide B_6	
Vitamin G	Anti-Pyrexin	Orchex	
Organic Minerals	Arginex	Ovex	
Cyrofood	Bio-Dent	Prostex	
Calsol	Cholacol II	Thymex	

Before Meals

Anti-Gastrin

Between Meals

Phosfood	Collinsonia	Potassium Bicarbonate
Carbamide	Di-Sodium Phosphate	Sodium Citrate
Chlorophyll (aqueous)		

On an Empty Stomach

Calcium Lactate

Note: Optima schedule for all Tissue Extracts should be taken as follows:

First Week	–	1 per day taken with the largest meal
Second "	--	2 per day taken one after lunch and one after dinner
Third "	--	3 per day taken one after each meal

Optima schedule for Cholacol is after meals

First Day	–	1 per meal
Second "	--	2 per meal
Third "	--	3 per meal
Fourth	--	none, repeat the process starting with day one over again on day five.

©1996 – 2010 International Foundation for Nutrition and Health, All Rights Reserved

NUTRITIONAL SOURCES OF WHOLE NATURAL FOODS

All patients respond better when using a healthy diet. The key to success is to get the patient to stop doing what has made them ill in the first place, clean up their diet. Having your patient keep a diet diary will help your overall success; support the foundational issues (digestion, sugar handling and liver biliary function).

VITAMIN A (Carotene, Fat Soluble)
- Alfalfa
- Fish-liver oils
- Butter
- Carrots
- Egg Yolk
- Dark green vegetables
- Beef liver
- Yellow & orange vegetables
- Dandelion greens

VITAMIN B COMPLES (Water Soluble for all B Vitamins)
- Brewer's yeast
- Desiccated liver
- Liver
- Wheat germ

VITAMIN B1 (Thiamine)
- Green peas
- Oranges
- Lean ham
- Muscle meats
- Nuts
- Lean pork
- Whole-grain products
- Soy beans

VITAMIN B2 (Riboflavin)
- Dried peas and beans
- Eggs
- Fish
- Liver
- Milk, cottage cheese & whey
- Brewer's yeast
- Muscle meats & tongue
- Mustard greens
- Oysters
- Soybeans
- Whole grain products

VITAMIN B6 (Pyridoxine)
- Molasses
- Eggs
- Ferment of yeast
- Fresh fruits & vegetables
- Seeds & nuts
- Soybean products & unpolished rice
- Whole-grain products

VITAMIN B12 (Cyanocobalamin)
- Cheese
- Egg yolk
- Kelp
- Liver
- Whole milk
- Yeast

VITAMIN B15 (Pangamic Acid)
- Brown rice
- Liver
- Pumpkin seeds
- Sesame seeds
- Sunflower seeds
- Rice bran

BIOTIN (B Vitamin)
- Cauliflower
- Eggs
- Organ & muscle meats
- Sardines & salmon
- Soybeans
- Unpolished rice
- Whole-grain products

VITAMIN C (Ascorbic Acid)
- Rose hips
- Citrus fruits
- Green leafy vegetables
- Green peppers
- Parsley
- Tomatoes
- Raw potato

CALCIUM
- Bone meal
- Cheese
- Fish
- Green leafy vegetables
- Milk
- Yogurt

CHLORINE (Mineral)
- Seaweed (Kelp, Dulse)
- Leafy green vegetables
- Claims
- Olives
- Oysters
- Sardines

CHOLINE (B Vitamin)
- Beans & peas
- Cabbage
- Eggs
- Liver
- Muscle meats
- Soybean products & nuts
- Spinach
- Yeast

NUTRITIONAL SOURCES OF WHOLE NATURAL FOODS

COPPER (Trace Mineral)
- Dried peas & beans
- Egg yolks
- Liver
- Prunes
- Shrimp
- Whole-grain products

VITAMIN D (Fat soluble)
- Fish liver oil
- Butter
- Eggs
- Liver
- Milk
- Saltwater fish

VITAMIN E (Fat soluble)
- Wheat germ
- Wheat germ oil
- Leafy green vegetables
- Sweet potato
- Sunflower seeds
- Nuts & legumes
- Vegetable oils
- Whole-grain products

VITAMIN F (Unsaturated Fatty Acids)
- Fish liver oil
- Golden vegetable oils
  (soy, corn, safflower)
- Avocados
- Nuts
- Salad dressings
- Sunflower seeds

FLUORINE (Trace Mineral)
- Bone meal
- Rose hips
- Seaweed
- Mineral water
- Ocean fish
- Sea salt

FOLIC ACID (Folacin, B Vitamin)
- Desiccated liver
- Green, leafy vegetables
- Legumes
- Liver
- Muscle meats

INOSITOL (B Vitamin)
- Blackstrap molasses
- Beef heart
- Cantaloupe
- Grapefruit
- Dried peas & beans
- Fruits & raisins
- Peanuts
- Yeast

IODINE MINERAL
- Seaweed (Kelp, Dulse)
- Dried beans
- Wheat
- Mushrooms
- Sea foods
- Spinach

IRON
- Blackstrap molasses
- Brewer's yeast
- Liver
- Wheat germ
- Soy beans
- Dried fruits
- Muscle & organ meats
- Oysters

VITAMIN K (Menadione K, Fat soluble)
- Fish liver oil
- Molasses
- Alfalfa, spinach, cabbage
- Green leafy vegetables
- Liver & eggs
- Soybeans

LECITHIN (Fatty substance)
- Cold-pressed oils
- Egg yolk
- Green leafy vegetables
- Liver & eggs
- Soybeans

MAGNESIUM
- Wheat germ & kelp
- Nuts & figs
- Pumpkin & Sunflower seeds
- Soybean products
- Whole-grain products

MANGANESE (Mineral)
- Beets
- Dried peas & beans
- Egg yolks
- Green leafy vegetables
- Sunflower seeds
- Whole-grain products

NIACIN (B Vitamin)
- Beef heart
- Fish
- Liver
- Muscle meats
- Mushrooms
- Peanuts
- Poultry
- Yeast

NUTRITIONAL SOURCES OF WHOLE NATURAL FOODS

VITAMIN P (Water Soluble, Bioflavonoids)
- Rose hips
- Grapes
- Foods high in Vitamin C
- Prunes
- White segment of citrus

PABA (Para-Aminobenzoic Acid, B Vitamin)
- Eggs
- Liver
- Milk
- Molasses
- Rice bran
- Rye
- Wheat Germ
- Yeast

PANTOTHENIC ACID (B Vitamin)
- Beans, dry
- Cheese
- Eggs
- Liver
- Mushrooms
- Peanuts
- Soybeans
- Yeast

PHOSPHORUS
- Bone Meal
- Dried peas & beans
- Eggs
- Meat & fish
- Nuts & Sunflower seeds
- Whole-grains

POTASSIUM
- Molasses
- Citrus fruits & figs
- Fish & meat
- Watercress
- Whole-grain products

PROTEIN AND AMINO ACIDS
- Brewer's yeast
- Wheat germ
- Dried peas & beans
- Milk, cheese & eggs
- Meats & fish
- Nuts & seeds
- Soybeans

SILICON
- White onion
- Oats
- Grasses
- Radishes
- Calmyrna figs
- Grains

SODIUM (Mineral)
- Kelp
- Beets & carrots
- Green leafy vegetables
- Sea foods
- Sea salt

SULPHUR
- Nuts & seeds
- Soybeans
- Sea foods
- Eggs
- Beans
- Cabbage

VANADIUM AND OTHER TRACE MINERALS
- Kelp & sea salt
- Brewer's yeast
- Bone meal
- Leafy green vegetables
- Salt-water fish

ZINC (Trace Mineral)
- Wheat germ
- Fish
- Liver
- Milk & eggs
- Poultry
- Sunflower seeds & nuts

This section on whole foods can help support patient compliance with lifestyle and diet recommendations. This is an excellent handout to put with the Page Food Plan. Dr. Page felt that success rotated around a good healthy diet and the use of supplements was only to get a patient started, unfortunately today were working with a different level of Pottenger's cats and our food supply is so compromised that you have to use both.

Recommended reading: Pottenger's Cat Study by France's Pottenger M.D. and Food and Behavior by Barbara Stitt.

©1996 – 2010 International Foundation for Nutrition and Health, All Rights Reserved

CLINICAL AND LABORATORY TESTS

CLINICAL DIAGNOSTIC POSSIBILITIES
Physical Examination Outline

A brief discussion of practical clinical tests which may be performed follows. Laboratory tests are also discussed from a clinical viewpoint. No attempt is made to discuss these tests at length, as this information is readily available from IFNH at ifnh.org. Many of these tests are part of the nutritional exam taught in the CCWFN program. For more information refer to website.

1. Postural Blood Pressure Test:

This test is made by taking the blood pressure in two positions, one with patient lying down and the other with patient standing. The difference between these two readings is a measure of the patient's ability to compensate for the hydrostatic effects of gravity. It is considered an approximation of the portal circulation as it is believed that in this area a significant amount of compensation occurs. This mechanism is under autonomic control and deviations are believed to be significant of sympathetic tone. The normal finding is for the blood pressure to be slightly higher (5 to 10 mm) in the standing as compared to the recumbent position. When the blood pressure fails to be higher when standing, this is considered to be a loss of sympathetic tone. Useful in: differentiating pathological from physiological low blood pressure; neurosthenic states; hypoadrenia; fatigue, tolerance indication; autonomic storms; and other neurocirculatory disorders.

2. Dilation and Concentration Test:

Complete instructions for this test are given in Arginex Bulletin. The ability of the kidney to concentrate and dilute urine is considered an important functional test for kidney function. It is an important consideration in determining the prognosis on any kidney case and is helpful in differentiating an infectious or inflammatory condition, from one involving degenerative changes.

3. Uristix (Trade Name):

These sticks are treated so as to show albuminuria and glycosuria by simply dipping them in the urine and comparing the color charts supplied with each bottle. The possibility of routine examination for these findings is considerably increased with this product. Note that a series of tests should be given as any one test may not prove significant.

4. Pulse Rate:

The pulse rate gives many indications of pathological possibilities. It may be <u>elevated</u> in the following conditions:
- *Marked in children in fever and toxemias, less marked in oldsters
- *Neurasthenia (psychogenic disorders)
- *Hyperthyroidism
- *Excessive coffee drinking
    - *Nephritis and other cardiovascular changes
    - *Seen after apoplexy
    - *Nervous hypertension
    - *Pathognomonic of thyrotoxicosis.

It may be <u>decreased</u> in the following conditions:
- *Heart block
- *Cardiac failure and in extreme toxic states
- *Long distance runners and others normally
- *Intracranial tension
- *Arteriosclerosis
- *Apoplexy
- *Congestive heart failure
- *Hypothyroidism
- *Hypopituitarism
- *Hypoadrenia

5. Ketosteroid Test:

While this test shows the hormonal output of the adrenal cortex, its significance may be extended to include the pituitary and sex gland as well, as these are often extenuating circumstances bringing about deviations in adrenal output.

CLINICAL AND LABORATORY TESTS

CLINICAL DIAGNOSTIC POSSIBILITIES
Physical Examination Outline

6. Liver Function Tests:
No one test for liver function is considered significant. The reserve capacity of the liver is the factor which obscures the findings in these tests, 80% failure often being required before liver function tests prove positive. See Betacol Bulletin for discussion.

7. Glucose Tolerance Tests:
The use of these tests in diabetes and in extreme hypoglycemia is well established. In transient sugar deviations, as most frequently found clinically, the test has less value. The significance in the later cases, is the RATE OF FALL off blood sugar which precipitates the attack, not necessarily the degree of fall. This change may occur in the diabetic as well as the hypoglycemic. The clinical test should be made under therapeutic circumstances, i.e., if the patient is relieved of his symptoms DURING AN ATTACK, the tentative diagnosis of dysinsulinism may be made. These attacks most generally accompany a sympathetic nervous system crisis which is lacking in most laboratory tests.

8. Basal Metabolism Test:
Although this is a valuable test, there are many more indications for its approximation than are usually practical in ordinary clinical practice. The most important indication of the B.M.R. that may be used clinically is the pulse rate. See discussion under "4., Pulse Rate" above.

9. Blood Sugar (Fasting):
A very valuable test which should be included in all lCBC's and especially where diabetes would be suspected as in boils, chronic infections, abnormal thirst, night sweats and chronic fatigue.

10. Reflex Tests:
These include various neurological reflex tests, such as the ta p of the facial nerve to determine alkalosis, patella and achilles reflex tests, gagging reflex tests and others. Generally speaking, these show involvements of the autonomic system, accentuated reflexes showing sympatheticotonia and decreased reflex, parasympatheticotonia. The gagging reflex (done with a tongue depressor) is particularly valuable. Where this is accentuated we generally find, photophobia, Dysphagia and tachycardia, also indicative of sympatheticotonia, where the gagging reflex is diminished, we generally find, nausea, stiffness of joints and bradycardia, also indicative of parasympatheticotonia.

11. Hypoproteinemia:
Albumin, Globulin, Total Protein, and A/G Ratio. Since albumin is lost easier than the larger molecule of globulin, shifts in A/G ratio are significant. The test is used in chronic nephritis, lipoid nephrosis, liver disease and malnutrition. The other significant factor is that many important nutrients are associated with blood levels of protein, two of the more important of which are ionized calcium and cholesterinase. (See Bulletins on Vitamin G Complex – Cataplex G, and Calcium Lactate.)

12. Blood Cholesterol:
Blood cholesterol may be elevated in many different conditions. In most of these conditions, the elevation is only an incidental finding. However, its significance would be considered important in coronary disease, hyperthyroidism, liver disease and keloids and in these cases, a blood cholesterol would be desirable.

13. Sulkowitch Reagent Test:
This test made on the urine, gives a reliable indication of blood calcium levels. The physiological reasoning behind this is as follows: There is a renal threshold for calcium – just as for glucose. This renal threshold is slightly below the normal blood calcium, so that in the normal subject, there is always a slight spillover of calcium into the urine. When equal parts of Sulkowitch Reagent and urine are mixed (filter unclear urine), the precipitant is observed as an opaque liquor. Perfectly clear specimens indicate low blood calcium, chalky or milky appearance indicates elevated blood calcium levels. The test is easily performed and is considered accurate. It is indicated specifically in tetany to determine if hypoparathyroidism is a possibility.

CLINICAL AND LABORATORY TESTS

CLINICAL DIAGNOSTIC POSSIBILITIES
Physical Examination Outline

14. <u>Therapeutic Tests:</u>

Various situations lend themselves particularly well to therapeutic tests. This is a test using the same remedy as that which would ordinarily be used for the correction of the condition. Generally, this procedure will either correct or aggravate the condition, and upon this basis a diagnosis is made. The following tests are useful:

HCL TEST	-See Bulletin on Zypan
THYROID TEST	-See Bulletin on Phosfood or Phosphade
ADRENAL TEST	-See Bulletin on Organic Minerals or Minaplex

Note also that side-reactions which may occur are usually significant for their diagnostic value and usually point to the basic condition involved. See "Side-Reactions" under the product concerned, also noting "Effects" as beneficial results are usually diagnostic as well and provide the means of fortifying an indicated situation.

15. <u>Breath-Holding Test:</u>

Dr. Brady, the popular newspaper medical columnist, for many years recommended the breath-holding test for alkalosis. The reasoning behind this is that in acidosis there is a deficiency of the bicarbonates and that without these the oxygen cannot be unloaded at the tissue levels. Clinical experience shows that it is an effective screen-test, inability to hold breath for at least 20 seconds without undue discomfort, is therefore considered a screen-test for acidosis.

16. <u>Urea Clearance Test:</u>

This is a test of function of the glomeruli of the kidneys and measures the ability of the kidneys to remove urea from the blood; urea clearance is decreased in kidney disease. The urea concentration of the blood and urine samples are measured.

17. <u>Bromthymol Blue Indicator:</u>

This is a color indication test which may be used on skin (sweat urine of feces specimens to show an alkaline colon, the most common finding in chronic constipation. The clinical picture generally improves when the pH is brought up to the acid side (Lactic Acid Yeast).

18. <u>Talquist Test:</u>

This is a color test of the blood, matching a blood stain to a fixed scale of dyes and offers a screen-test for possible anemia. The test is crude and does not provide technical information possible from a blood count.

19. <u>Tetany Test (Blood Pressure):</u>

When the blood pressure cuff is placed on the patient's arm and the pressure maintained at just above the diastolic level for 2 or 3 minutes, in the tetany prone patient, the hand will clamp and discomfort will be felt. This does not happen in the normal subject.

20. <u>Creatinine Test:</u>

Creatinine is derived from the breakdown of muscle creatine phosphate and increased secretion is indicative of disorder of kidney function or muscle tissue breakdown.

21. <u>Protein Bound Iodine Test (P.B.I.):</u>

This is a measure of thyroid function, thyroxin being a protein, the amount of protein-bound iodine present being the amount of thyroid hormone present.

22. <u>Papanicolaou Test:</u>

Microscopic tests for malignant cells, usually taken on female genital tract but also includes other areas such as bronchial, esophageal, rectal and colonic washings, nipple secretions, etc.

CLINICAL AND LABORATORY TESTS

NORMAL PHYSIOLOGICAL DATA

TEMPERATURE AND PULSE OF THE BODY:

Average temperature:
- Adult 98.6° F.
- Children 98.8° F.
- Aged 99° F.

1 to 1.5° F. fluctuation daily normally occurs, the maximum temperature being reached between 5 and 7 p.m.

A variation of one degree of temperature, above 98° F. is approximately equivalent to a difference of ten beats in the pulse, thus:

- Temperature of 98° corresponds with a pulse of 60.
- Temperature of 99° corresponds with a pulse of 70.
- Temperature of 100° corresponds with a pulse of 80.
- Temperature of 101° corresponds with a pulse of 90.
- Temperature of 102° corresponds with a pulse of 100.
- Temperature of 103° corresponds with a pulse of 110.

The pulse is generally more rapid in females, by 10-14 beats per minute; faster during digestion or mental excitement and in the morning. It is less rapid in phlegmatic temperaments. The pulse rate variations in health are as follows.

In the fetus in utero	140-150
Newborn infants	130-140
During first year	115-130
During second year	100-115 (Carpenter)
During third year	95-105
From 7th to 14th year	80-90
From 14th to 21st year	80-85
From 21st to 60th year	75-80
In old age	75-80

RESPIRATION RATES:
- First year: 25-35 respirations per minute
- At puberty: 20-25 respirations per minute
- Adult: 16 to 18 respirations per minute

AVERAGE NORMAL BLOOD PRESSURES:

Age	Systolic	Diastolic	Pulse Pressure
10 years	103	70	33
15 years	113	75	38
20 years	120	80	40
25 years	122	81	40
30 years	123	82	41
35 years	124	83	41
40 years	126	84	42
45 years	128	85	43
50 years	130	86	44
55 years	132	87	45
60 years	135	89	46

CLINICAL AND LABORATORY TESTS

CLINICAL DIAGNOSTIC POSSIBILITIES
Physical Examination Outline

There are approximately 200 diseases commonly found in the United States, 23 less physical abnormalities and 6 essential laboratory tests. These serve as keys to the diagnosis of most of these ills. The following outlines this situation.

I. **MAJOR ETIOLOGICAL DISEASE GROUPS**
 1. Infectious diseases.
 2. Premature decline of some important body function because of degeneration.
 3. Trauma (and atmospheric poisons).
 4. Metabolic and nutritional disturbances.
 5. Allergies.
 6. Inadequacy of adaptive function of personality.
 7. Disturbance related to generative capacity.
 8. Congenital and acquired anomalies and malformations.
    (Altered structure and function of the major anatomic system)

II. **COMMON SYMPTOMS**
 According to etiological history:
 1. Weakness (or loss or gain of weight).
 2. Discharge of pus or blood.
 3. Fever, chills or sweat.
 4. Sense of uneasiness or worry.
 5. Inability to get along with people.

 According to regional history:
 6. Headache.
 7. Fainting (coma or convulsions).
 8. Earache or tinnitus.
 9. Sneezing, nasal drip or sore throat.
 10. Cough, shortness of breath or precordial pain.
 11. Dyspnea, indigestion or changes in bowel movements.
 12. Cramps or abdominal soreness.
 13. Menstrual disturbances.
 14. Frequency of urination or nocturia.
 15. Lameness or backache.
 16. Itching or rash.

III. **LEADING PHYSICAL ABNORMALITIES**
 A. General Inspection
 1. Discolored or altered complexion.
 2. Cutaneous sores or blemishes.
 3. Stiffness (impaired motion or posture).
 4. Hoarseness.
 5. Unsteady gait, ataxia, tremors, twitches, paralysis.
 6. Vaso-motor instability (blood pressure).

CLINICAL AND LABORATORY TESTS

CLINICAL DIAGNOSTIC POSSIBILITIES
Physical Examination Outline

    B. <u>Implemented Examination</u> (including auscultation)
       7. Fever, loss or gain of weight.
       8. Pulse or blood pressure variation, cardiac murmurs.
       9. Dental abnormalities, inflamed or abnormal mucous membranes.
      10. Rales, rubs, squeaks.
    C. <u>Palpation of Neck, Abdomen and Extremities</u>
      11. Masses of tenderness or edema.
      12. Impaired motion, vascular abnormalities.
    D. <u>Rectal and Pelvic Examination</u>
      13. Inflamed or abnormal mucous membranes.
      14. Masses or tenderness
      15. Displaced and relaxed structures
    E. <u>Neurological Examination</u>
      16. Hyper-reflexion or hypo-reflexion.
      17. Paralysis.
      18. Defective vision or hearing.
    F. <u>Psychiatric Examination</u>
      19. Retarded, accelerated or bizarre animations.
      20. Abnormal emotional response.
      21. Fixed ideas.
      22. Suspiciousness or spread of meaning.
      23. Forgetfulness or disorientation.

IV. **ESSENTIAL LABORATORY TESTS**
    1. Urinalysis.
    2. Sedimentation rate.
    3. Hemoglobin.
    4. Occult blood in feces.
    5. Gerology.
    6. P/A Chest X-Ray (standing at 6').

V. **ADDITIONAL CLASSIFICATIONS**
   <u>Groups of Major Diseases</u>
    1. Medical emergencies.
    2. Diseases of skin.
    3. Diseases of oral cavity.
    4. Diseases of respiratory passages.
    5. Pulmonary diseases.
    6. Cardiac diseases.

CLINICAL AND LABORATORY TESTS

CLINICAL DIAGNOSTIC POSSIBILITIES
Physical Examination Outline

>Groups of Major Diseases

7. Gastro-Intestinal disturbances.
   A. Dyspepsia.
   B. Changes in bowel movements.
   C. Passing of blood in stool
      1. Severe anemia or blood dyscrasia including leukemia or purpura.
      2. Vitamin K or C deficiency.
      3. Lesions of blood vessels including hypertension, varicosities, angiomas, aneurysms and forms of atherosclerosis.
   D. Abdominal soreness, cramps or colic.
   E. Nausea, vomiting or altered appetite.
8. Liver and biliary tract diseases.
9. Urinary tract.
10. Disease of the breast.
11. Diseases of female reproductive organs.
12. Diseases affecting habitus and endocrine system.
13. Traumatic postural and congenital disorders of the musculo-skeletal system.
14. Infectious and degenerative diseases of the musculo-skeletal systems.
15. Peripheral vascular diseases.
16. Neurologic diseases.
17. Diseases of the eye.
18. Diseases of the ear.
19. Miner psychogenic disorders.
20. Psychoneurosis and congenital psychopathological states.
21. Anemias and blood dyscrasias.

CLINICAL AND LABORATORY TESTS

GROVER DIAGNOSTIC CHART

As evidenced by relationships between systolic and diastolic pressures and pulse rates.

How to use chart: Systolic pressures from 60 to 280 mm. are shown on the horizontal line at the top of the chart. Diastolic pressures from 10 to 170 mm are in the vertical right hand column. Underlined figures are pulse rates. The starred figures behind the pulse rates are the key numbers to the diagnosis.

Example: Systolic 112, Diastolic 50, Pulse Rate 50

Systolic 112 is in the horizontal line, third section, and diastolic 50 is in the vertical column, fourth section from the top. Follow down and across these two sections till they converge at the pulse rate 50. The starred key number "2" is the diagnosis.

Systolic Pressures Read Across	Between 60 & 90 mm.	Between 92 & 110 mm	Between 112 & 140 mm.	Between 142 & 190 mm.	Between 192 & 280 mm	Diastolic Pressures Read Down
				50-70 – 4* 70-86 – 4* 88-120 – 5*	50-70 – 4* 70-86 – 4* 88-120 – 5*	Between 110 & 170mm
			72-86 – 13* 88-120 – 1*	50-72 – 2* 72-86 – 9* 88–120 – 5*	50-70 – 4* 72-86 – 4* 88-120 – 5*	Between 90 & 110mm
		72-86 – 6* 88-120 – 7*	Normal	50-70 – 10* 72-86 – 10* 88-120 – 14*	50-70 – 10* 72-86 – 10* 88-120 – 14*	Between 74 & 90mm
		90-120 – 8	50-70 – 2*	72-86 – 15* 120-150 – 12*	50-72 – 2*	Between 50 & 72 mm
	50-70 – 11*	50-70 – 11* 92-120 – 8*	60-80 – 3*	15*	15*	Between 10 & 50 mm

1* Suggests a poor myocardium; incipient dilatation.
2* Suggests an overworked heart; incipient hypertrophy.
3* Suggests aortic insufficiency. The diastolic is failing in its effort to compensate for the increased cardiac effort.
4* Intracranial tension. Suggests vascular changes seen in arteriosclerosis cardiorenal diseases, etc. Points to apoplexy.
5* Suggests a failing myocardium, a possible nephritis and other cardiovascular changes. Seen after apoplexy.
6* A reading often seen in neurasthenia, neurosis, etc.
7* Cardiac insufficiency. Suggests tuberculosis or other infection.
8* Suggests abnormal relation of the components of the blood as seen in anemias, cardiac weakness; possible tuberculosis. A reading seen in typhoid, septic endocarditis, etc.
9* Cardiovascular strain: incipient cardiorenal disease.
10* Hyperpiesia (essential hypertension), a condition of areterial tension existing prior to cardiovascular changes a reading often present in neuritis, climacteric period, mental overwork, worries, etc.
11* Suggests that patient is extremely toxic; precedes cardiac failure.
12* Suggests thyroid intoxication. Endocrine dysfunction.
13* When long continued, it points to kidney dysfunction with or without albuminuria.
14* Nervous hypertension. Look for psychic causes.
15* When persistent, it points to failing heart.

This chart will simplify diagnosis to a considerable degree, and should be helpful to the practitioner who requires a quick method in order to start immediate treatment before the laboratory findings are available. The findings should be corroborated through the patient's subjective and objective symptoms, and ultimately be a differential laboratory check-up.

CLINICAL AND LABORATORY TESTS

THERAPEUTIC TEST FOR FUNCTIONAL
STATUS OF THYROID AND ADRENAL GLANDS

Calcium, potassium and phosphorus, each have a definite effect upon the autonomic nervous system and must be in balance for its normal function. When one of these is in excess or deficiency symptoms of autonomic unbalance are evident.

These minerals are all specifically under the influence of the thyroid and adrenal glands (plus sodium, which has little effect upon the autonomic system).

Therefore, if this information is applied to clinical situations, an estimate of the activity of the gland can be fairly accurately made.

It is essential that the following chart be used in the interpretation of such reactions.

GLAND STATUS	MINERAL TOLERANCE	NEED FOR TEST SHOWN BY
HYPERTHYROID	LOW TO PHOSPHORUS HIGH TO CALCIUM	TACHYCARDIA
HYPOTHYROID	HIGH TO PHOSPHORUS LOW TO CALCIUM	STIFFNESS OF JOINTS, NAUSEA, BRADYCARDIA
HYPERADRENIA	LOW TO SODIUM HIGH TO POTASSIUM	HYPERTENSION, EDEMA MASCULATION
HYPOADRENIA	LOW TO POTASSIUM	HYPOTENSION, ASTHENIA, NEUROSIS

Thus, by supplying the concentrate of the mineral concerned above, the symptoms shown will be aggravated or relieved and the functional state of the gland concerned is determined. The following chart shows the concentrated mineral supplements which may be used for such therapeutic tests.

Potassium Source	–	Organic Minerals	– Minaplex
Calcium Source	–	Calcium Lactate	
Phosphorus Source	–	Phosfood Liquid	– Phosphade Liquid
Sodium Source	–	Sodium Citrate	

When the glandular status has been determined, either by deliberate testing as above, or by reactions in the course of other programs, the following schedules should be applied.

Hyperthyroid	–	Calcium Lactate and Organic Iodine
Hypothyroid	–	Vitamin F Perles – Eflex and Thyroid Cytotrophin
Hyperadrenia	–	Adrenamin – Adrenaplex and Organic Iodine and Calcium Lactate
Hypoadrenia	–	Adrenamin or Adrenaplex and Sodium Citrate

CLINICAL AND LABORATORY TESTS

DRUG INDUCED NUTRITIONAL DEFICIENCIES

Type Medicine	Nutrient Deficiency
Analgesic (pain relievers) aspirin	Vitamin C
Antacids	Vitamin B1 & Calcium
Antibiotics	Vitamin K & Most of the B Vitamins
Chloramphenicol	Phenylalanine (amino acid)
Isoniazid	Vitamin B6 and other B Vitamins
Neomycin	Vitamins A, B12, D, E, & K
Para-Aminosalicylic Acid	Vitamins B12 & Folic Acid
Sulfonamides	Folic Acid, Vitamin K & other B Vitamins
Tetracycline	Vitamins C, B6, B12, Calcium & Pantotheni Acid
Blood pressure lowering agents	
Hydralazines	
Cholesterol lowering agents	Vitamin B6
Diuretics	Vitamins A, D, E & K
Thiazides	
Oral Hypoglycemic Agents	Potassium, Vitamin C, & Other B Vitamins
Laxatives	Vitamin B12
Mineral Oil	Vitamins A, D, E & K plus prevents absorption of
Phenolphthalein	many other nutrients.
Sedatives	
Glutethimide	Vitamin D and multiple other Vitamins

CLINICAL AND LABORATORY TESTS

COMPLETE BLOOD COUNT

SUGGESTED NUTRITIONAL SUPPLEMENTS FOR BALANCING INSUFFICIENCIES

	Increased	Decreased
HEMOGLOBIN:	Phosfood—60 – 90 drops daily Spleen—One three times a day, after meals A & F with Betafood—Two before each meal	Ferrofood—One before each meal Chlorophyll—Two before each meal Complex T—Once twice a day before meals
R.B.C.:	Same as Hemoglobin	Same as Hemoglobin
W.B.C.:	Thymex—Two three times a day before meals Complex A & C—Three, three times a day before meals Calcium Lactate—Three, three times a day before meals	R.N.A.—One three times a day Thymex—Two three times a day after meals Spleen—One three times a day after meals

SHILLING DIFF.

P.M.N.:	Thymex—Two, three times a day before meals A & C Complex—Three, three times a day before meals. Calcium Lactate—Three, three times a day before meals.	
EOSINOPHILS:	Allergy Antronex—One, three times daily Allerplex—Two, three times a day Parasites Zymex—Two, three times a day Wheat Germ Oil—One, three times daily Salt Water Enema—Three times a week	
BASOPHILS:	Complex T—One, three times a day before meals Spleen—One, three times a day before meals Ostogen—One, three times a day before meals Betaine HCl—One, three times a day with meals	
LYMPHOCYTES:	Congaplex—Two, three times a day after meals Thymex—Two, three times a day after meals Complex A & C—Two, three times a day after meals	Thymex—Two, three times a day after meals Complex A & C—Two, three times a day after meals Complex C—Two, three times a day after meals
MONOCYTES:	Spleen—One, three times a day after meals Betacol—One, two times a day after meals Complex A-C-P—Three, three times a day after	
GLUCOSE:	Diaplex—Two, three times a day after meals Vitamin B—One, three times a day after meals Multizyme—One, three times a day after meals	A & F with Betafood—One tablet between meals Drenamin—One tablet between meals Protefood-One between meals Zypan—One tablet with meals (if the patient feels bloated after meals)

CLINICAL AND LABORATORY TESTS

COMPLETE BLOOD COUNT
SUGGESTED NUTRITIONAL SUPPLEMENTS FOR BALANCING INSUFFICIENCIES

	Increased	Decreased
B.U.N.:	Renatrophin—One, three times a day after meals Arginex—One, three times a day after meals Comfrey Pepsin E_3—Two, three times a day after meal	Betacol—One to three a day taken after meals Inositol—One, three times a day after meals Choline—Two, three times a day after meals Nutrimere—Three, three times a day after meals
CREATININE:	Albaplex—Two, three times a day after meals Arginex—Two, three times a day after meals Cardiotrophin—One, two times a day after meals after meals after meals Complex A & C—One, three times a day	Neurotrophin—One, two times a day after meals Calcifood Wafer—One, two times a day after meals Super-EFF—One, three times a day after meals Circuplex—One, three times a day after meals Inositol—Three, three times a day
CHOLESTEROL: (total serum)	Phosfood—15 drops in water or tomato juice after meals Linum B_6—Two, three times a day A & F with Betafood—Three in Hot water before breakfast Cyruta—One, two times a day after meals	Drenamin—Three, three times a day before meals Betacol—Start with one a day and increased to three a day before meals
THYMOL TURBIDITY:	Betacol—One, two times a day after meals Ostogen—One, two times a day after meals A & F with Betafood—Two, three times daily after meals Thymex—Two, three times a day after meals	
URIC ACID SERUM:	Comfrey-Pepsin E3—Two, three times a day after meals (this is to funish the end product of uric acid into allantoin via the uricase enzyme) Betaine HCl—If patient is running a globulin over 2.7 Organic Minerals—If patient's serum sodium is above normal.	Cyro-Yeast—One, three times a day between meals Vitamin B_{12}—Three, three times a day between meals Drenamin—Two, three times a day between meals
PHOSPHORUS:	Renatrophin (Kidney PMG)—One, three times a day after meals. Thytrophin (Thyroid PMG)—One, three times a day after meals Vitamin D Complex—One, three times a day after meals	(Inorganic Serum) Ostogen (Bone PMG)—One, three times a day before meals Calcifood Wafers—One, three times a day before meals Complex F—One, three times a day before after meals

CLINICAL AND LABORATORY TESTS

COMPLETE BLOOD COUNT
SUGGESTED NUTRITIONAL SUPPLEMENTS FOR BALANCING INSUFFICIENCIES

Increased	Decreased

CALCIUM: (Total Serum)

    Thyrtophin (Thyroid PMG)—One, three times a day after meals   Multizyme—One, two times a day before meals and at bedtime

    Protefood—One, two times a day after meals   Vitamin D Complex—One, two times a day before meals and at bedtime

    Complex F—One, three times a day after meals

    Betaine H.C.L.—One or two, three times a day   Calcium Lactate—Three, four times a day before meals and at bedtime

PROTEIN BOUND IODINE: (P.B.I.)

    Complex D—One, three times a day after meals thyroid   Complex F—One tablet three times a day before meals

    Thyroid-Thytrophin—One, three times a day before after meals   Thyroid-Thytrophin—One, three times a day meals

    Betacol—One, three times a day after meals   Symples F or M—One daily before meals

    Thymex—Two, three times a day after meals

IODINE: (Inorganic)

    Complex F—One, three times a day before meals   Drenamin—Two, three times a day before meals

    Chlorophyll Perles—Three, three times a day before meals

BILIRUBIN:
(DIRECT)

    A & F with Betafood—Three, three times a day before meals   Ferrofood—One, three times a day before meals

    Choline—Three, three times a day before meals   Super-EFF—One, three times a day before meals

(INDIRECT)   Thymex—Two, three times a day before meals

    Ferrofood—One, three times a day before meals

(BOTH)

    Betacol—One, three times a day before meals

    A & F with Betafood—One, three times a day before meals

    Hepatotrophin (Liver)—One, three times a day before meals

ALKALINE PHOSPHATASE:

    Ostogen—One, two times a day before meals   Thytrophin (Thyroid)—One, daily before meals

    Bio-Dent—Two, three times a day before meals   Ferrofood—One, two times a day before meals

    Betacol—One, two times a day before meals   Cyroplex—One, three times a day before meals

    Cardioplus—Two, three times a day before meals   Super-EFF—One, three times a day before meals

TRANSAMINASE:

    SGO: (A) Onset-Normal   SKP TEST   True Cardiac attack before EKG, Phono, or other for: Coronary Attack

    8 hours—begins to rise

    4 days—Normal

    (A) Supplements: Note: Increased in any Heart, Liver, Kidney or muscle condition

    Cardiotrophin—One, three times a day before meals

    Wheat Germ Oil Perles—One, three times a day before meals

CLINICAL AND LABORATORY TESTS

TRANSAMINASE:
    SGO: (B)   HEPATIC CIRRHOSIS
    SGP: SGO: 43 – 300 Units

    SGP: 20 – 250 Units

(B)   Supplements
Livaplex—One, three times a day
Protefood—One, two times a day
Thymex—Two, three times a day
Units
    SGP: 500 – 2500 Units   Hepatitis

    SGO: 40 – 200 Units
    SGP: 50 – 300 Units   Obstructive Jaundice

    Supplements same as in (B) above

LACTIC ACID DEHYDROGINASE: (L.D.H.)
    Normal: 100 – 350 Units
    Borderline: 350 – 550 Units

    Serum: Myocardial Infarct
    Cardiotrophin – One a day

    Cardioplus – Three, three times a day

    Pulmonary Embolism:
    Pneumotrophin – Three, three times a day

    Cyruta Plus – Three, three times a day

    Vitamin C Complex – One tab three times a day

    Hepatic Necrosis:
    Livaplex – Two, three times a day

    Protefood – One, two times a day

    Thymex – Two three times a day

    Note: All of the above on empty stomach

SUBJECT INDEX
Instructions for the Use of this Index

The numbers assigned below represent page numbers; the capitalized words in the index refer specifically to Laboratory and Clinical Tests. The remainder of the Index is concerned with information listed under Clinical Considerations.

Abdomen
    Flabby, 155
    Pain in, 71
Vein prominence, 5, 65
Abortion, 181
Accomodation defects, 107
Achlorhydric, 17
Acholic stool, 15, 103
Acid-Alkaline balance, 191
Acid-base disorders, 147
Acidosis, 1, 81, 91
ACID PHOSPHATASE, 151
Acid rebound syndrome 101, 143
Acne, 61, 71, 89, 167
Addison's Disease, 199
Adenasine triphosphate, 165
Adrenal glands, 97
    Hormones, 19
    Hyperactivity, 167
    Insufficiency, 53, 91, 125
Aged,
    Irritability of, 149
ALBUMINURIA, 41, 43, 45, 71
Alcoholism, 5, 127
Allergic reactions, 7, 19, 73, 93, 95, 163, 165, 167
Alkalosis, 19, 21,
Alopecia, 89
Altitude discomfort, 129
Amenorrhea, 97, 135
Amino acids, 27, 19, 133, 155
Anemic, 17, 19, 21, 47, 71, 97, 99, 157, 165
Angitis, 41
Angina pectoris, 57, 65
Angioneurotic edema, 47
Ankles, swollen, 155
Anoxia, 1, 47, 81, 97, 183, 185
Antibiotic therapy, 187
Apathy, 47
Appetite,
    Changes, 17
Decreased, 51, 65, 83, 121, 155, 165
    Excessive, 149
Apprehension, 65
Arms, flabby flesh, 155
Arteriosclerosis, 19, 21, 71, 77, 85, 99, 161
Arthritis, 11, 21, 27, 71, 133, 153
    Osteo, 21
    Rheumatoid, 27, 85, 95, 97, 133, 167
Ascites, 7, 11, 65, 103, 155, 157

Asthma, 57, 93, 95, 147
Atrophy, 165, 171
    Muscular, 37, 139,155
Autonomic unbalance, 61, 95, 145
Axial,
    Swelling of, 163

Back pain, 139, 157
Balance ability, 123
BASAL METABOLIC RATE, 115, 145, 149, 177
Bed sores, 55, 71, 97
Betaine, 15
BILE AND BILIRUBIN, 75
Biliary stasis, 57
Biliousness, 11, 77, 91, 187
BIOST, powder, 19
"Black and Blue Spots, 85, 125, 185
Bladder,
    Disease, 71
    Dysfunction, 9
    Irritation, 41, 43, 71
    Pain, 45, 71
    Symptoms, 1
BLOOD CHOLESTEROL, 15, 85, 115
BLOOD COAGULATION, 71, 143
BLOOD COUNT, 47, 163
Blood,
    Dyscrasias, 19, 21, 71, 163
    In stool, 189
    In urine, 157
    Iodine, 115
    Blood pressure changes, 183
BLOOD PRESSURE, 7, 11, 19, 41, 65, 77, 85, 95, 103, 125, 183
    Postural, 29, 93
Blood sugar imbalance, 93
Blood sugar regulation, 195
BLOOD SUGAR TEST, 139, 145
BLOOD VOLUME, 7
Body odor, 9, 71, 109, 187
Boils, 167
Bone,
    Deformities, 19, 21
    Diseases, 47
    Disorders, 55
    Infections, 167
    Marrow, 19
    Nutrients, 19
    Pain in, 135
    X-Ray of, 137
Bowel movements,
    Frequency of, 7, 73, 77
Bradycardia, 143

Brain trauma, 119
Breasts,
    Disorders of, 163
    Swelling of, 111
BREATH HOLDING TEST, 185
    Breath odors, 109
    Breathlessness, 129
BROMTHYMOL BLUE TEST, 109, 187
Bronchitis, 55, 95, 147
Bruises, 196
Bruising easily, 85, 125, 185
Bursitis, 161
Burns, 69, 71
    Industrial, 179
    X-Ray, 179
Burning sensations, 11, 121
Bursitis, 19, 161
Calcium,
    Loss, 115
    Metabolism, 27, 133, 137
    Stored in bone, 59
    Utilization, 61, 161, 183, 185
CALCIUM TEST, 55
    Blood discussion, 29
Calf muscles,
    Tenderness of, 51
Cardiac neurosis, 57
Cancer, toxemia in, 187
Canker sores, 163
Capillaries,
    Engorgement, 125, 185
    Fragility, 53, 85, 87, 183
    Stasis, 77
Carbohydrates,
    Digestion of, 73
    Metabolism, 37, 103
Caries, 19, 21
Cataracts, 71
Cellulitis, 53
CEPHALIN FLOCCULATION, 11, 77, 103
Chest,
    Pain in, 57,143
    Vein prominence, 5, 65
Children,
    Underdeveloped, 141
Cholesterol, 179
CHOLESTEROL TEST, 149 161,
CHOLINESTERASE, 65
Chromosomes, 165
CHVOSTAK'S SIGN, 19

SUBJECT INDEX

Cigarette cough, 147
    Circulation, 43
    Circulatory disorders, 27, 37, 43, 85, 133
Colds, 39, 43, 45, 83, 81, 93, 95, 147
Cold extremities, 173
Cerebral pressure,
    Symptoms of, 7
CERVIX UTERI SMEAR, 181
"Charley-horse,", 185
Colic, intestinal, 77
Colitis, , 57, 71, 83, 101, 123, 145, 189
    Ulcerative, 87
Complexion, blotchy, 39, 83
CO_2 Combining Power, 19, 185
CONCENTRATION-DILUTION TEST, 41, 43
Connective tissue changes, 19, 27, 135
Constipation, 11, 15, 73, 75, 77, 91, 109, 123, 151, 187, 189
    Spastic, 129
Coordination, loss of, 1
Coronary disease, 1, 165
    Sclerosis, 71
Cortisone, 19
Costiveness, 109, 123
Coughs, 29, 93, 143
    Chronic, 147
Cramps, 19, 21, 29, 55, 143, 161, 185
    Esophageal, 129
    Menstrual, 115
    Muscular, 83, 115
CREATINE, 155, 159
    Test, 165
    Urine, 1, 37
"Cross-eyes," 107
Cryptorchism, 127
Cystitis, 41, 71
Cysts, uterine, 181
Dandruff, 179
Debilitation, 47, 155, 171
Deficiencies, 83
Dehydration, 197, 199
Demineralization, 17
Dental problems, 21
Depression, 47, 161
Dermatitis, 69, 93, 95, 121, 179
Developmental
    Characteristics, 141
Diabetes, 71, 105
    Cholesterol elevation, 15
    Toxemia in, 187
    Traumatic, 119
DIAGNEX (Squibbs) Test, 17
Diarrhea, 17, 73, 101, 109, 123, 145, 187, 189
Digestive complaints, 65, 145, 161

Disc lesions, 21
Diseases,
    Chronic, 39, 83
    Degenerative, 39, 83
Dizziness, 99, 189
Drowsiness, 97
    After eating, 51
Drug addiction, 7, 187
Dysmenorrhea, 135, 137
Dysovarism, 135, 137
Dysphagia, 97, 129, 145
Eclampsia, 7
Eczema, 179
Edema, 1, 7, 9, 11, 19, 51, 103, 143, 155, 157, 163
Electrical burns, 89
Emaciation, 19, 21, 99, 139, 155, 159, 161, 165
Encephalitis, 149
ENCEPHALOGRAPH, 119
Endocrines, insufficiency of, 97
ENDOCARDIOGRAPH, 37, 57, 95, 143, 183
Endocervicitis, 173
Energy mechanisms, 37, 165
Enlargement,
    Liver, 103
    Spleen, 103
Enzyme,
    Bone, stored in, 19
    Content, 61, 133
    Deficiency, 19
ENZYME TESTS, 139
Epidermis, 179
Epilepsy, 7
    Toxemia in, 187
Epistaxis, 55, 71
Epithelial cells, 41
    Kidney, 43
    In urine, 45
Erysipelas, 53
Exercise tolerance, 37, 183
Exhaustion, 95
Exostosis, 19, 21,
Eye complaints, 107
    Conditions, 41
    Disorders of, 41, 43, 45
    Night blinders, 41
    Symptoms, 65
Faintness, 5
Farsightedness, 107
Fatigue, 47, 85
    Chronic, 19, 21, 39, 83, 93, 183, 185
    Mental, 145
Fatty acids, unsaturated, 179
Fatty degeneration, 77
Fats,
    Absorption of, 75
    Digestion of, 73, 91
    Intolerance of, 5, 15, 77, 161
    Metabolism, 103

Febrile diseases, symptoms, 123
Feet,
    Burning of, 15
    Redness of, 65
Fermentation,
    Intestinal, 51, 73
Festers, 145
Fever, 17, 29, 43, 45, 159
    Blisters, 61, 163
    Recurrent, 189
Fibrillations, 51, 95
Fibroids, 181
Fibrotic lesions, 149
Flabbiness, 155
Flatulence, 11, 15, 73, 83, 101, 189
Flora, intestinal, 73
Flu, 39, 43, 45, 83, 95, 147
    "Intestinal," 123
Fluid balance, 1, 157
Foods, undigested, 73
"Frightened" face, 149, 173
Frigidity, 135, 137
Frothy urine, 75

Gallbladder, 5, 105
    Disease, 5,
    Irritation of, 71
    Symptoms, 15, 75, 77, 161
GALACTOSE TOLERANCE, 11, 77, 103
Gas,
    Pains of, 77
    Foods producing, 77
Gastric secretions, 17
GASTRIC ANALYSIS TESTS, 17
Gastritis, 1, 41, 47, 53, 65, 71, 101, 123, 145
Gastrointestinal,
    Environment, 187
    Mobility, 57
Gingivitis, 71, 87, 97
Glandular disorders, 39, 41, 43, 45, 83
Glossitis, 97
Glucose-glycogen, 37
GLUCOSE TOLERANCE TEST, 15
Goiter, 141
Gout, 1, 71, 123
Grave's disease, 171
Grippe, 147
Groin, swelling of, 163
Gums,
    Bleeding of, 21, 29, 53, 71, 83, 133, 185, 189

    Reabsorption of, 19
    Receding, 27, 135
    Sore, tender, 19, 27, 135
Gynecomastia, 7, 127

SUBJECT INDEX

Hair,
    Brittle, 115
    Falling, 63
    Integrity of, 61
Halitosis, 71
Hands, redness of, 5, 65
Hands and feet,
    Coldness of, 159
Headaches, 1, 5, 7, 11, 27, 97, 107, 133
    Migraine, 43, 87
    Morning, 85, 185
Head,
    Feeling of band, 51
    Tightness in, 83
Healing, 53, 69, 71, 145
    Delay of, 55
    Mechanisms, 165
    Processes, 85
    Reactions, 139
Heartburn, 101, 123
Heart failure,
    Congestive, 1, 147, 183
Heart,
    Degeneration, 195
    Enlargement, 51
    Symptoms, 51
Hemoglobin, 53
Hemopoietic system,
    Nutrient, 19
Hemorrhage, 29, 53, 55, 71, 97
Hepatitis, 5, 103
Hives, 93, 163
Hormones, 103
Hot flashes, 63
Hydrochloric acid,
    Loss of, 17, 19
Hyperacidity, 19, 73
    Gastric, 143
Hyperadrenia, 19, 167
Hypercholesterolemia, 15, 63
Hyperglandular activity, 167
Hyperglycemia, 93
Hyperirritability, 1, 9, 21, 51, 55, 57, 63, 81, 83, 99, 125, 129, 149, 185
Hyperperistalsis, 77, 83
Hypertension, 7, 39, 41, 57, 71, 77, 83, 85, 93, 143, 157, 161
Hyperthyroid, 7, 61, 167, 177
    Differentiation, 129
Hyperthyroidism, 41, 115, 171
Hyperventilation, 19
Hypoadrenia, 95
Hypochlorhydria, 77
Hypoglycemia, 5, 15, 139
HYPOPROTEINEMIA, 19, 65
Hypotension, 39, 83, 93, 95, 97, 161
Hypothyroidism, 63, 105, 159

ICTERUS INDEX, 11, 77, 103
Impotency, 99
Indigestion, 5, 11, 17, 73, 77, 143
    Nervous, 65
    Symptoms, 57, 75, 101, 103, 123
INDICAN, 71, 187
Infantilism, 135, 137
Infections, 29, 43, 45, 53, 167
    Susceptibility to, 39, 83, 163
Inflammation, 11, 53, 69, 71, 85, 145, 163
    Of blood, 41
    Of lymph vessels, 41
Inorganic iodine, 115
Inositol, 21
Insomnia, 7, 19, 21, 29, 39, 55, 57, 83, 99, 115, 143
Intestinal colic, 77
Intestinal toxemia, 73, 103
Iodism, 141
Irritability, 19, 97,
Itching sensations, 11
Jaundice, 15, 77, 103
Joints,
    Creaking, 19
    Inflammation, 95
    Pain in, 27, 133, 153
    Stiffness, 161
17-KETOSTEROID TEST, 93, 95, 127, 135, 145, 151
Kidney, 1, 9, 11, 45, 71, 103
    Disease, 41, 43
    Stones, 41
Lactation, 111
Lactic acid
    Decrease, 109
    Excess, 51
Lecithin, 179
Legs, weakness of, 51
Leukopenia, 171
Leukorrhea, 181
Leukocytosis, 103
Libido, loss of, 97, 151, 153
Ligaments, 19, 21, 27, 113, 133, 149
Lipotropic, factors, 103
Liver,
    Cirrhosis, 127
    Disease, 5, 7, 9, 77, 79, 105
    Function, 15
    Dysfunction, 39, 103, 157
    Inability to metabolize carotene, 41
    Inflammation, 71
    Insufficiency, 15
LIVER FUNCTION TESTS, 15
Lung conditions, 55
Lymph node congestion, 43, 45, 163, 165, 167
Lymphocytes, 171
Lymphocytosis, 163

Malnutrition, 39, 83, 109
Malassimilation,
    Calcium, iron, protein, 17
    Weight loss, 109
Male, climacteric, 127
Mammary glands, 111
Mastitis, 111, 167
Mastoiditis, 167
Meat, loss of taste for, 155
Melancholia, 51, 65, 121, 125
Memory, loss of, 85, 99, 119
Menopause symptoms, 19, 83, 135, 137
Menorrhagia, 137
Menstruation,
    Excessive, 29, 71
    Scanty, 63
    Symptoms, 19, 181
Mental activity, 119
    Changes, 19, 21
    Depression, 125
    Dullness, 173
    Instability, 177
    Slowness, 47
    Stress, 145, 173
Mental symptoms, 65, 99, 161
Metabolism,
    Cell, 37
    Disorders, 27, 133, 145
    Fat, 5, 77
    Systems, 27, 133
    Waste products, 71
Metabolic rate
    Increased, 29, 61, 115, 129
    Decreased, 143, 161, 185
Metrorrhagia, 135, 137
Milk, allergy to, 167
Mineral, 19
Motility, lack of, 19
Mouth, soreness of, 189
Mucous colitis, 189
Mucous membranes, 97
Muscle control, loss of, 65
Muscle,
    Cramps, 83
    Integrity, 37
    Spasms, 55
    Stiffness, 143
    Tone, 51
Muscular,
    Atrophy, 1, 155
    Dystrophy, 1, 105
    Symptoms, 83
    Weakness, 155, 171, 183
Myasthenia gravis, 171
Myositis, 143, 161, 165
Nausea, 5, 11, 15, 75, 77, 143, 161, 165, 189
Nasal secretions, diminished, 149
Nearsightedness, 107

SUBJECT INDEX

Neck, swelling of, 163
Nephritis, 41, 43, 45, 53, 97, 157, 165
Nephrosis, 195
"Nervousness,"
    Complaints, 93
    Exhaustion, 145
    Tension, 7, 57, 115, 125
Neuralgia, 97
Neurasthenia, 55, 93, 95, 121, 129
Neuromuscular disorders, 35, 165
Nipple, disorders of, 111
Nocturia, 151, 153
Nosebleed, 29, 55, 71
Numbness, 65
Nutritional
    Governor, 39
    Response, 39

Obesity, 145
Observation, 15, 27, 127, 133
Oliguria, 103
Orchitis, idiopathic, 127
Orthnopnea, 183
Osteoarthritis, 19, 143
Osteomyelitis, 27, 133
Osteoporosis, 19, 27, 133
    Of aged, 19
Ovarian
    Dysfunction, 137
    Irritability, 137
    Poisoning, 137
Oxygenation, 53, 115
Pain,
    Abdominal, 41, 45, 71, 189
    Back, 61, 115
    Bladder, 41
    Gas, 83
    Head, 85
    Joints, 11, 71
    Leg, 151
    Nutritional aspects, 153
    Tooth extraction, 69
Pallor, 77, 97
Palpation, 15, 41, 43, 103, 127
Palsy, 57
Paralysis, 1, 65
Paresthesias, 39, 65, 83, 121
Pellegra symptoms, 125
PELVIC EXAMINATION, 181
Periarteritis, 41
Perspiration,
    Deviations, 1
    Diminished, 129
    Excessive, 129
Peristalsis, 77
Personality, stability of, 173
Petechiae, 71
    Phonocardiograph, 11, 29, 65, 77, 93, 103

Phosphorus, stored in bone, 19
Photophobia, 129, 145
Phagocyte, 53
Pneumonia, 45, 93, 95, 147
Polio, 149
Polycythemia, 163
Polyuria, 41, 43, 45
Portal Hypertension, 15
POSTURAL BLOOD PRESSURE, 7, 95
POSTURAL EXAMINATION, 19
Posture, stooped, 19, 21
Potassium,
    Excess, 53,
    Reactions, 93
    Sodium ratio test, 93
    Tolerance, 93
Pregnancy, 17
Prickling sensation, 121
Prolapse, 37
Prophylaxis, 39
Prostate disease, 61, 149, 151, 153
PROTEIN BOUND IODINE, 61, 115, 149, 177
Protein,
    Deficiency, 19, 21
    Digestion, 73, 139
    Metabolism, 27, 53, 103, 133, 157
    Protection, 53
    Serum, 19
    Stored in bone, 19
    Test, 55, 61, 149
PROTHROMBIN TIME, 71
Pruritis, 165
    Ani, 189
PSYCHIATRIC EXAMINATION, 119, 121, 125
Psychoneurosia, 119
    Delayed, , 135, 137
PULSE RATE, 29, 41, 43, 45, 57, 125, 149, 167, 177, 183
Purpura, 71, 77, 85, 125, 185
Putrefaction, intestinal, 73
Psoriasis, 167
Ptosis, 65
Pyhorrea, 185
Pyloric spasms, 33
Radiation,
    Injury, 87
    Therapy, 19
Rashes, 7, 47, 95, 179, 189
Recuperation, 93, 155,
Redness of hands, 11
REFLEX TESTS, 29, 143, 149, 161
Repetitiousness, 85, 105
Resistance, lowered, 5, 39, 43, 55, 73, 83, 95, 159, 163
Respiration,
    Irregular, 129
    Rapid, 19
    Rate of, 29

Respiratory disorders, 93, 95
Restlessness, 19, 21, 33, 55, 143
Saliva,
    Diminished, 149
    Excessive, 29, 143,
Salivary disorders, 141
Salt,
    Craving for, 93
    Diets, 1, 19
Scar formation, 89
Scurvy, 53
Secretions diminished, 149
Sedentary occupations
    Heart failure, 37
SEDIMENTATION RATE, 1
Senility, 99
    Premature, 135, 137
SERUM ALBUMIN TEST, 103
Sex,
    Secondary characteristics, 127
Sighting, 129, 185,
Sinusitis, 71, 93, 95
Sinus drainage,
    Increased, 29
Skin,
    Bronzing of, 199
    Color of, 11
    Disorders of, 41, 43, 45, 61, 71, 95, 167, 179,
    Dryness of, 61, 115
    Irritated, 179
    Lesions, 1, 125
    Moisture of, 173
    Pallor of, 71, 97
    "Salty," 9
    Rashes, 7
    Thick, dry, 63
Sleep, restlessness in, 189
Smoking, excessive, 71
Sneezing attacks, 93
Soda, 19
Sodium balance, 53, 93
Sodium bicarbonate, 19
Sodium retention, 19
SOCIUM-POTASSIUM RATIO, 93, 95
Spasticity, 57
SPECIFIC GRAVITY, URINE, 45
SPERM COUNT, 127
Spermatogenesis, 127
Sphincters,
    Control of, 57
    Spasms of, 33, 77
Spinal lesions, 19, 21
Stamina, 51, 95, 99
Sterility, 181
Stiffness of joints, 19, 143
Stomach,
    Pain "ache," 189
    Delayed emptying, 33

SUBJECT INDEX

Stones, salivary, 141
Stool,
    Clay-colored, 75, 91
    Dry, 109
    Foul smelling, 109
pH of, 109
    Variations, 11
Strabismus, 107
Stress, 17, 97, 171
    Intolerance, 63
Suffocation symptoms, 129
SULKOWITCH REAGENT, 29, 33, 55, 143, 161
Sun,
    Burn, 61, 179
    Exposure to, 61, 63
Sun blistered lips, 61
Sunlight, sensitivity to, 121, 179
Sweat glands
    Activity of, 1, 149
    "cold" type, 129
    Excess of, 173
    Increased, 29
    Night occurring, 65
Swelling, 11, 43, 45
Synapse, 57
Tachycardia (under this heading products are listed by name and page number for convenience)
    Vitamin A complex, 41
    Vitamin A & C Complex, 43
    Vitamin A & F with Betafood, 5
    Adrenamin, 93
    Anti-Coryza, 81
    Anti-Pyrexin, 7
    Vitamin B Complex, 51
    Vitamin B_{12}, 47
    Calcium Lactate, 29
    Carbamide, 1
    Wheat Germ Oil Perles, 185
    Chlorophyll Capsules, 71
    Di-Sodium Phosphate, 91
    Vitamin E Complex, 59
    Super-EFF (F_2), 165
    Vitamin F Complex, 61
    Ferrofood, 97
    Organic Minerals, 129
    Organic Iodine, 149
    Pituitary Cytotrophin, 145
    Thyroid Cytotrophin, 173
    Zymex, 187
TALQVIST SCALE, 47
Teeth,
    Gnawing of, 189
    Loose, 19, 27, 133
Telangiectasia, 11, 71, 77, 85
TEMPERATURE, 29, 45, 167
    Elevated, 43
    Lowered, 173
Tendons, 19, 21

Testicles,
    Atrophy, 127
    Involution, 127
    Undescended, 141
Tetany, 55
THERAPEUTIC TEST, 115
Throbbing sensations, 85
Thymocytes, 171
Thyroid, 141, 145, 167, 173
    Disorders, 41
Tinnitus, 85, 97
Tongue, tremors of, 173
Tonsillitis, 167
Tonus, 37
Tooth extraction, 69
Toxemia, 7, 9, 71, 97, 103, 157, 187
Toxic manifestations, 39, 83
Tremors, 5, 61, 115, 149, 155, 177
Tyrosinase, 53

Ulcer syndrome, 1, 55, 71, 145, 167
Ulcers,
    Diabetic, 139
    Leg, 69, 143
Uremia, 9, 71, 187
URIC ACID, BLOOD, 123
URINALYSIS, 19, 41, 45, 71, 157
URINARY 55-KETOSTEROIDS, 137
URINE, BILE TEST, 11, 103
Urine, blood in, 157
Urination,
    Burning, 71
    Diminished, 1, 9, 77, 103, 129
    Increased, 29, 45
    Symptoms, 157
URISIX (albuminuria) Test, 41
Urticaria, 47
VAGINAL SMEAR, 135, 137
Vaginitis, 69, 71, 181
VAN DEN BERG REACTION, 11, 77, 103
Varicose veins, 11, 27, 79, 133
Vascular changes, 11, 71
Veins, prominence of, 5, 15, 103
Venous congestion, 7, 11, 15, 27, 65, 77, 79, 103, 133
Vertigo, 85, 173, 189
Vitamin, 127, 171
Vomiting, 17, 19, 143, 189
Water balance, 1, 11, 103
"Water-brash," 101
Weakness, 39, 83
    Cardiac, 37
    Muscular, 1, 37
Weight,
    Gain, 173
    Instability, 73
    Loss, 61, 109, 115, 149, 155, 159, 177
WHITE LINE TEST, 95
Wrinkles, 63

X-RAY EXAMINATION, 15, 19, 27, 57, 101, 133, 135, 161
Yawning, 185

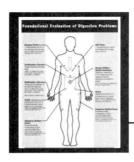

INTRODUCTION AND OVERVIEW OF THE NUTRITIONAL EXAM

We would like to take this opportunity to introduce you to the International Foundation for Nutrition and Health (IFNH). IFNH is a non-profit educational organization supporting the healthcare professional.

The Nutritional Exam in this section is just one part of the 100-hour certification in whole food nutrition (CCWFN). This program was introduced by IFNH to help doctors make a transition from a disease-based practice to a wellness model. IFNH incorporated many parts of the physical exam taught by medical schools in the 1940s and 1950s which we now call the Nutritional Exam. This includes many quick and easy tests that look at function vs. pathology. Postural Hypotension and the Barnes Thyroid Test are just a few of the many diagnostic tools covered in the program. Other physical tests such as the Riddler Points, Murphy's Signs, Chapman Reflex Points and the Lowenburg's Tissue Calcium Test are also included in the Nutritional Exam.

The purpose of the certification program and Nutritional Exam is to help guide the practitioner through a systematic approach to implement nutrition in his/her practice. This is accomplished by presenting a verifiable overlay of information.

The certification program is laid out in a organized systematic manner with modules on digestion, sugar handling problems, musculoskeletal issues, hormonal dysfunction, immune allergy concerns, nutritional biochemistry as well as practice management.

Without a complete understanding of how digestion, as well as sugar handling issues affects the patient is the most common cause of protocol failure. Why do we say this? Because the average North Americans consume 140 lbs or more of sugar per year, whereas man in his natural state consumed less than one pound per year.

This course and its supporting materials can help the beginner or veteran build a sound foundation to integrate nutrition into his or her practice. The following pages consist of a compilation of some of the copyrighted materials from the 100-hour CCWFN certification that has been taught throughout the United States and Europe since 1994.

The CCWFN course is a distance learning program which includes appropriate study materials in a DVD/CD format, study manuals, and is supported by weekly teleconferences. The following pages will give you a snapshot of the course. For further information visit our website at www.ifnh.org or call IFNH at (858) 488-8932.

It is IFNH's mission to keep the spirit of Dr. Royal Lee and the Lee Foundation alive. IFNH was given the responsibility and custodianship of the many copyrighted works of the Lee Foundation for Nutritional Research. In that endeavor, IFNH strives to republish many of these original copyrighted works held in trust by the Lee Foundation. It is our belief that these classic works are as important today as when they were first published.

NUTRITIONAL EXAM

Patient Name _____ Date _____

Age _____   Male   or   Female   Height _____   Weight _____

DIGESTION

___HCL Point	*Zypan*
___Enzyme Point	*Multizyme, Lact-Enz*
Gallbladder	*A-F Betafood, Betafood*
___Murphy's Sign	*Choline, Cholacol*
___Right Thumb Web	
Large Intestine	*Zymex, Lactic Acid Yeast*
___Palpate Large Intestine	*Spanish Black Radish*
___Palpate Iliotibial Band (ITB)	*Zymex II, Fen-Cho*
Small Intestine	*Cholacol II, Lact-Enz*

TISSUE CALCIUM

_____ **Cuff Pressure**

CALCIUM SOURCE	HORMONAL
Calcium Lactate	*Symplex F or M*
Calsol	*Ovex*
Cal-Ma Plus	*Prost-X / Utrophin PMG*
Calcifood	*For-Til B₁₂*
Biost	OTHER FACTORS
DIGESTION	*Cataplex D / G*
Zypan	*Biost*
Cal-Amo	*Organic Minerals*
Betaine Hydrochloride	Allorganic Trace Minerals
ESSENTIAL FATTY ACIDS	*Min-Tran*

ESSENTIAL FATTY ACIDS

_____ **Oral pH**   _____ **Urine pH**

ESSENTIAL FATS
- *Linum B₆*
- *Cataplex F Tablets*
- *Cataplex F Perles*
- *Black Currant Seed Oil*
- *Sesame Seed Oil*
- *Wheat Germ Oil*

CO-FACTORS
- *A-F Betafood*
- *Betafood*
- *Choline*
- *Cholacol*

SUGAR HANDLING

Cataplex B, Paraplex, Diaplex

Adrenals   *Drenamin, Desiccated Adrenal, Drenatrophin PMG, B₆-Niacinamide*

___Postural Hypotension:
BP_____ Supine_____ Standing_____
___Paradoxical Pupillary Reflex
___Inguinal Ligament tenderness
___Posterior Ilium / Short Leg

Pancreas   *Pancreatrophin PMG, Cataplex GTF*
___Palpate Pancreas for tenderness
___Right Thenar Pad tenderness

Liver   *A-F Betafood, Livaplex, Hepatrophin PMG*
___3rd Rib tender to palpation 3" right of sternum

Zinc Test___   *Chezyn, Trace Minerals B12*
Histamine Point___   *Antronex, Cal-Amo*

SYMPTOM SURVEY   ACG

Primary Health: Nutritec findings: ACG Findings:
Concerns:
1.   1.   Allergies
                                Vitamin B
2.   2.   Protein Metabolism
                                Vitamin E, Calcium, EFA
3.   3.   Digestion
                                Adrenal Fatigue
4.   4.   Liver/Gallbladder congestion
                                Kidney congestion
5.   5.   Mineral imbalance
                                Oxygen utilization

VERTEBRAL INDICATORS*

___C1	Food Sensitivity	*Antronex, A-F Betafood, Spanish Black Radish*
___C2	Sinus	(see T5)
___C3	Diaphragm	*Ligaplex II, Cyruta Plus, Cal-Ma Plus*
___C4	Thyroid	*Symplex F or M*
	Hypo	*Thytrophin PMG, Circuplex, Cataplex F Tablets*
	Hyper	*Thytrophin PMG, Antronex, Min-Tran*
___C5	Sugar Handling	*Diaplex, Cataplex B, A-F Betafood*
___C6	Gastric	(see T5)
___C7	Hepatic	(see T8)
___T1	Heart	*Cardio-Plus*
___T2	Myocardium	*Vasculin*
___T3	Lungs & Bronchi	*Allerplex, Cal-Amo*
___T4	Gallbladder	*A-F Betafood, Choline, Cholacol*
___T5	Stomach	*Multizyme, Gastrex*
___T6	Pancreas	*Diaplex, Cataplex B, A-F Betafood, Multizyme*
___T7	Spleen/Immune	*Immuplex*
___T8	Liver	*Livaplex*
___T9	Adrenals	*Drenamin*
___T10	Small Intestine	*Multizyme*
___T11/12	Kidneys	*Albaplex*
	Acidic	*Organic Minerals*
	Alkaline	*Cal-Amo*
___L1	Iliocecal Valve	*Chlorophyll Complex, Antronex, A-F Betafood*
___L2	Cecum	*Ostarplex, Lact-Enz*
___L3	Endocrine	*Symplex F or M, Chlorophyll, Wheat Germ Oil*
	Constipation	*Fen-Cho, Choline, Spanish Black Radish*
	Diarrhea	*Cholacol II, Zymex*
___L5	Prostate/Uterus	
	Male	*Prost-X, Immuplex*
	Female	*Utrophin, Min-Chex*
P1	Ilium Adrenal Stress	*Drenamin*
AS	Ilium E Deficiency	*Cataplex E, Wheat Germ Oil*

Chiropractic Nutrition by Nicolai Lennox, D.C.

An example of some of the tests used in the Nutritional Exam and CCWFN certification program are now available in the white pages of this manual.

Foundational Evaluation of Sugar Handling
(Adrenal, Liver, Pancreas)

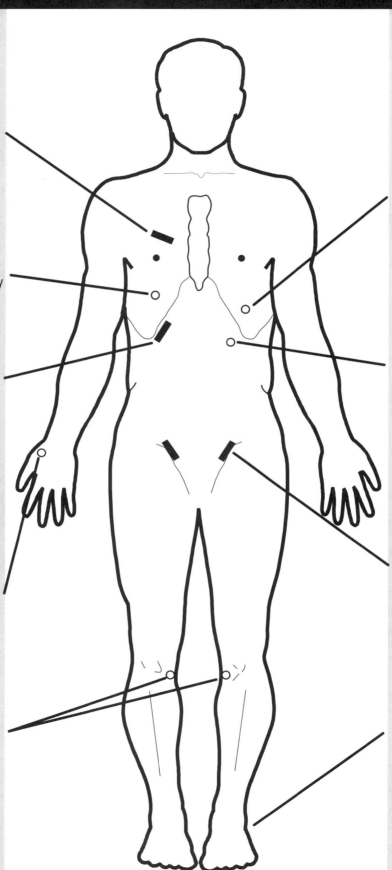

Liver Point
On the 3rd rib, 3" to the right of Sternum, at the Costochondral junction. Press anterior to posterior.
Need for: A-F Betafood (6-15) or Livaplex (3-6)

Chapman Reflex (Liver and Gallbladder)
6th Intercostal, Mid Mammillary
Need for: A-F Betafood (6-15) or Livaplex (3-6)

Murphy's Sign (Liver and/or Gallbladder)
Under ribs at anatomical location of the Gallbladder and Liver.
Need for: A-F Betafood (6-15), Severe cases consider: Choline, Inositol, Phosfood, Cataplex G, or Multizyme

History of Gallstones: Betafood instead of A-F Betafood
Gallbladder removed: Cholacol

Right Thenar Pad
Pancreas indicator when tender
Need for: Cataplex B (9), Paraplex (6), A-F Betafood (6), Pancreatrophin PMG (3), Cataplex GTF (3)

Medial Knee
The insertion of the Sartorius muscle at the Pes Anserinus. An Adrenal indicator when tender.
Need for: Drenamin (6) or Drenatrophin (3) depending on blood pressure

Chapman Reflex/ Pancreas
7th Intercostal, Mid-Mammill
Need for: Cataplex B (9), Paraplex (6), A-F Betafood (6), Pancreatrophin PMG (3), Cataplex GTF (3)

Head of Pancreas
Palpate for tenderness or guarding in the left upper quadrant of the abdominal region. Located 1/2 to 2/3 of the way between the umbilicus and the angle of the ribs.
Need for: Cataplex B (9), Paraplex (6), A-F Betafood (6), Pancreatrophin PMG (3), Cataplex GTF (3)

Inguinal Ligament Tenderness
Unilateral tenderness to palpation is an Adrenal indicator.
Need for: Drenamin (6-12), Whole Desiccated Adrenal (2-3), Cyruta-Plus (6), B6-Niacinamide (6)

Chronic Short Leg Due to Posterior-Interior Ilium (PI)
Adrenal indicator when confirmed with Postural Hypotension and Paradoxica Pupillary Response.
Need for: Drenamin (6) or Drenatrophin (3) depending on blood pressure

© 1996-2010 International Foundation for Nutrition and Health   All Rights Reserved

Barnes Thyroid Test

Patient Name _____

Date _____ **Re**-evaluation _____

Tracking dates	Time	Temperature
Day 1		
Day 2		
Day 3		
Day 4		
Day 5		

This test is an excellent way to determine thyroid function using basal body temperature (the body's temperature at rest). If the thyroid is running low, the body's temperature will drop below normal while the body is at rest or asleep. This test is performed by measuring the underarm temperature upon waking after a night's sleep. For accuracy, the test is conducted five mornings in a row and then the mean average is calculated. The test is performed with a basal (or ovulating) thermometer; the instructions for performing the test are as follows:

Recording Underarm Temperature in the A.M. for 5 Days

1. The night before, shake down the thermometer (an oral glass thermometer only), and set it on the nightstand next to the bed.
2. Immediately upon waking, without raising your head from the pillow, place the thermometer under the arm.
3. Leave thermometer under arm for 10 minutes.
4. Move as little as possible in this process; you must remain flat on your back during this entire time — otherwise the thyroid gland will be activated and a false reading will be taken.
5. After 10 minutes, remove thermometer and record temperature.
6. The test is invalidated if you expend any energy just before recording the temperature, i.e. getting up for any reason, shaking down the thermometer, etc.

A mean average temperature of between 98.2°F and 98.8°F is considered normal.

To figure average: Total_____ divided by 5 = _____.

©1996 – 2010 International Foundation for Nutrition and Health, All Rights Reserved

Iodine Patch Test

NAME: _____ DATE: _____

Why are Iodine levels important? Each Endocrine gland requires certain minerals to balance and respond readily to each other. For proper thyroid function, iodine is required; two thirds of the body's iodine is found in the thyroid gland. With low levels of iodine, certain signs and symptoms are noticeable; irregular heartbeats, mental sluggishness, difficulty losing weight, frequent urination and fatigue just to name a few. The following instructions are simple and easy tests to check iodine in the body.

Step I: Go to the pharmacy and pick up a solution called *TINCTURE OF IODINE*.

Step II: At night, before going to bed, paint on your skin a 3" x 3" square, filled in, with the tincture of iodine, using the enclosed stick. The patch is applied to the inside of either thigh or arm.

Step III: In the morning, upon rising, note the color and check off as follows:

- [ ] Bright yellow-orange (as it was the night before)
- [ ] Pale yellow
- [ ] Grayish colored
- [ ] No color left at all
- [ ] Other _____

IF THERE IS *NO* COLOR LEFT, YOUR TEST IS DONE.

IF THERE IS *ANY* COLOR REMAINING, GO ON TO STEP IV.

Step IV: For the remainder of the day, check the patch every few hours. Note the time that all of the color disappears. If color still remains at bedtime, you may consider the test completed.

- [ ] Color was gone by 12:00 noon
- [ ] Color was gone by 4:00 pm
- [ ] Color was gone by 8:00 pm
- [ ] Color was gone by bedtime
- [ ] Some color still remained
- [ ] Other _____

Please feel free to make any comments or notes on the back side and bring this in at your next visit.

©1996 – 2010 International Foundation for Nutrition and Health, All Rights Reserved

DIRECTIONS FOR USE OF ZINC TEST

Zinc test is a solution of zinc sulfate.
Put two teaspoons (10 ml.) in a cup.

To use, have your patient hold solution in the mouth for 10 seconds,
then expectorate (not harmful if swallowed).

Ask patient if there was any taste.
If so, ask to describe the taste he/she experienced.

Taste Response	*Indications*
Grade 4 – No taste	Severe deficiency
Grade 3 – Slight taste or delayed slight taste	Deficiency
Grade 2 – Moderate, unpleasant taste	Mild deficiency
Grade 1 – Immediate, strong unpleasant taste	Adequate zinc status

---

Because of the deficiencies in the North American diet, clinical experience indicates
that most Americans suffer from some degree of zinc deficiency.
It is common for nearly all new patients to fail this test.
Testing your current patients will assess how well your current approach
is addressing your patient's zinc challenge.

©1996 – 2010 International Foundation for Nutrition and Health, All Rights Reserved

Postural Hypotension Test
(Ragland's Test)

This is one of the most valuable tests of the FNT course. The nutritional exam taught in the course along with the symptom survey software and with theACG can dramatically change a nutritional practice.

Step 1   For your baseline temp; take the patient's systolic and diastolic blood pressure readings in a sitting position. It is preferable to have the cuff approximately level with the heart.

Step 2   Have the patient lie down on a table and rest for 60 seconds or longer. Take the systolic and diastolic pressure reading while the patient is in the supine position.

- With the patient still in the supine position, pump up the cuff again to approximately 20 millibars above the systolic supine reading.

Step 3   Have the patient immediately stand, taking care to guide the patient in case he/she becomes light-headed or begins to wobble. Immediately take the systolic and diastolic pressure when the patient reaches the standing position.

- Promptness in taking the standing pressure reading is paramount because the test is measuring a transitory event.

Notes

- Normally, the sitting to supine systolic reading will drop 6 to 10 mm from the sitting baseline.

- If the supine systolic reading increases more than 10 mm over the sitting baseline, this could be an indication of kidney issues. Those with an Endocardiograph or an ACG, can use them to confirm this information.

- A positive Adrenal response is when a patient's tests from supine to standing systolic BP reading drops from 10 mm to 40 mm. A normal reading should see a rise of 6 to 10 mm from the supine to standing position. (A patient who drops over 20mm should be considered chronic hypoadrenia and followed up with the pupil eye response test from the Nutritional Exam.)

- The greater the drop, the greater the degree of hypoadrenia.

- If the systolic reading drops more than 20 mm, it might be appropriate to use Whole Desiccated Adrenal (one tablet three times per daily for a maximum 30 days).

- If blood pressure is lower than 110/70, it is recommended that Drenatrophin PMG be considered instead of Drenamin.

If a patient fails this test check the Nutritional Exam sugar handling section for other tests, such as Paradoxical Papillary Reflex etc. The key to this test and that of the other tests is the systematic overlaying of information that confirms the direction of your support.

Foundational Evaluation of the Spine

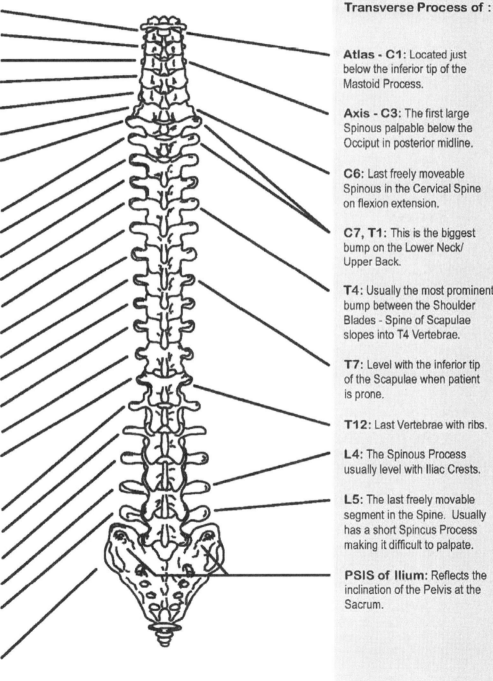

VERTEBRAL INDICATORS

- C1: Food Sensitivity
- C2: Sinus
- C3: Diaphragm
- C4: Thyroid
- C5: Sugar Handling
- C6: Gastric (T5)
- C7: Hepatic (T8)

- T1: Heart
- T2: Myocardium
- T3: Lungs and Bronchi
- T4: Gallbladder
- T5: Stomach
- T6: Pancreas
- T7: Spleen/Immune
- T8: Liver
- T9: Adrenals
- T10: Small Intestines
- T11/12: Kidneys

- L1: Ileocecal Valve
- L2: Cecum
- L3: Endocrine
- L4: Colon
- L5: Prostrate/Uterus

Ilium

VERTEBRAL LOCATORS

Transverse Process of :

Atlas - C1: Located just below the inferior tip of the Mastoid Process.

Axis - C3: The first large Spinous palpable below the Occiput in posterior midline.

C6: Last freely moveable Spinous in the Cervical Spine on flexion extension.

C7, T1: This is the biggest bump on the Lower Neck/Upper Back.

T4: Usually the most prominent bump between the Shoulder Blades - Spine of Scapulae slopes into T4 Vertebrae.

T7: Level with the inferior tip of the Scapulae when patient is prone.

T12: Last Vertebrae with ribs.

L4: The Spinous Process usually level with Iliac Crests.

L5: The last freely movable segment in the Spine. Usually has a short Spincus Process making it difficult to palpate.

PSIS of Ilium: Reflects the inclination of the Pelvis at the Sacrum.

Nutritional Support for Common Cardiovascular Problems

**All amounts indicate number to be taken per day.
In general, take supplements in equal portions throughout the day.
(Example: 6/daily = 2 tablets 3 times per day with meals)**

CARDIOVASCULAR SUPPORT

General support   6 Cardio-Plus
Normal to high BP: 6 Linum B_6

High blood pressure:
- 6 to 9 Magnesium lactate
- 9 AF Betafood
- 3 Choline

Low blood pressure:
- 6 Vasculin
- 6 Linum B_6

Note: With chest tightness add: 6-8 Cataplex E_2. Consider additional Cardio-Plus or Vasculin (4-6 per day) as the case warrants.

ANGINA

If acute:
- 6 Cardio-Plus
- 6-12 Cataplex E_2

Preventative maintenance: 6 Cataplex E_2

HIGH CHOLESTEROL

- 9 Cholaplex
- 4 Black Currant Seed Oil
- 4 Linum B_6

Note: Reduce stress if possible and increase the consumption of green leafy vegetables.

LOW HDL CHOLESTEROL

- 1-2 Copper Liver Chelate
- 4 Magnesium Lactate
- 6 Cataplex GTF
- 4 Super-Eff

Note: Aerobic exercise is recommended. Low cholesterol shows stressed immune system, and is a marker for neoplasm.

ROULEAUX PHENOMENA

6 Linum B_6 or 6 Zypan

Note: If acute: 10-15 drops Phosfood Liquid (twice per day) Phosfood Liquid is a short-term therapy

Nutritional Support for the Common Underlying Causes of Hypertension

Remember – address the basics <u>first</u> and you may never need this page again:
- Hydrochloric Acid
- Liver/Gallbladder
- Adrenals
- Essential fatty acids/Calcium
- Need for Vitamin B or G
- Digestion

©1996 – 2010 International Foundation for Nutrition and Health, All Rights Reserved

HYPERTENSION (HPT)

Adrenal
    Hypoadrenia: 3 Desiccated Adrenal

Note: Use Adrenal (Desiccated) when postural blood pressure falls over 10 points, never dose at more than 3 per day.
    OR
    Hyperadrenia: (rare)   6-9 Drenamin
                                           6 Drenamin
                                           6 Min-Chex

Note: Take Min-Chex on an empty stomach.

Hepatic-Portal Congestion: 9 Livaplex
                                               12 A-F Betafood
                                               6 Antronex

Renal: 9-12 Renafood

Emotional: 6 Min-Chex per day (and as needed, on an empty stomach)

*Benign Essential Hypertension   *Excerpted from Blood Chemistry Manual, pp. 58-60
                                                                 6 Diaplex
                                                                  6 Organically Bound Minerals
                                                                  3 Protefood
                                                                  3 Cal-Ma Plus
                                                                  9 Albaplex

For Elevated Diastolic add: 6 Cataplex EB_2
                                                                  6 Renafood

For Elevated Systolic add: 6 Cholaplex

Arteriosclerotic: 2-4 Cyruta

Sympathetic Dominance: 4 Organically Bound Minerals
                                                                   4 Calcium Lactate

STROKE – There are two kinds of strokes:
    Hemorrhagic: 6-15 Cyruta-Plus (for capillary fragility)

    Thrombolytic or Occlusive: 6 Linum B_6
                                                                  6 Cataplex G
                                                                  6 Cataplex B
                                                                  3 Cyruta

    Stroke: General Protocol: 2-3 Circuplex
                                                                  2-3 Cyruta-Plus
                                                                  1 Protefood

Note: Rule out need for Zypan or EFA

CARDIOVASCULAR MAINTENANCE   3 Catalyn
                                                                                           2-4 Cardio-Plus
                                                                                           2-4 AF Betafood

Nutritional Support for Common Digestive Problems

**All amounts indicate number to be taken per day.
In general, take supplements in equal portions throughout the day.
(Example: 6/daily = 2 tablets 3 times per day with meals)**

HEARTBURN INDIGESTION OR BELCHING

For short-term Symptomatic relief:	1-2 Gastrex Capsules (as needed for relief)
To promote healing of existing damage:	6 Okra Pepsin E3 6 Multizyme 8 Chlorophyll Complex Perles
To correct underlying problem:	6-9 Zypan with meals (Heal stomach lining first if Zypan is painful on empty stomach.)

Note: Heartburn, indigestion or belching is normally the result of insufficient acidity in the stomach. This sounds like a contradiction, but it's not. The stomach needs hydrochloric acid (HCL) to digest food properly. When the stomach becomes HCL-deficient, the result is the putrefaction of food. This produces organic acids, which cause heartburn and indigestion. Antacids, such as Tums, are effective in alleviating these symptoms because they neutralize the organic acids. However, they only aggravate the underlying problem by increasing the alkalinity of the stomach.

GALLBLADDER SYMPTOMS

Bloating, fat intolerance:	6-15 A-F Betafood
If severe add:	6 Choline
If light-colored stool:	6 Cholacol

GALLBLADDER REMOVED

6 Cholacol
6 Betafood

FLATULENCE

6 Zymex
6 Zypan

BOWEL DETOX

6 Zymex
6 Spanish Black Radish
3-6 Chlorophyll Complex Perles

Note: If tends to constipation:	6-9 Fen-Cho
If tends to diarrhea:	6-9 Cholacol II
If history of dairy use:	6-9 Lact-Enz on empty stomach

Diet recommendations: Use Page Food Plan or Low Stress Diet
Always drink a lot of water. (should consume at least ½ body weight in ounces per day)

Systemic Detox add:	6-9 Livaplex 6 Parotid PMG

BOWEL FLORA – Always after antibiotic therapy.

6 Lact-Enz
6 Lactic Acid Yeast

©1996 – 2010 International Foundation for Nutrition and Health, All Rights Reserved

IRRITABLE BOWEL

        9 Gastrex (use initially while acute to relieve symptoms; then switch to 9 Okra Pepsin E3)
        6 Zymex
        6 Lact-Enz
        6-12 Antronex

Note: In acute cases, consider increasing Antronex up to 20 per day. Diet recommendations: For 30 days eliminate all grains (except brown rice), milk and milk products, and refined carbohydrates.

- Identify and eliminate other allergic foods if possible.
- Rule out essential fatty acid deficiencies.
- Rule out need for Zypan, Multizyme and A-F Betafood.

CONSTIPATION

        6 Zypan
        6 Multizyme

Note: If persistent, add one 6 Cholacol at a time until cleared

        6 Choline
        6 A-F Betafood

Alternative   9 Fen-Cho

Note: Fen-Cho acts as a natural laxative to provide relief. The above protocol deals with the underlying causes of constipation. <u>General Note:</u> Patients should drink at least 8 glasses of water daily.

DIARRHEA

Take until symptoms abate: 12 Cholacol II (4 tablets 3 times daily between meals)
After symptoms abate: 6 Zymex

YEAST

        6 Zymex
        3 Spanish Black Radish
        3 Lact-Enz
        3 Cal-Amo

Note: Non-dairy users should also use 3 Lactic Acid Yeast per day. Diet recommendations: For 30 days eliminate all milk and milk products, canned foods, high-carbohydrate fruits and vegetables, and all grains except brown rice. (Use the Page Food Plan; download free patient handout "www.ifnh.org")

PARASITES

        12 Zymex II (2-3 times daily on an empty stomach)
        3 Cal-Amo
        3 Spanish Black Radish

Note: This protocol must be continued for eight weeks even if symptoms are gone. To prevent re-occurrence, rule out need for Zypan. Homeopathic enhancement: Para Solve

HEMORRHOIDS

        6 Collinsonia Root (between meals with water)
        6-15 A-F Betafood

FOOD POISONING

        3-6 Gastrex Capsules (as needed for relief)

Nutritional Support for Common Endocrine and Female Hormonal Conditions

All amounts indicate number to be taken per day.
In general, take supplements in equal portions throughout the day.
(Example: 6/daily = 2 tablets 3 times per day with meals)

GENERAL ENDOCRINE SUPPORT
- 6 Symplex F or M
- 4 Trace Minerals- B_{12}

Note: Check digestion, EFA (essential fatty acids), tissue calcium levels and adrenal function.

FEMALE FERTILITY
General endocrine support:
- 6 For-Til B_{12}
- 4 Ovex or Ovex P
- 6 Wheat Germ Oil

Chronic miscarriages, add:
- 4 Utrophin PMG
- 4 Chlorophyll Complex Perles

DIFFICULT MENOPAUSE.
- 4 Ovex or Ovex P
- 6 Symplex F
- 1 Organic Iodine

Note: Rule out adrenal fatigue, support decreased adrenal function

MENORRHAGIA/HEAVY FLOW
General endocrine support:
- 6 Ovex or Ovex P (may increase to 15 in acute cases)
- 6 Utrophin PMG

SCANTY MENSES/AMENORRHEA
General endocrine support:
- 6 Ovatrophin PMG

Note: Rule out EFA need and anemia. Need to enhance blood quality: 2 Immuplex or 1 Ferrofood

DYSMENORRHEA/PAINFUL MENSES
General endocrine support: 3 Cal-Ma Plus
Acute symptoms: 6 or less Cal-Ma Plus each hour, crushed in warm water

Note: Check tissue calcium cuff test, calcium level, rule out hypoglycemia, need for EFA, magnesium, anemia and digestive support.

PMS/PRE-MENSTRUAL SYNDROME
- 6 Utrophin PMG
- 6 Min-Chex

Note: Testosterone is precursor to estrogen. Address digestion, liver and adrenals.

OVARIAN CYSTS
- 3 Ovex or Ovex P
- 12 Cataplex A-C-P
- 3 Lact-Enz
- 3 Chlorophyll Complex Perles

Note: Reduce or eliminate dairy products, caffeine, and chocolate.

FIBROID
1. Get them off all alkaloids (coffee, chocolate, tea, cola, etc.).
2. Give a Protomorphogen of tissue involved, i.e. mammary, uterus.
3. Give them General Endocrine Support. (Symplex F and Trace Minererals B_{12})
4. Rule out yeast.
5. If fibroid is painful when palpated, use Zymex.

ENDOMETRIOSIS
- 6 Cataplex D
- 9 For-Til B_{12}
- 6 Ribonucleic Acid (RNA)

Note: Take off all alkaloids and treat like a Fibroid.

BREAST TENDERNESS
- 6 Zymex
- 3 Spanish Black Radish

Note: Rule out liver, gallbladder, sugar problems, and synthetic thiamine use.

DIMINISHED SEX DRIVE
- 6 For-Til B_{12}
- 6 Min Chex

Nutritional Support for Pharmaceutical HRT

Clinical notes: (This approach can be extremely helpful when a patient requests support in weaning themselves from a pharmaceutical program of Hormonal Replacement Therapy.) The most successful approach to HRT is through emphasizing the impact of today's lifestyle and diet and its relationship to sugar handling (liver, pancreas, and adrenals), digestion, and liver/biliary function. Most patients need some form of nutritional support to be successful. The use of the Page Food Plan can make a major difference.

Step 1 For the first six weeks (weeks 1-6) of treatment, maintain the full dose of HRT. At the same time, begin using Symplex F or M (6/day), Tribulus (2/day), Wild Yam Complex (4/day), Drenamin (4/day) and Catalyn (6/day). The patient should check with his/her doctor about lowering the dosage.

Step 2 For the next six weeks (weeks 6-12) of treatment, continue on Symplex F, Tribulus, Wild Yam Complex, Drenamin and Catalyn at the same dosage as above. Many doctors will reduce the dosage of HRT to ½ the original dosage. After 12 weeks, the patient should again check with his/her doctor about lowering the dosage.

Step 3 For the next six weeks (weeks 13-18), continue on Symplex F, Tribulus, Wild Yam Complex, Drenamin and Catalyn at the same dosage as above. Many doctors reduce the dosage of HRT by ¼ - ½ of the original. After 18 weeks, the patient should check with his/her doctor about lowering the dosage.

Step 4 At week 19, it is possible to discontinue HRT entirely. If asymptomatic, reduce dosage of herbs to maintenance doses of Symplex F (3/day), Tribulus (2/day), Wild Yam Complex (3/day), and Catalyn (3/day).

Nutritional Support for Basic Pre-Natal Care

The nutrition list addresses the common complaints of pregnancy. Regardless of symptoms, the following nutrition guide is recommended for the development of a healthy baby:

- 2 Folic Acid-B_{12} (take 2 per day for entire pregnancy)
- 4 Calcium Lactate Tablets (a source of easily assimilated calcium)
- 2 Bio-Dent (calcium and minerals to build strong bones and teeth)
- 4 Cyrofood Tablets (a multivitamin concentrated from whole food)
- 1 Ferrofood (iron and blood building factors)
- 1 Immuplex (supports immune function)
- 1 Protefood (essential amino acids)
- 1 Nutrimere (from a whole protein complex)
- 2 Cataplex GTF (promotes proper sugar handling by the mother during fetal development)
- 2 Trace Minerals B_{12} (provides essential trace minerals)

This program is for the 1st Trimester. Increase amounts for the 2nd Trimester, and again for the 3rd Trimester until the infant is weaned.

Nutritional Support for Common Discomforts of Pregnancy

MORNING SICKNESS — Primarily the result of compromised digestion. The underlying problem exists prior to pregnancy. With the added digestive challenge of pregnancy, the problem becomes symptomatic.

To control vomiting: Phosfood Liquid – 15 drops in water, as often as needed then:
Sick, but not vomiting:
- 6 A-F Betafood
- 6 Zypan
- 6 Multizyme

If condition persists, add one at a time until cleared
- 6 Cholacol
- 6 Choline
- 6 Cataplex G
- 6 Inositol

HEARTBURN OR INDIGESTION — Generally a result of insufficient acidity in the stomach. This sounds like a contradiction, but it is not. The stomach needs hydrochloric acid (HCL) to digest food properly. When the stomach becomes HCL-deficient the result is the putrefaction of food. This produces organic acids, which cause heartburn and indigestion. Antacids, such as Tums, are effective in alleviating these symptoms because they neutralize the organic acids. However, they only aggravate the underlying problem by increasing the alkalinity of the stomach.

For short-term
Symptomatic relief: 1-2 Gastrex Capsules (as needed for relief)
To correct underlying problem: 2 Zypan (with each meal)
To promote healing 6 Okra Pepsin-E_3
Of existing damage: 6 Multizyme

FATIGUE — Excessive fatigue is often the result of adrenal insufficiency. The added physical demands of pregnancy along with stress are very trying on the adrenal glands. This can also be an indication for iron need (see Basic Pre-natal Nutritional Program on other side)

10 Drenamin (one per hour from rising)

Note: Check for anemia

SLEEPLESSNESS

Trouble falling asleep:
    4 Cataplex G
    4 Min-Chex   (before bed)

Note: Min-Chex is a combination of natural vitamins, minerals, and nutritional factors that promote relaxation and sleep.

Trouble staying asleep:
    4 A-F Betafood   (before bed)
    1 Protefood   (before bed)

CONSTIPATION — Like morning sickness, it is the result of a compromised digestive system.
    6 Zypan
    6 Multizyme   (2 tablets ½ hour before meals)
    6 Trace Minerals B_{12}

Note: Trace Minerals B_{12} is the precursor to hydrochloric acid.

If persistent, add one   6 Cholacol
at a time until cleared   6 Choline 6 A-F Betafood

LEG AND MUSCLE CRAMPS – The body needs extra calcium during pregnancy to build the fetal bones. If sufficient dietary calcium is not available, tissue stores are recruited and insufficient tissue calcium results in leg and muscle cramps. (Milk is a poor source of dietary calcium. Compared with other countries, the U.S. has a very high rate of consumption of dairy products and a very high incidence of osteoporosis.)

Occurring during activity: 6 Cataplex E_2
Occurring during inactivity: 6 Calcium Lactate Tablets   (on an empty stomach)
    6 Cataplex F Tablets
    6 Trace Minerals B_{12} (until relief; 3 thereafter)

VARICOSE VEINS AND HEMORRHOIDS — Result from loss of vascular integrity and are almost always associated with liver congestion.
    6 Collinsonia Root   (with warm water, between meals)
    6 A-F Betafood
    6 Cataplex A-C-P   (bioflavonoids)

EXCESSIVE WATER RETENTION

Note: Check adrenals, digestion and anemia

SWOLLEN ANKLES OR FEET (EDEMA) —This is an indication of poor adrenal function.
    10 Drenamin   (1 per hour from rising)

BACKACHE — This is an indication of a need for Vitamin E.
    6 Cataplex E and/or
    6 Wheat Germ Oil Perles
    6 Trace Minerals B_{12}

FAINTNESS OR DIZZINESS — Usually the result of adrenal insufficiency.
    10 Drenamin   (1 per hour from rising)

Note: Rule out kidneys (Cataplex A-C) and Anemia (Ferrofood)

YEAST INFECTIONS
    6 Zymex   (if diet does not include dairy products add)
    3 Lact-Enz   (add if diet includes dairy products)

POOR MEMORY
    6 Ribonucleic Acid (RNA)
    2 Ginko Synergy

NURSING PROBLEMS

      6   Mammary PMG

Note: Rule out blood quality problem, EFA and thiamine need. Check mother's digestion.

POST-PARTUM DEPRESSION

    10 Drenamin
    3 Cyruta Plus

TOXEMIA

    3   Arginex
    3   Zymex
    3   Protefood

ANEMIA

    2   Immuplex
    3   Zymex
    3   Protefood

Nutritional Support for Infants

BABY FORMULA

    ½tsp Cyrofood Powder
    ½tsp Calcifood Powder
    1   Thymus PMG

Note: Infants have started vitamin therapy as early as two weeks old. (*Vitamin News* page 128 Vol-7 1939)

FEVER

    3   Calciun Lactate
    3   Thymex

Note: Children over two years of age dosage 1 to 2 every hour until fever breaks.

*These nutrients are food concentrates provided to upgrade the quality of the diet
in order to support normal physiology and biochemistry function*

*****

Nutritional Support for Common Immune Problems

All amounts indicate number to be taken per day.
In general, take supplements in equal portions throughout the day.
(Example: 6/daily = 2 tablets 3 times per day with meals)

CHRONIC IMMUNE DEFICIENCY

- 6 Immuplex
- 6 Livaplex
- 9 Thymex
- 6 Cataplex A-C
- 6 Sesame Seed Oil

ACUTE INFECTIONS

When associated with sore throat, ear symptoms, fever:
- 20 Congaplex
- 4-10 Cal-Amo

Note: Should be on protocol for a minimum of three weeks or one week after symptoms are *completely* gone.

Remember to address acute adrenal hypofunction.
Alternative protocol:
- 10 Congaplex
- 10 Immuplex
- 4-10 Cal-Amo

EARACHE IN CHILDREN

No sign of infection: 20 Antronex
Ear infection: 20 Congaplex

Note: If sure of infection:
- 20 Congaplex
- 20 Antronex

Note: If nursing, treat mother. If under 6 years old – 1/3 of protocol above.
If 6 to 12 year old – 2/3 protocol
If over 12 years old – full protocol

EPSTEIN-BARR VIRUS (E.B.V.)

- 10 Immuplex
- 3 Betacol   (take all for 6-12 weeks)
- 15 Cyruta-Plus

Always rule out digestive insufficiency first.

These nutrients are food concentrates provided to upgrade the quality of the diet in order to support normal physiology and biochemistry function

*****

Nutritional Support for Common Musculo-Skeletal Problems

All amounts indicate number to be taken per day.
In general. Take supplements in equal portions throughout the day.
(Example: 6/daily = 2 tablets 3 times per day with meals)

SOFT TISSUE TRAUMA

Healthy person with   9   Ligaplex I
simple trauma: 6   Multizyme

Inflammation protocol: *see below*
If severe: 20 Zymex II (5 tablets 4 times per day on empty
(stomach)

CHRONIC LAXITY OF LIGAMENTS – (Usually a sick person)

     9   Ligaplex II
     6   Collagen C

Note: Rule out gallbladder problem; manganese uptake is biliary dependent.

OSTEO ARTHRITIS – CALCIUM METABOLISM ——40% advanced to be diagnosable by X-ray.

McDougall's Medicine. Worldwide population studies show the higher the dairy use in a country, the higher the incidence of osteoarthritis.

Treatment: Essential Fatty Acids – Calcium Utilization

     6   Cataplex F Tablets
     3   Cal-Amo   (acidify system, calcium absorption)
     6   Drenamin   (for adrenal hormone support)

OSTEO POROSIS

     6   Biost
     3   Cal-Ma Plus   (all for 3 months)
     6   Cataplex F Tablets

For maintenance/   3   Biost
Prevention   6   Calcifood
     6   Cataplex F

BROKEN BONES

     6   Biost
     6   Cal-Ma Plus

Note: Reduces healing time to 50%. Homeopathic enhancement: NET Remedy #9 ER911

INFLAMMATION

     5   Cyruta-Plus (to avoid digestive upset start with 2-3 in middle of meal and work up to 5 per meal)
     9   Drenamin
     6   Black Currant Seed Oil

To soothe muscles, add: 6   Cal-Ma Plus (optimum) or 6 Calcium Lactate

Note: When tissue is destroyed ie surgery, crushing wounds; add: 20 Zymex II (5 tablets 4 times per day on empty stomach)

BONE SPURS

     6   Cal-Amo
     6   Biost

BURSITIS

      6 Black Currant Seed Oil (Calcium metabolizer and anti-inflammatory)
      6-8 Drenamin (adrenal hormone support)

Secondary to calcification
As a result of alkalinity add: 6 Cal-Amo (systemic acidifier)
      30-90 drops Phosfood Liquid (Calcium normalizer)

Note: Rule out gallbladder and HCL need.

FIBRO MYALGIA

As a result of a real thiamine deficiency: 9 Cataplex B

Note: Usually secondary to a sugar handling problem or excessive use of synthetic B vitamins.

If sugar handling problem   15 Calsol ruled out: 5 Cal-Amo Plus
      6 Cataplex A-C-P (take all for 3-12 weeks)
      6 Spanish Black Radish
      6 Immuplex

Note: For maintenance   6 For-Til B_{12}
prevention: (take both for life)   2 Cataplex F Perles

HOT DISC

      6 Ligaplex II
      6 Cal-Ma Plus
      15 Cyruta-Plus (to avoid digestive upset start with 2-3 in middle of meal and work up to 5 per meal)

MUSCLE CRAMPS

Nocturnal: 8 Calcium Lactate (on empty stomach)
      6 Cataplex F

On exercise: 6 Cataplex E

JOINT STIFFNESS UPON RISING — Need for organic Phosphorus to utilize the calcium.

      6 Circuplex
      15 A-F Betafood

MUSCLE STIFFNESS WORSE WITH ACTIVITY

      15 A-F Betafood
      3 Betacol (anti-stiffness factor; Wulzen factor)

Note: Often need to address patient constipation (see digestive protocols)

RHEUMATOID ARTHRITIS — This is not a musculoskeletal problem; it is a metabolic problem. Since 1984 various papers have been published in peer review literature implicating amoebas, parasites, diet and food sensitivity in many cases of rheumatoid arthritis. Current information also indicates grains (except brown rice) and all milk products should be eliminated from the diet for a period of time to determine if improvement is noted.

      6 Rumaplex
      9 Thymex
      3 Zinc Liver Chelate (The zinc and copper should be used at separate times)
      2 Copper Liver Chelate (Times: e.g. zinc in the a.m. & copper in the p.m.)

(Continued Next Page)

RHEUMATOID ARTHRITIS (Continued from previous page)

      6 Lact-Enz
      6 Organically Bound Minerals
      2 Trace Minerals-B12
      8 Zymex II (on empty stomach)

HEBERDEN'S NODES

      3 B_6-Niacinamide

Note: eating a handful of raw pecans at least once a day can be helpful.

Nutritional Support For Nail Problems

Note: Using finger nails and hands for diagnosis has been a major part of Oriental medicine for centuries. This next section is extremely helpful for any practitioner using nutrition in their practice for it also gives you the signs and symptoms of each deficiency.

PROTEIN: Soft, tear or peel easily, opaque white lines

      2 Protefood   (after protein meals)
      6 Calcifood Wafers

CALCIUM: Dry, brittle, break easily, horizontal or vertical ridges (hypothyroidism may be a contributing factor)

      6 Calcifood Wafers
      6 Cataplex F
      6 Calcium Lactate (on an empty stomach)

IRON: Thin, flat, spoon-shaped, white or yellow nail beds (white nail beds or white coloration near the cuticle with dark coloration near the tip can also indicate chronic liver/kidney disease)

      3 Ferrofood
      6 Zypan

ZINC: White spots or bands on nails or nail bed (can also indicate liver/kidney disease or appear consequent on fasting or menstruation)

      3 Chezyn

VITAMIN E: Yellow nail bed, poor or no growth (also indicates possible lymphatic or respiratory congestion)

      9 Cataplex E

VITAMIN B_{12}: Darkened nail beds

      2 Cataplex B_{12}

Note: Impaired circulation to the extremities, as in Reynaud's phenomenon, phlebitis, etc., can cause any of the above symptoms. Dry, brittle nails can also be caused by excessive exposure to solvents, detergents, nail polish and nail polish remover. Always rule out digestive insufficiency first

*These nutrients are food concentrates provided to upgrade the quality of the diet
in order to support normal physiology and biochemistry function*

*****

Nutritional Support for Common Sugar Handling Problems

All amounts indicate number to be taken per day.
In general, take supplements in equal portions throughout the day.
(Example: 6/daily = 2 tablets 3 times per day with meals)

BLOOD SUGAR issues are the root cause of almost all complaints your patients are faced with today. To ignore these issues of sugar handling and their impact on digestion and liver biliary function will guarantee failure. Use the Nutritional Exam daily as it is your guarantee for success.

BLOOD SUGAR IMBALANCE (REACTIVE HYPOGLYCEMIA)

Primary:
- 6 A-F Betafood
- 9 Cataplex B
- 6 Drenamin
- 6 Paraplex

Additional support:
- 3 Protefood
- 3 Cataplex GTF

Note: Always check digestion with sugar handling problems

CRAVES SWEETS

Primary:
- 6 Inositol
- 6 Cholacol (1-2 bottles only)

Maintenance: Inositol as needed

DIABETES

Primary:
- 9 Diaplex
- 9 Multizyme
- 6 B_6-Niacinamide
- 6 Cataplex GTF

Additional support:
- 3 Immuplex
- 6 Cataplex B

If on insulin:
- 6 Cyruta-Plus

Note: Any patients on this protocol must monitor blood sugar closely, as the need for insulin may decrease dramatically.

TROUBLE STAYING ASLEEP AT NIGHT

Before going to bed:
- 1 Protefood
- 4 A-F Betafood

SLEEPY AFTER MEALS

- 6 Cataplex B
- 6 Zypan (2 with each meal)
- 10 Antronex

Always rule out digestive insufficiency first.

These nutrients are food concentrates provided to upgrade the quality of the diet in order to support normal physiology and biochemistry function

*****

©1996 – 2010 International Foundation for Nutrition and Health, All Rights Reserved

Standard Process Glandular Products

Protomorphogens

Biost = *bone, marrow, spinal cord*
Cardiotrophin PMG = *heart*
Dermatrophin PMB = *epithelial*
Drenatrophin PMG = *adrenal*
Hepatrophin PMG = *liver*
Hypothalamus PMG = *hypothalamus*
Mammary PMG = *mammary*
Myotrophin PMG = *heart muscle*
Neurotrophin PMG = *brain*
Oculotrophin PMG = *eye*

Orchic PMG = *testis*
Ostrophin PMG = *bone, marrow, spinal cord*
Ovatrophin PMG = *ovary*
Pancreatrophin PMG = *pancreas*
Parotid PMG = *parotid*
Pituitrophin PMG = *pituitary*
Pneumotrophin PMG = *lung*
Prostate PMG = *prostate*
Renatrophin PMG = *kidney*

Spleen PMG = *spleen*
Thymus PMG = *thymus*
Thytrophin PMG = *thyroid*
Utrophin PMG = *uterus*
Paraplex = *pituitary, thyroid, adrenal, pancreas*
Symplex F = *pituitary, thyroid,*
(female)   *adrenal, ovary*
Symplex M = *pituitary, thyroid,*
(male)   *adrenal, testis*

Special Formula Products & Key Protomorphogens

Albaplex = *kidney*
Allerplex = *lung, adrenal*
Cardio-Plus = *heart*
Diaplex = *pancreas, pituitary*
Drenamin = *adrenal*
Emphaplex = *lung, adrenal*

Immuplex = *spleen, thymus*
Iplex = *eye*
Livaplex = *liver*
Myo-Plus = *muscle*
Neuroplex = *brain, pituitary*
Ostarplex = *bone*

Paraplex = *pancreas, adrenal, pituitary, thyroid*
Renafood = *kidney*
Rumaplex = *bone*
Vasculin = *heart*

Cytosol Extracts

Hypothalmex = *hypothalamus*
Orchex = *testis*
Ovex = *ovary*
Prost-X = *prostate*
Thymex = *thymus*

Whole Desiccated Products

Adrenal, Desiccated = *adrenal*
Cal-Ma Plus = *parathyroid*
E-Manganese = *anterior pituitary*
Neuroplex = *hypothalamus, anterior pituitary, spleen*
Spleen, Desiccated = *spleen*

Selected Products Containing Cytosol Extracts

Albaplex = *thymus*
Cataplex B_{12} = *adrenal*
Betacol = *adrenal*
Cardio-Plus = *adrenal*
Cholaplex = *orchic, adrenal*
Circuplex = *adrenal*
Congaplex = *thymus*
Cyruta = *adrenal*

Cyruta-Plus = *adrenal*
Diaplex = *spleen, pancreas*
Cataplex E2 = *adrenal*
Folic Acid-B_{12} = *adrenal*
Cataplex GTF = *pancreas, adrenal*
Immuplex = *thymus*
Iplex = *adrenal*
Ligaplex I = *adrenal*

Ligaplex II = *adrenal*
Livaplex = *adrenal*
Min-Chex = *orchic*
Myo-Plus = *adrenal*
Vasculin = *adrenal*
Zypan = *pancreas*

The Three Types of Glandulars

- Protomorphogens
- Cytosol Extracts
- Whole Glands (concentrates or desiccates)

✓ These three clinical tools are as different as a hammer, a screwdriver and a saw.
✓ Success in using glandulars depends on using the correct one for the job at hand.
✓ Only Standard Process makes all three.

Protomorphogens

"Promotes healing over time"

Protomorphogens are extracts of the nucleic acids from the nucleus of the cell. The nucleic acids, of course, control the function of the cell. Many doctors use the terms protomorphogens and glandulars interchangeably. While not strictly accurate, the protomorphogen is the fundamental type of glandular product, and the principal source of the reputation earned over many decades for clinical results, especially in chronic cases.

Examples:
Drenatrophin PMG = adrenal
Ovatrophin PMG = ovary
Pancreatrophin = pancreas

Made only by Standard Process because only Standard Process has the technology, invented and produced by Dr. Royal Lee, that can create protomorphogens. The Protomorphogens are used widely in the well-known Special Formula Products.

Examples:
Drenamin = Drenatrophin PMG
Symplex F = Ovatrophin PMG
Diaplex = Pancreatrophin PMG

Cytosol Extracts
"Provides function — and relief — right away"

Cytosols are extracts from the cytoplasm of the cell. In the cytoplasm is found the unique and critical outputs of the cell. Cytosol extracts are undoubtedly the next most important type of glandular and the principal source of the reputation that glandulars have for really dramatic clinical results, especially in acute cases.

Examples:
Adrenal Cytosol
Ovex
Pancreas Cytosol Extract

Cytosol extracts are used widely in the S.P. line, and are crucial to the success of many of the best-known S.P. products.

For Example: Zypan contains Pancreas Cytosol Extract, and Ligaplex I and II contain Adrenal Cytosol Extract.

Cytosol extracts and protomorphogens are only produced by Standard Process.

Whole Glands
"Provides the nuts and bolts that make up the gland"

Whole glands are the easiest to manufacture and are available from everyone. It is interesting to note that the type of glandular with the narrowest range of uses is the one most widely offered to the doctor. At the same time, in the special case when it is the proper tool, only then does it produce the desired result.

Examples:
Whole Desiccated Adrenal
Whole Desiccated Spleen

©1996 – 2010 International Foundation for Nutrition and Health, All Rights Reserved

Nutritional Support for Specific Glands

ATM – Trace Minerals for the Endocrine Glands

Manganese	→	Pituitary
Iodine	→	Thyroid
Copper	→	Adrenal
Chromium	→	Pancreas
Zinc	→	Prostate/Uterus
Selenium	→	Testes/Ovaries

Specific Support for the Endocrine and Related Organs

Pituitrophin PMG E-Manganese	→	Pituitary
Thytrophin PMG Organic Minerals Iodomere Organic Iodine Cataplex F	→	Thyroid
Drenatrophin PMG Drenamin Adrenal, Desiccated Copper – Cataplex C B_6-Niacinamide	→	Adrenal
Cataplex GTF (Chromium) Pancreatrophin PMG Multizyme	→	Pancreas
Prost-X Prostate PMG	→	Prostate
Utrophin PMG	→	Uterus
Orchex Orchic PMG	→	Testes
Ovex Ovatrophin PMG	→	Ovary
Cal-Ma Plus	→	Parathyroid

TYPES OF ADRENAL SUPPORT

	80%		20%	
Whole Gland (Emergency Use)	**Protomorphogen (Normal Use)**		**Cytosol Extract**	**Via Autonomics**
	Healing over time			
Whole Desiccated Adrenal	Drenatrophin PMG		Cyruta Plus 6 / day	B6 Niacinamide 6 / day
2-3 per day	**Drenamin**			
	• Drenatrophin PMG			
	• Cataplex C			
	• Cataplex G			
	6-12 per day			
Always with food			*Always with food*	
Rule of thumb:	Rule of thumb:		Rule of thumb:	Rule of thumb:
Use **Whole Desiccated Adrenal** when systolic drop is greater than 15. 2-3 per day, 1 per meal, usually for 1 or 2 bottles. Graduate to **Drenamin** or Drenatrophin PMG when drop is adequately improved or as indicated by adrenal reflex response to nutrition.	**Drenamin** If low BP: **Drenamin** + Cataplex B		Acute adrenal emergency or defensively during a period of stress	Usually used short term. Graduate to **Drenamin**.

These nutrients are food concentrates provided to upgrade the quality of the diet
in order to support normal physiology and biochemistry.
*****
This information is provided by the International Foundation for Nutrition and Health
As part of the CCWFN program for the educational use of health care professionals.

The Protomorphogen

The hallmark of Standard Process is its glandular supplements, especially the protomorphogen (PMG). The uniqueness of the protomorphogen stands on its own. For more in depth information the International Foundation for Nutrition and Health (IFNH) carries many of the publications from the old Lee Foundation for Nutritional Research, such as <u>An Introduction to Protomorphology</u> a 24 page booklet. <u>Applied Protomorphology</u> is a collection of articles and bulletins by Dr. Royal Lee, and Standard Process laboratories supporting the uses and application of protomorphogens. <u>Protomorphology-The Principles of Cell Auto Regulation</u> published by Dr Royal Lee and William Hansen in 1947 are just a few of the educational materials available at <u>ifnh.org</u>.

The following excerpts are from <u>Applied Protomorphology</u>, by Royal Lee: A protomorphogen (PMG) is that component of the cell chromosome that is responsible for morphogenetic determination of cell characteristics. It is the smallest unit of the cell blueprint assembly. It is the smallest unit of the gene system that guides the cell into its hereditary form as it grows, develops or repairs itself. Without sufficient protomorphogen in its chromatin, the cell degenerates, de-differentiates, becomes senile and dies. The protomorphogen level in the cell is regulated by the fact that, while normally more is constantly being created by the cell nucleus, it is antigenic and promotes the formation of antibodies (in the mammalian organism) which in turn controls the level of extra cellular protomorphogen in blood and lymphatic system.

Throughout the years, we have periodically pioneered remarkable "*firsts*". These "firsts" have not all been immediately accepted by the consensus of opinion. No method of measuring the effectiveness of protomorphogen by laboratory means has been discovered, just as was the case for many years with vitamins. The clinical response, however, can be demonstrated in a matter of minutes by an instrument such as the Endocardiograph.

Cytotropic Extracts are manufactured under the US patent # 2,374,219 which states the purpose of this patent is to provide an improved method of "producing a sterilized dry substance from a juice." This sterilization takes place below pasteurization temperature of a juice, thus the synergistic agents, such as amino acids and enzymes are not destroyed. Cytotropic extracts are not drugs. They are composed of the mineral fractions of animal tissue which is found associated in the protein molecule. Nutritionally this would be considered in the category of meat extracts. No food products are subject to, or restricted by the Experimental Drug Law.

Extracted from another section of this manuscript: It may be assumed that this specific growth factor (the cellular blueprint known as protomorphogens (PMG) that are constantly being secreted by each cell into its surrounding fluids) are prevented from traveling very far by the influence of the specific antibodies, known as natural tissue antibodies (NTA). They must be destroyed, if allowed to build up in any concentration; they would promote cell growth and mitosis. Only if any specific organ becomes subject to overwork and consequent inflammation in some degree does this occur. A kidney doubles in size in six months after its partner has been removed, just as muscles grow if sufficient demand is made on their ability.

Where disease has damaged an organ such as tuberculosis in the case of lungs, or where the heart has hypertrophied by overwork, the ingestion of heart or lung PMG, as the case may be, may at first create adverse reactions of a toxic nature (malaise, tiredness), apparently by a reason of the immediate proteolytic destruction of the ingested PMG by antibodies in the blood stream, that are present in higher amounts than normal, by reason of the long-standing inflammation of the specific organ.

Cardio graphic recordings will show that within a few minutes after ingestion of the cardiac PMG, the heart action changes for the better. It is hard to explain this reaction other than by assuming that the excess heart tissue antibody in the circulating blood has been reduced by combination with the ingested heart PMG. This is probably done without danger of stimulating the formation of more heart tissue antibody, since alimentary ingestion normally does not permit proteins to act as antigens. Parenteral introduction of such materials is another matter.

Other factors that assist in controlling natural tissue antibodies are allantoin, betaine, (probably be a depolymerizing affect), and the hormones of the gonads, thyroid, thymus and adrenal. Thymus acts by promoting colloidal dispersion that physiologically opposes cortisone, which flocculates antigens into particulate dimensions that permit their ingestion by phagocytes (and then antibody formation.) The thymus during the development age prevents this and keeps PMG's available for growth stimulation and ultimate enzyme digestion and renal elimination.

Thyroid hormones split PMG's off the chromatin reserve of the cell, or from absorbed stores in connective tissue. That is why thyroxin accelerates tadpole metamorphosis. It is also the reason why thyroxin increases the metabolic rate. The released PMG stimulates cell activities.

The Multiple-Vitamin Products

CATALYN: *The original product formulated by Dr. Royal Lee*

CATALYN is the concentrated multiple vitamin, trace mineral and enzyme product. It was designed to contain all of the vitamin and trace minerals, both known and unknown. Because it is made from natural sources (liver, wheat germ, etc.) it contains all of the trace elements found in nature as well as the major minerals (calcium, iron, and phosphorus). **CATALYN** is analyzed each time a new trace element, enzyme or other micro nutrient is discovered – and the substance is always found to be present in **CATALYN**. The unique effectiveness of supplements derived directly from nature is due to the trace elements they contain.

* * * The All-Purpose Multiple * * *

CYRO-YEAST:
    Is CATALYN
    Plus LACTIC ACID YEAST in a chewable wafer

    For all the benefits of CATALYN plus extra natural B vitamins from yeast.

* * * Especially for the Adult Male * * *

E-POISE:
Specially formulated for Standard Process by Dr. George Goodheart, based on the research of James P. Isaacs, M.D. on the body's electron poising system.

    Is CATALYN
    Plus FERROFOOD
    Plus CHLOROPHYLL from the herb Tillandsia.

    For all the benefits of CATALYN plus FERROFOOD and CHLOROPHYLL for the blood.

* * * Especially for Adolescent and Adult Females * * *

CYROFOOD TABLETS:
A multi-vitamin, multi-mineral, multi-enzyme **high fiber** supplement derived from the same broad array of raw whole foods as CATALYN, but specially processed so as to leave the fiber in. In addition, CYROFOOD is one-third CALCIFOOD POWDER, raw veal bone flour.

    For all the benefits of a **high-fiber** CATALYN plus CALCIFOOD for bones and teeth.

* * * Especially for Children and the Elderly * * *

These nutrients are food concentrates provided to upgrade the quality of the diet
in order to support normal physiology and biochemistry

IFNH Recommended Clinical Reading List

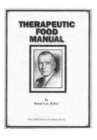

Therapeutic Food Manual - Royal Lee, DDS Dr. Lee's "Personalized" treatment protocols. After some introductory material, it presents an alphabetical list of most illness by classifications. Included under each listing are: a general description, a treatment protocol, physiological consider-nations, synergistic products and coordination suggestions. A highly recommended "source" for the practitioner developed by the "nutritional genius" himself. This manual looks at disease and pathology, where as the symptom survey manual looks at signs and symptoms. These manuals complement each other. [#1541 $39.95]

Mastering Nutrition with the Symptom Survey - IFNH The Symptom Survey is a must for any healthcare practitioner learning nutrition. This complete workbook consists of several sections including over 224 signs and symptoms giving a full description and commentary on the primary cause and secondary cause as well as the primary and secondary proto-col in Standard Process and MediHerb. Additional sections and information for using the Symptom Survey and supporting whole food nutrition are included. Contemporary research and commentary for this manual is due largely to the contributions of Jeremy Kaslow, MD Leo Roy, MD, ND Michael Dobbins, DC James Murphy, DO Robert Curry, DC Robert J. Peshek, DDS Jay Robbrins, DC [#2701 $35.00]

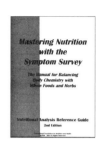

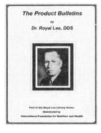

The Product Bulletins - Royal Lee, DDS The original guideline articles for the Standard Process core products developed by Dr. Lee. It gives an in-depth presentation on each of the products. Included under each listing are: a treatment protocol, physiological considerations, synergistic products and Clinical coordination suggestions. This useful work helps us understand the background of Dr. Lee's approach to clinical treatment with nutrition. One of the Royal Lee Library selected manuals. [#1542 $34.95]

Clinical Reference Guide - An updated guide to Standard Process product line. The descriptive sketches by long-time Standard Process biochemist, John Courtney are done in a conversational tone. Mr. Courtney worked with Dr. Lee and directed research and development after Dr. Lee's death. It has a section for each product that provides the following information: formulation, indications for use, synergists, The final section covers additional topics that support the practitioner in using the individual products, including a treatment protocol guide, best known as "the gray pages," and tests from the Nutritional Exam and the FNT course. [#1601 $19.00]

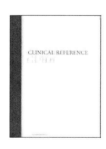

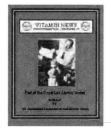

Vitamin News - Royal Lee, DDS   NEW RELEASE - WITH ALL THE MISSING ARTICLES & REFERENCES A compilation of all the newsletters published by the Vitamin Products, Co. Milwaukee, Wisconsin. These monthly newsletters provide useful information to support the practitioner. They offered a wide range of topics Dr. Lee thought were necessary to understand nutritional therapy during the 1930's, 40's, and 50's. At last with a table of contents and index. You will love this book! Remember the references in this book is when real food was used for research, [#1546 $39.95]

Visit our website for more information and our complete list of Practitioner and Patient Support materials and handouts: www.ifnh.org or call (858)488-8932